Ruools, Eugene S., Yoga For beauty and health
Y/0 West Nyack, N.Y. : Parker 1982

Gupta, Yogi., Yoga and Yogic Powers, New York, Yogi
Gupta, New York Center: 1987

Promoting Exercise and Behavior Change in Older Adults

Interventions With the Transtheoretical Model

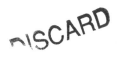

Patricia M. Burbank, DNSc, RN, is a professor in the College of Nursing at the University of Rhode Island and faculty member in the Rhode Island Geriatric Education Center. Currently, she directs the Gerontological Clinical Nurse Specialist concentration. She received her bachelor's degree from the University of Rhode Island and her masters and doctoral degrees from Boston University. Her clinical background has been in the area of community health nursing and gerontology. Research and publications have been in the areas of meaning in life among older adults, including collaborative crosscultural research in Korea, and health behavior change of older adults. She is currently a member of the interdisciplinary research team of the SENIOR project, an NIH-funded study examining exercise and nutrition behavior change among a diverse group of older adults using the Transtheoretical Model.

Deborah Riebe, PhD, FACSM, obtained her BS degree from Springfield College in Physical Education, her MS degree from the University of Rhode Island in Exercise Science and her PhD from the University of Connecticut in Exercise Physiology. She is currently an Associate Professor in the Department of Physical Education and Exercise Science and a member of the Health Promotion Partnership at the University of Rhode Island. Dr. Riebe is a Fellow in the American College of Sports Medicine and is currently the President of the New England Chapter of American College of Sports Medicine and serves on the Executive Committee of the Rhode Island Prevention Coalition. Her research interests include the role of physical activity in primary and secondary disease prevention, weight management, and thermoregulation.

Promoting Exercise and Behavior Change in Older Adults

Interventions With the Transtheoretical Model

Patricia M. Burbank, DNSc, RN
Deborah Riebe, PhD, Editors

 Springer Publishing Company

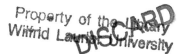

Springer Publishing Company, Inc.
536 Broadway
New York, NY 10012-3955

Acquisitions Editor: Helvi Gold
Production Editor: Jeanne Libby
Cover design by Susan Hauley

01 02 03 04 05 / 5 4 3 2 1

Library of Congress Cataloging-in-Publication Data

Promoting exercise and behavior change in older adults : interventions with the transtheoretical model / Patricia M. Burbank, Deborah Riebe, editors.
    p. cm.
    Includes bibliographical references in index.
    ISBN 0-8261-1502-0
    1. Physical fitness for the aged.   2. Aged—Psychology.   3. Aging—Psychological aspects.   4. Exercise for the aged.   5. Psychotherapy.   I. Burbank, Patricia M.
II. Riebe, Deborah.
RC953.8.E93 P76 2002
613.7'0446—dc21
                                             2001049756
                                                CIP

Printed in the United States of America by Maple-Vail Book Manufacturing Group.

This book is dedicated in love and gratitude
to the very special older adults
in our lives:

Ruth Balluff
Richard Lamb
Jack & Lolly Fitts
Doris Berry
Jean Browell

And in loving memory of

Virginia Balluff
John Browell

Contents

Possible intros (handwritten)

Contributors

Bryan Blissmer, PhD, is currently an assistant professor in the Department of Physical Education & Exercise Science at the University of Rhode Island. His research interests are centered around exercise psychology, focusing on both the determinants and consequences of engaging in regular physical activity, particularly within an elderly population. He has coauthored several articles and chapters in the area of exercise psychology.

Gary J. Burkholder, PhD, is currently a senior research analyst at the Institute for Community Research in Hartford, CT. He holds adjunct faculty positions at the Rhode Island School of Design and University of Massachusetts at Amherst. His areas of research interests are health psychology, HIV/AIDS risk reduction, substance abuse among adolescents and young adults, and longitudinal statistical modeling methods.

Kerry E. Evers, PhD, is director of health behavior change programs at Pro-Change Behavior Systems, Inc., a company founded by James O. Prochaska, PhD, which is committed to enhancing the well-being of individuals and organizations through the scientific development and dissemination of Transtheoretical Model-based change management programs.

Carol Ewing Garber, PhD, FACSM, is associate professor of Cardiopulmonary and Exercise Science in the Bouvé College of Health Sciences, School of Health Professions, at Northeastern University, Boston, MA and a clinical associate professor of medicine at the Brown University School of Medicine. She is a clinical exercise physiologist with particular expertise in exercise evaluation and physical activity training in persons with chronic illness and disability.

Mark Hirsch, PhD, is assistant professor in the Department of Physical Medicine and Rehabilitation at Johns Hopkins University and chair of the Department of Motor Therapy and Motor Control at St. Mauritius Therapienklinik, Germany. His main research interest is the effect activity has on brain plasticity and functional independence in persons with Parkinson's disease, stroke, and traumatic brain injury.

Patricia J. Jordan, PhD, is a Postdoctoral Fellow with Behavior Change Consortium at the National Institutes of Health. She has approximately 15 years of experience in the marketing, advertising and public relations industry, and her primary areas of expertise include behavior change, health psychology, measurement development, and eating disorders.

Diane Martins, MEd, MS, RN, is assistant professor at the University of Rhode Island, College of Nursing. She is a nursing volunteer for the Minority Health Project and the Homeless Medical Outreach Service, Travelers Aid Societies Medical Van Project in Providence, RI. Her primary research interest is the health care experiences of homeless persons and racism in health care.

Claudio Nigg, PhD, is assistant professor, the Department of Public Health Sciences, Johns A. Burns School of Medicine, at the University of Hawaii at Manoa. His areas of interest and expertise include health and exercise psychology, theories of behavior change, and design/methodology for the motivation to engage in health behaviors, specifically exercise.

Cynthia A. Padula, PhD, RN, CS, is presently an associate professor at the University of Rhode Island, College of Nursing. Her research interests include aging and family issues, health promotion, and older adults. She has numerous publications in the areas of aging couples, health promotion, and application of the Transtheoretical Model to nutrition and exercise behaviors.

Sandra D. Saunders, MPH, MS, is an assistant professor in the Department of Human Development and Family Studies, and director of Dental Hygiene Programs at the University of Rhode Island. She is also program coordinator of the SENIOR Project, an NIH-sponsored exercise and nutrition behavior change research study targeting older adults and based on the Transtheoretical model (TTM), where she manages and coordinates the site office and intervention programs.

Foreword I

Older people tell you that "aging is not for sissies." Aging, and especially advanced old age, almost inevitably brings with it unwanted bodily changes, changes in function and changes in thinking. These changes contribute to older peoples' feelings of loss of control over themselves and their environment, and bring on thoughts of impending mortality.

Health care professionals continuously seek to "frame" age changes in such a way that older adults can come to grips with the aging process and achieve an acceptable quality of life. Whether for the active older adult who seeks ways to remain vigorous and independent, or for the frail nursing home resident desirous of going to the dining room, quality of life in old age is almost inevitably tied to functional capacity.

It is therefore no surprise that, with great fanfare, exercise has entered the armamentarium of health care professionals as a tool to improve the quality of life of older adults. Studies strongly support the idea that exercise plays an essential role in keeping people healthy, slowing the slope of aging declines, and raising the functional capacity and spirit of older people who suffer from both physical and mental disabilities. Information about exercise is available in numerous books for the lay public. And increasingly, older people expect an exercise prescription from their health care professional, along with advice on medications and diet.

Yet even when highly motivated, most of us know first hand how hard it is to start, attain, and maintain a program of regular exercise. This can be especially true for today's older adults, for whom exercise has never been a part of their daily routine. And as health care professionals, few if any of us received information about exercise in our professional schools. It is in filling these gaps that health care practitioners will find Patricia Burbank and Deborah Riebe's book so helpful.

Burbank and Riebe provide health care professionals with a road map for examining exercise behavior. By translating the Transtheoretical Model for the health care worker in the field, this book helps practitioners gain confidence in advising older adults about exercise. Highly practical, the chapters lead practitioners through a carefully laid out process. This book should help health care professionals increase their comfort in initiating and staging an exercise program. In turn, provider confidence will help assure that older clients appreciate, and thus adopt behavioral changes that will improve their lives. By applying the contents of this book in their clinical practice with older adults, health care professionals will have the satisfaction of seeing improved outcomes based on a shared understanding of the goals of care, a hallmark of a quality patient/provider relationship.

MATHY MEZEY, EDD, RN

Foreword II

The Transtheoretical Model is dedicated to enhancing the quality and quantity of life for entire populations by generating health promotion programs that can be tailored to the needs of as many people as possible. This book is dedicated to enhancing the well-being of older adults by teaching health professionals how the Transtheoretical Model can help maximize exercise in this special growing population.

The field has known for decades that the leading causes of chronic disease and death are all behaviors. Inactivity is one of the major killers and cripplers of our time. In spite of this knowledge, health care systems have not treated high-risk behaviors seriously.

More recently research has begun to focus on the costs of these chronic behaviors. The cost of health care in the United States in 2001 is projected at $1.2 billion. Double-digit inflation has returned, in part, because managed care has spent a great deal of effort on cutting costs, but very little on preventing costs. Pharmaceuticals account for only about 10% of total costs while behavior accounts for about 60%. The way behavior medicine is currently practiced, less than 5% of those costs are treated effectively.

Leading health care systems are now starting to ask how they can impact the major killers, cripplers, and cost drivers on a population basis. This book is one of the first to present a method of treating a major health risk behavior, not just on an individual patient basis, but with entire older populations.

Why should professionals care? Why should they make the effort to master the wisdom in this work? If professionals are to change their practices, they need to follow the same principles of progress that are applied when changing patient populations. The first principle of progress is that one must become aware of the benefits of behavior change. This text presents information about the multitude of benefits that can accompany exercise with aging and the unmet needs of the growing number of sedentary people in our society.

The second principle of progress is that the cons of changing must decrease. This text presents the challenges of increasing exercise in subpopulations faced with physical, psychological, social, and environmental barriers to regular exercise. This knowledge can guide the development of programs that can reduce or remove many of the barriers to exercise in older adults.

The third principle involves increasing awareness of *how* to change. We present a state-of-the-science description of the Transtheoretical Model and the growing body of science that supports it from research on a broad range of behaviors, and focus on the specific research relating the Transtheoretical Model to exercise. In both cases we need to be aware of the limitations of the model as well as its successes. I kid my doctoral candidates that they are ready to pass their PhD comprehensive exams when they can differentiate between what they don't know and what the field doesn't know.

Increasingly, there is a requirement for evidence-based treatments. This *should* involve an evaluation of the evidence that goes into developing interventions as well as the outcome evidence that are produced by the interventions. Historically, health prevention programs have been based primarily on clinical judgment: What does a clinician believe will be helpful to patients? All too little science informed such treatments and all too little science flowed from these treatments. Today, the standard must be higher and this book demonstrates how research can and should serve as the foundation for state-of-the-art and state-of-the-science behavior medicine.

Another principle of progress is doing the right thing at the right stage of change. The authors teach us how to tailor exercise programs for older adults at each stage of change, but we cannot tailor if we cannot tell what stage people are in. Sensitive assessments are included, followed by examples of intervention materials tailored to each stage of change.

Fortunately, the authors add to the Transtheoretical Model and teach us how to tailor exercise interventions across a health and illness continuum. Physical limitations can be seen as reasons to be sedentary or as a basis for creativity, as we develop programs for populations with a variety of chronic diseases.

This book also prepares us to meet the challenges of older adults from diverse socioeconomic and ethnic backgrounds. Again, the challenge is to our creativity: We need to find activities that are consistent with the cultural values and practices of diverse populations.

The Transtheoretical Model is based on the belief that no single theory of counseling, therapy, or behavior change is always correct. Each leading perspective can contribute to our understanding of how people change and our ability to help people change. The Transtheoretical Model is designed to combine the most important processes and principles of change from across diverse theories, hence the term *transtheoretical*. This book continues that tradition by drawing from multiple models and from perspectives on illness and adult development.

The result for the reader is a broad-ranging yet systematic approach to promoting exercise in older adults. The Transtheoretical Model is designed to go beyond eclecticism and to help create integration across leading theories. In the post-information age it is being recognized that information is not knowledge. The integration of information is knowledge. This book seeks to provide an integrative guide for enhancing exercise in inactive older adults.

Another challenge for enhancing exercise in the elderly is that progress often requires changing the beliefs and behaviors of family caregivers and professional caregivers. As with patient populations, more caregivers can be helped to change if health promotion programs are tailored to their needs as well. Understanding the needs of caregivers can cut through considerable resistance to change and help motivate many more to sustain exercise promotion as one of their important priorities.

I hope these few words have given you a glimpse of what you can learn from the multidisciplinary group of scientists, practitioners, and teachers who have contributed to this work. But be forewarned—their intention is to change your behavior so that you can help many more older people exercise than you ever imagined possible.

JAMES O. PROCHASKA, PhD

Preface

Nearly every book about older adults begins with a statement of the problem, citing demographics that describe the rapidly growing population of those aged 65 and over. Barring an epidemic or natural disaster that alters those demographics, this prediction will become a reality—the largest age group in the United States will soon be older adults. Depending on the purpose of the book, emphasis then shifts to the complex set of problems this will bring, the stresses it will cause for families and caregivers, on finances (especially Social Security and Medicare), the need for resources to care for those with physical and cognitive impairments, a call for new and improved drugs, and the strain placed on an already failing health care system. Usually, a bleak picture emerges of looming masses of older people, chronically ill, confused, and unable to care for themselves. The reader is enticed into the book by a sense of urgency and by an opportunity to take action and make a difference in the quality of the lives of these older adults of the future. This image of being called to help solve problems and improve the lives of a vulnerable population group is a powerful one.

This book takes a different approach. Although the demographics are sound—if trends continue as they have, there will be 70 million older adults comprising 22% of the population by the year 2030 (Federal Interagency Forum on Aging-Related Statistics [FIFARS], 2000), the proposed image is a different one. Imagine 70 million healthy, vibrant older adults enjoying life and making significant contributions to families, jobs, and communities. If Americans changed their sedentary lifestyles and became physically active, significant progress toward this image could be achieved. Although illnesses may not be prevented in many instances, functional capacity can be retained much longer with regular exercise. Although younger people must adopt regular exercise programs for this to occur, exercise, whether begun late in life or as part of a daily routine throughout life, opens the door to new possibilities for a healthier old age.

The Transtheoretical Model (TTM) of behavior change holds great promise as a tool for helping people change their behaviors. It is a stage-based model that incorporates concepts from multiple theoretical perspectives to identify the methods that work best for individuals at each stage of change. It has been used with a wide variety of behaviors ranging from smoking cessation to weight management to sunscreen use, and most recently is being tested in organizational change situations. The TTM helps people change by tailoring interventions to stages of change, working to help people identify their reasons for not changing and their feelings about themselves as people who can change, and empowering them to make the changes themselves.

The focus of this book is to help bridge the gap between theory and practice. In every practice profession there are academicians and researchers as well as practitioners. Although some individual people cross the boundaries and function in both capacities, most spend the majority of their time and energy in one area or the other. A commonly cited problem is the research-practice gap, characterized by a lack of communication between researchers and practitioners. The problem has been how to get the research findings to the practitioner for application to improve practice. Most often the problem is defined as difficulty going from theory and research to practice. The reverse—lack of communication from the practitioner to the researcher—is also problematic. No mechanism exists for communication back to the researcher about clinical problems that need to be solved, or about how research-based interventions worked when applied. This book makes progress in bridging the gap by providing practitioners with the knowledge necessary to apply the TTM in their care of older adults, especially to help them change their exercise behavior. Practical information about older adults, including summaries of research findings about exercise, is provided. The TTM is described thoroughly in order to make the entire model accessible for application by the practitioner. Research using the TTM with a wide range of behaviors including exercise is summarized to give the practitioner a basis for understanding how the TTM has been used in the past and the strengths and limitations of the model as a whole. Efforts have been made to use case histories throughout to make the linkages between theory, research, and practice clearer. Lastly, practitioners are encouraged to keep anecdotal records of their experiences using the TTM. These could be shared with other practitioners and researchers to foster knowledge development and serve as the basis for new outcome-based research studies.

This book is not a book of exercises for older adults, nor does it discuss types of exercise programs suitable for older people with different chronic conditions. There are numerous books available on exercises for older people and exercise physiologists and physical therapists are skilled at planning programs of exercise designed to meet these special individualized needs. Instead, this book discusses the effects of exercise on healthy older adults (chapter 1) and the challenges that must be confronted when considering exercise programs for older adults (chapter 2). A complete description of the TTM including historical development, stages, and major concepts is given in chapter 3, while chapter 4 provides a comprehensive review of research using the model with behaviors other than exercise, including a discussion of limitations of the model. Research studies are summarized in tables for each behavior at the end of the chapter. Chapter 5 summarizes the research literature applying the TTM to exercise behavior with special emphasis on applications with older adults. Questions for determining stage of change are included here. Chapter 6 gives a clear description of how the TTM is applied to healthy older adults and specific guidelines for interventions using examples to illustrate each process of change. Application of the model with physically and cognitively impaired older people (chapter 7), those of diverse ethnic groups and low socioeconomic status (chapter 8), and with family caregivers and health care staff (chapter 9) complete the description of how the model can be used in these special situations. Case examples are used throughout to illustrate application of the model in more detail. Chapter 10 summarizes the main ideas of the book and provides the reader with resources for learning more about exercise and older adults.

This book is written for health care professionals of all kinds including nurses, exercise specialists, administrators, program directors, physicians, social workers, physical therapists, and even family caregivers—anyone who works with older adults and is committed to helping them change behavior and be healthier. Those who wish to use the TTM to change behaviors other than exercise and in populations other than older adults will also find this book useful. Chapters 3, 4, and 6 are general enough for the reader to take information about the TTM and apply it successfully to any behavior in diverse populations.

New territory is charted here. Research applying the TTM to older adults is emerging, including that currently being conducted by the editors' research team. Knowledge gained from this experience is incorporated into the complete description of the application of the TTM to change exercise behavior among older adults provided here. Chapters 4 and 5 are among the most comprehensive reviews of the research literature on the TTM available at this time. One of the unique features is a discussion of applying TTM principles to those older adults who are physically or cognitively impaired or frail. A criticism of the TTM has been its limited application to low income and minority groups. This issue is addressed in chapter 8, citing examples and suggestions from the authors' research and program experiences. Lastly, application of the model with caregivers and with the patient/caregiver dyad functioning as a team is described in chapters 7 and 9. A summary chapter, chapter 10, also lists resources for the health care provider who needs additional information or specifics on exercise programs suitable for older people. The goal is to give health care professionals and caregivers the best tools available to help older adults incorporate exercise into their daily lives. Active older adults have the potential to change the image of aging in America.

REFERENCE

Federal Interagency Forum on Aging Related Statistics. (2000). *Older Americans 2000: Key indicators of well-being.* Hyattsville, MD: Author.

CHAPTER 1

Setting the Stage for Active Older Adults

Deborah Riebe, Patricia M. Burbank, and Carol Ewing Garber

> "If exercise could be packed in a pill, it would be the single most widely prescribed and beneficial medicine in the nation."
>
> ~Robert N. Butler

Americans idolize youth. Products that promise to make people look young and feel young are best sellers. Those over 40 whisper their age for fear that others will consider them "over the hill." But this obsession with youth is not reflective of what is really happening in the United States. The population is, in fact, getting older at a rapid rate.

The fastest-growing minority in the United States today is older adults (conventionally defined as those who reach or pass the age of 65). Presently, there are approximately 36 million elderly people in the United States. It is estimated that this number will climb to 70 million, or 22% of the population, by the year 2030 (Federal Interagency Forum on Aging-Related Statistics [FIFARS], 2000;

American College of Sports Medicine [ACSM], 1998a; Geographic Profile of the Aged, 1993). People 85 years and older are projected to be the fastest growing segment of the population, increasing from 3.1 million in 1990 to approximately 17.7 million by the year 2050 (FIFARS, 2000; Geographic Profile of the Aged, 1993; National Center for Health Statistics, 1997). Refer to Figure 1.1.

Why are we experiencing such a rapid growth in the elderly population? Since the mid-19th century, the life expectancy (the number of years a newborn baby can expect to live) of the United States population has nearly doubled from 40 to almost 80 years. Life expectancy at age 65 is also increasing. Those who live to age 65 can now expect to live an additional 17 to 18 years (National Center for Health Statistics, 1997), and the baby boom generation is advancing toward old age. Baby boomers were born between 1945 and 1965 and represent one third of the United States population (Geographic Profile of the Aged, 1993). This generation will approach retirement age in large numbers, especially during the years 2010 to 2020.

The fact that life expectancy is increasing sounds appealing, but other factors associated with an increased life span must be considered. Aging refers to the normal yet irreversible biological changes that occur throughout a person's lifetime (Table 1.1). These biological changes often result in increases in disease along with decreases in functional ability and independent living. The National Center

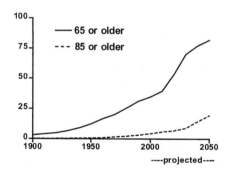

FIGURE 1.1   Total number of persons age 65 or older, by age group, 1900 to 2050, in millions.

Source: U.S. Census Bureau, Decennial Census Data and Population Projections.

TABLE 1.1   Physiological Changes Associated with Aging

- Aerobic capacity decreases by 10% per decade
- Pulmonary function decreases
- Percentage of body fat increases
- Muscular strength is reduced
- Muscle mass is substantially reduced
- Bone mass decreases
- Size and number of muscle fibers decrease
- Maximal stroke volume decreases
- Maximal cardiac output decreases
- Movement time and reaction time decrease

Points to Remember:

- With aging, there is a natural deterioration in physiological function. This decline is compounded by the fact that aging is often accompanied by a sedentary lifestyle.
- Regular exercise appears to slow age-related decrements in physiological function.
- Research indicates that older adults adapt to exercise. They have the ability to increase cardiovascular endurance, muscular strength, and flexibility.

for Health Statistics (1997) estimates that among the population of adults aged 65 and over, 30% of their remaining time will be impaired by disabilities, injuries, and/or disease. Approximately 90% of older adults have at least one chronic health condition (FIFARS, 2000; Hoffman, Rice, & Sung, 1996).

The changes that accompany aging are not all due to biologic aging, genetics, and/or cumulative diseases. Lifestyle factors such as smoking, obesity, and poor nutritional habits contribute to the aging process. A key ingredient for healthy aging is regular physical activity (U.S. Department of Health and Human Services [USDHHS], 1996; Institute of Medicine, Division of Health Promotion and Disease Prevention, 1990). A significant portion of the deterioration attributed to aging can be explained by the tendency for people to become less active as they age. Disuse has debilitating effects on the entire human body, including the cardiorespiratory system, bones, and muscles, resulting in premature aging.

Older adults have much to gain by being active. They can improve their ability to perform the activities of daily living, increase strength levels, decrease body fat, increase cardiorespiratory fitness, and improve their quality of life. They can decrease their risk for numerous diseases including heart disease, cancer, diabetes, osteoporosis, bone fractures, and high blood pressure (Nieman, 1999). They can better manage arthritis. They have fewer problems with depression. Data on individuals who have taken part in physical activity throughout life indicate that they maintain a higher level of functional capacity and do not experience the typical declines associated with aging to the same extent as inactive people. To this end, the American College of Sports Medicine (1998a) has stated that participation in a regular exercise program is an effective intervention to reduce or prevent a number of functional declines associated with aging.

With so much to gain from physical activity, one would expect that most older adults would choose to be active. In reality, however, just the opposite is true. The Behavioral Risk Factor Surveillance System, a national survey that asked questions about the physical activity habits of Americans, found that older people tend to avoid physical activity, particularly at older ages (USDHHS, 1996). In this health surveillance, 36.6% of women and 33.2% of men aged 65 to 74 reported no participation in leisure-time physical activity. This increased to 50.5% of women and 38.2% of men in those over age 75. In addition to those who are not physically active, many other individuals are inadequately active—they participate in some activity, but not enough to reap the benefits of exercise. Less than 25% of older adults exercise regularly at a level sufficient to gain physical and health benefits.

Research has shown that people who stay active throughout their lives appear to significantly slow down the aging process, but what about those older adults who have not been active? Is it worth it for them to start an exercise program? The answer is yes! Older adults adapt to exercise in a manner that is similar to younger individuals (ACSM, 1998b; Nieman, 1999). If they start to participate in regular exercise, even at an older age, elders can improve the strength, decrease their risk of falls, improve cardiorespiratory fitness, and improve their ability to live independently.

The quality of life for older adults is closely related to their physical fitness. Physical fitness, from a health perspective, is defined as the ability to carry out daily tasks with alertness and vigor, without undue fatigue, and with enough reserve to meet emergencies or to enjoy

[handwritten: How do]

leisure time pursuits (Anderson, 1986). To improve all aspects of physical fitness, exercise for the elderly should emphasize aerobic, strength, flexibility and balance training. This chapter will review the age-related changes that occur in various aspects of physical fitness along with the benefits older adults can achieve from participating in regular exercise. *[handwritten: what program should include]*

THE MUSCULOSKELETAL SYSTEM

Muscular Strength

The highest strength levels for men and women are usually reached between the ages of 20 and 30. After age 30, strength in most muscle groups declines steadily. The decline progresses slowly at first, and then more rapidly after middle age (ACSM, 1998a, 1998b; McArdle, Katch, & Katch, 1996). By age 65, a 20% decrease in strength usually occurs. After age 70, the losses in strength are even more dramatic. Muscular strength declines by approximately 15% in the 6th and 7th decades and about 30% thereafter (ACSM, 1998a, 1998b; Harries & Bassie, 1990; Larsson, 1978).

The loss of strength that accompanies advancing age and inactivity is problematic. Adequate strength is necessary for even the most basic activities of daily living, whether it be carrying groceries, vacuuming the rugs, getting in and out of the bathtub, or even rising from a chair. Strength is also important in preserving the ability to participate in social activities such as dancing or travel, and to continue with hobbies such as wood working or gardening (Spiraduso, 1995). Furthermore, a loss of strength in the lower body is associated with an impaired ability to walk and an increased risk of falls (Tinetti, Doucette, & Claus, 1995).

It is important to maintain strength with increasing age because it is vital to health, functional abilities, and independent living. The following examples illustrate how the loss of strength affects the activities of daily living. In the Framingham study it was found that 40% of women aged 55 to 64 years, 45% of women aged 65 to 74 years, and 65% of women aged 75 to 84 years were unable to lift 10 pounds. Many of these women reported that they were unable to perform some aspects of normal household work (Jette & Branch,

1981). Another study measured the ability of middle-aged and older adults to open the lid of a jar that had a set resistance. Almost all of the men and women aged 40 to 60 were able to open the jar. However, after age 60, the failure rate increased dramatically. By the time these individuals reach the age of 71 to 80, only 32% will be able to open the jar (Saltin, 1990; Wilmore & Costill, 1994).

The age-related loss of strength results primarily from the substantial loss of muscle mass that accompanies aging and an inactive lifestyle. Total muscle mass decreases by 40 to 50% between the ages of 25 and 80 years (ACSM, 1998a, 1998b; Booth, Weedem, & Tseng, 1994; Brooks & Faulkner, 1994; Doherty, Vandervoort, Taylor, & Brown, 1993). This is accompanied by a dramatic increase in stored body fat. The decrease in muscle mass is due to changes in muscle fibers. As individuals age, there is a decrease in the number and size of individual muscle fibers (Doherty et al., 1993; Frontera, Meredith, O'Reilly, Knuttgen, & Evans, 1988; Larsson, 1982; Lexell, Henriksson-Larsen, Winbald, & Sjostrom, 1983). It is estimated that about 10% of the total number of muscle fibers are lost per decade after age 50 (Lexell, Taylor, & Sjostrom, 1988). The decline is more apparent in Type II fibers, which are used during high-intensity, short-duration movements such as lifting heavy objects or sprinting, although some of this apparent loss is due to motor unit remodeling (shift to Type I fibers) and changes in the innervation of muscle fibers (Doherty et al., 1993).

In addition to inactivity, inadequate dietary protein may contribute to the loss of muscle mass in the elderly. The American College of Sports Medicine's Position Stand on Exercise and Physical Activity for Older Adults (1998) suggests that the protein intake for older adults should be 1.0 to 1.25 grams of protein per kilogram of body weight per day. This is slightly above the U.S. Recommended Dietary Allowance for adults (0.8 to 1.0 grams of protein per kilogram of body weight per day). A survey completed in Massachusetts found that 50% of individuals over the age of 60 consumed less than the recommended amount of protein, with 25% consuming substantially less (Hartz, 1992).

Neural and hormonal changes in the elderly may also be responsible for some of the strength loss. Studies have shown that aging is accompanied by substantial changes in the nervous system's ability to activate muscles. Specifically, aging affects the ability to detect a stimulus and process the information to produce a response (Wilmore & Costill, 1994). Movements are slowed with aging, although people who remain physically active have better movement times than younger, inactive individuals (Spiraduso, 1975). Anabolic hormones such as testosterone and growth hormone help stimulate the development of muscle tissue. Typically, anabolic hormone concentration increases after a workout, stimulating muscle growth (Kraemer et al., 1993; Kraemer et al., 1991). Studies of older men and women demonstrated that testosterone and growth hormone do not increase in response to resistance training suggesting that the endocrine system may be compromised with age (Hakkinen & Pakarinen, 1995; Hakkinen & Pakarinen, 1993). More research is needed in this area.

Resistance Training

Long-term involvement in resistance training appears to offset the magnitude of strength loss that accompanies aging. Everyone will experience a decline in strength with increasing age, including competitive weight lifters, but the situation is not hopeless. Individuals who participate in resistance training throughout their lives peak at a much greater strength level and undergo a slower rate of decline compared to inactive individuals.

For many older adults, it may have been many years since they lifted weights; some may have never participated in any type of resistance training. Numerous studies have demonstrated that older men and women can increase strength by participating in a resistance training program. The gains they make are similar, or in some cases, more dramatic than those of younger adults. Frontera et al. (1988) trained previously sedentary men between the ages of 60 and 72 for twelve weeks at 80% of their one repetition maximum. At the end of the study there were large increases in strength. Knee flexion (prime mover: hamstring) strength had increased by 107% and knee extension (prime mover: quadriceps) strength was enhanced by 227%. These improvements in strength were accompanied by a significant increase in muscle size. There was a 27.6% rise in the size of fast-twitch fibers and a 33.5% increase in the size of slow-twitch fibers.

In a landmark study, Fiatarone et al. (1990) used high-intensity resistance training with frail elderly patients in a nursing home. The subjects, ranging in age from 86 to 96, underwent eight weeks of lower body resistance training. Strength increased 174% and the size of the thigh muscles increased 9%. There were also several functional gains made by these patients. Gait speed, assessed by a six-meter walk, improved 48%. Two subjects no longer used canes to walk at the end of the study and one of three subjects who could not initially rise from a chair without the use of the arms was able to do so. Unfortunately, when the study was over, the subjects returned to their sedentary lifestyle. After just four weeks of detraining, strength decreased 32%, illustrating the need to continue with exercise, once it has been adopted.

Daily energy expenditure decreases with age, primarily due to the loss of muscle mass. If resistance training can increase muscle mass, there may be a concomitant increase in the metabolic rate. Campbell, Crim, Young, and Evans (1994) studied men and women ages 56 to 80 before and after a 12-week resistance training program. Following the program, participants gained about 3 pounds of muscle, lost 4 pounds of fat, increased their resting metabolic rate, and needed to eat 370 more calories per day to maintain their body weight. The ability to eat more without gaining weight is important for older adults. Caloric requirements necessary to maintain body weight generally decrease with age in part because of a decline in physical activity and in part due to the decline in metabolic rate associated with the loss of muscle mass. Many older adults maintain their weight by consuming smaller amounts of food, often having extremely low caloric intakes. Accompanying the low caloric intake is a reduced nutrient intake, which may contribute to the development of nutritional deficiencies.

Bone

Osteoporosis is characterized by decreased bone mass and structural deterioration of bone tissue, leading to bone fragility and increased susceptibility to fractures (USDHHS, 1996). Osteoporosis is a common condition afflicting 25 million Americans. Because bone mass and strength progressively decline with advancing age, it is a particularly significant health problem for older adults. Osteoporosis causes an estimated 1.5 million bone fractures each year in those over the age of 45. Among those that live to be 90, 33% of women and 17% of men will suffer hip fractures (USDHHS, 1996). Of the elderly experiencing a hip fracture, 18 to 33% will die within one year, and most have a deterioration in the quality of life (Ross, 1996; Wolinsky, Fitzgerald, & Stump, 1997).

There is no cure for osteoporosis, but the National Osteoporosis Foundation recommends that diet, estrogen and other medications, and exercise are important steps for slowing its progress. Exercise can play a role in both the prevention and treatment of osteoporosis (ACSM, 1995).

Mechanical stress is important to keep bones healthy. Bones respond to mechanical loading by becoming bigger and denser (Chilibeck, Sale, & Webber, 1995; Nieman, 1999). Therefore, each time an individual takes a step or pushes against something, forces work on the bones, helping to keep them strong. When there is no stress, bone mass is lost. For example, healthy individuals who undergo bed rest can lose 1% of bone mineral content per week (Bloomfield, 1997). Due to the gravity-free environment of space, astronauts have lost between 1 and 4% of bone in 1 month (Zernicke, Vailas, & Salem, 1990). Physical activity is essential in maintaining the normal structure and functional strength of bone.

Individuals who are active stress their bones more than their sedentary counterparts and usually have greater bone mass (ACSM, 1995). Comparisons between athletes and inactive individuals have consistently shown that athletes have greater bone density (Dook, James, Hendersen, & Price, 1997; Hutchinson, Whalen, Cleek, Vogel, & Arnaud, 1995). This is especially true when the activity they perform is weight-bearing (walking, running, weight lifting) rather than non-weight bearing (swimming, cycling; Lee et al., 1995). Individuals who remain active throughout life will build stronger bones, reducing the risk of fractures later in life.

Participation in physical activity increases bone density after menopause, although it is difficult for many women to exercise at an intensity level needed to achieve this benefit (ACSM, 1995; Chow, Harrison, Brown, & Hajek, 1986; Dalsky et al., 1988). Nelson and colleagues (1994) found that one year of high-intensity strength training increased the bone mineral density of the femur and lumbar spine (as well as muscular strength, muscle mass, and balance) of 39 postmenopausal women. During the same one-year period, the inactive control subjects experienced a decrease in bone mineral density. Walking, jogging, and climbing stairs also improve bone density in postmenopausal women (Kohrt, Snead, Slatopolsky, & Birge, 1995). In this study, some women were treated with exercise only, some with estrogen only, and some with both exercise and estrogen. The greatest improvements in bone were found in the women who received both exercise and estrogen, suggesting that exercise enhances the efficacy of estrogen treatment. However, exercise itself was responsible for 33% of the improvements in bone.

THE CARDIORESPIRATORY SYSTEM

Cardiorespiratory Fitness

The body's ability to use oxygen is the key to cardiorespiratory (aerobic) fitness. All of the major body systems are involved. The lungs get oxygen into the body from the atmosphere, the blood carries oxygen, and the heart pumps blood so that oxygen is delivered to all parts of the body and the muscles use the oxygen to make energy for movement.

The best measure of cardiorespiratory fitness is maximal oxygen consumption (VO_2max). VO_2max represents the greatest amount of oxygen that can be used by the body per minute of physical activity and can be accurately measured in a laboratory. VO_2max decreases 5 to 15% per decade after the age of 25 years (ACSM, 1998b; Heath, Hagberg, Ehsani, & Holloszy, 1981). Why does VO_2max decrease with age and tend to be low in older adults? Declining physical activity along with changes in body composition appear to be the major factors. Two major studies of almost 2000 men and women determined that nearly half of the age-related decline in cardiorespiratory fitness was due to the loss of muscle mass, the accompanying increase in fat mass, and reduced physical activity (Jackson et al., 1995; Jackson et al., 1996).

Even athletes who exercise vigorously throughout their lifetimes experience a decline in VO_2max as they get older (ACSM, 1998b). Not all of the age-related decrease in cardiorespiratory fitness and cardiovascular function can be prevented. Some physiological changes are unavoidable and contribute to the age-related decline in VO_2max even when an individual stays active. A person who has been active throughout his life, however, begins with a much higher VO_2max, so even with a decline, there is still a relatively high base level of fitness. In fact, active older men and women have the same cardiorespiratory fitness levels of sedentary individuals half their age (Heath et al., 1981; Warren et al., 1993).

The age-related decrease in VO_2max is due to changes in the cardiovascular system, primarily from decreases in maximal cardiac output, heart rate, and stroke volume (Fleg et al., 1995; Ogawa et al., 1992; Stratton, Levy, Cerqueira, Schwartz, & Abrass, 1994; Wiebe, Gledhill, Jamnki, & Ferguson, 1999). Cardiac output is the total amount of blood ejected from the heart each minute. Cardiac output is the product of heart rate (the number of times the heart beats each minute) and stroke volume (the amount of blood pumped from the heart with each beat). Decreases in heart rate are primarily responsible for lowering the cardiac output, although a lower stroke volume also contributes.

The average resting heart rates of older adults are not significantly different than those of young adults. However, maximum heart rate, the highest rate at which the heart can beat during heavy exercise, decreases 6 to 10 beats per decade (Fleg et al., 1995; Ogawa et al., 1992; Stratton et al., 1994; Wiebe et al., 1999). It is this decrease in maximum heart rate that has a significant effect on lowering cardiac output, hence lowering VO_2max.

The decrease in VO_2max with age is of particular concern because there is a level of cardiorespiratory fitness that must be maintained for a full independent life. Individuals whose level falls below this threshold are unable to carry out normal daily functions. The minimum level for independent living is 13 ml/kg/min (Spiraduso, 1995), although some researchers suggest this level is too low. Paterson, Cunningham, Koval, and St. Croix (1999) found the minimal level for men to be 17.7 ml/kg/min and for women 15.4 ml/kg/min. Despite minor disparities in the exact level necessary for independent living, the decline in VO_2max with age leaves many of the least fit older adults below this minimum level. Many other inactive adults are very near this point, and may have difficulty in completing at least some common tasks. Although active individuals experience a decrease in VO_2max over time, they begin at a higher level and are unlikely to fall below minimum requirements. The good news is that inactive older adults respond to endurance training and can increase their VO_2max by 10 to 20%; enough of an improvement, in most cases, to surpass the minimal level.

Effects of Physical Activity

Individuals who are physically active do not experience the same declines in cardiovascular fitness as those who are unfit. Although exercising cannot stop all the changes that accompany aging, it slows them considerably.

Consider the study of active and inactive older men conducted by Kash, Boyer, Van Camp, Verity, and Wallace (1990). The VO_2max of the exercisers was almost twice that of the non-exercisers (38.6 vs 20.3 ml/kg/min). The decrease in VO_2max between the ages of 50 and 68 was only 13% in the active group compared to 41% in the inactive group. This suggested that about one third of the loss in VO_2max resulted from aging while two thirds of the loss came from inactivity and the body composition changes that accompany aging. Blood pressure and body weight were also significantly lower in the active group.

Similar results have been reported in women. A study of highly conditioned women in their late 60s revealed that they had a VO_2max that was 67% higher than an age-matched group of sedentary women and was similar to sedentary women aged 35 (Warren et al., 1993).

Trainability of Older Adults

As reported earlier, many older adults do not participate in regular exercise. Although it was once thought that the elderly did not respond to aerobic exercise, research has suggested otherwise (ACSM, 1998a, 1998b). When older adults participate in regular aerobic exercise such as walking, they undergo physiological changes that make the body more efficient in its ability to use oxygen. These changes occur throughout the body, including the heart, lungs, blood, and muscles.

Warren et al. (1993) placed women over the age of 70 on a walking program and found that they improved VO_2max 12.6% in just 12 weeks. Another study of men and women between the ages of 70 and 79 found that higher intensity exercise (walking and jogging) increased VO_2max by 22%. These findings have been replicated in many other studies suggesting that older adults do benefit from regular aerobic exercise (Hagberg, Graves, et al., 1989; Hagberg, Montain, Martin, & Ehsani, 1989; Kohrt et al., 1991). It is important to note that little research has been completed in the area of cardio-respiratory fitness in those over the age of 85.

Cardiovascular Disease

Cardiovascular disease is the major cause of death in the elderly. Research has shown that even moderate amounts of exercise reduce the risk of heart disease. Exercise has preventive benefits for healthy individuals and provides remedial benefits for those with cardiovascular disease by reversing symptoms and improving the quality of life (Spiraduso, 1995). Therefore, the effect of cardiorespiratory training on the risk factors for cardiovascular disease is extremely important to this population.

Blood pressure increases with age. Major blood vessels increase in rigidity, causing those arteries to accept cardiac stroke volume less rapidly, causing an increase in systolic blood pressure (Spiraduso, 1995). At least 40% of people over age 65 have hypertension (systolic blood pressure over 160 mmHg and/or diastolic blood pressure over 95 mmHg; Vokanas, Kannel, & Cupples, 1988). This is a major concern since 65 to 70% of cardiovascular events occur in those with hypertension (Klag, Whelton, & Appel, 1990). Although blood pressure increases during exercise, the long-term effect of chronic exercise is to lower resting systolic and diastolic blood pressure by about 10 mmHg. These favorable effects have been demonstrated in older adults (Cononie et al., 1991; Hagberg, Montain, et al., 1989; Motoyama et al., 1998). It appears that low-to-moderate intensity exercise is more effective at lowering blood pressure than vigorous exercise in older hypertensive adults (Hagberg, Montain, et al., 1989).

Regular exercise results in favorable changes in body composition. Studies suggest that older adults decrease their percentage of body fat from 1 to 5% as a result of participation in regular aerobic exercise (Hagberg, Graves, et al., 1989; Hagberg, Montain, et al., 1989). Schwartz et al. (1991) found that intra-abdominal fat decreased by 25% with intense endurance training, even though the subjects only lost about 5 pounds. This is extremely important since fat stored on the trunk is especially associated with cardiovascular disease (ACSM, 1998).

The effect of exercise training on blood lipids has not been widely studied in the older adult population. Available data suggest that older adults with high levels of cardiorespiratory fitness have better lipid profiles than non-exercisers (Haddock, Hopp, Mason, Blix, & Blair, 1998). After adopting exercise, the elderly improve their lipid profiles in a manner similar to younger adults (Katzel et al., 1995; Seals, Hagberg, Hurley, Ehsani, & Holloszy, 1984). That is, triglyceride levels decrease and HDL cholesterol increases. Increases in HDL cholesterol are desirable as they help to rid the body of LDL cholesterol.

Regular exercise can play a major role in the prevention and control of Type II diabetes, a major risk factor for heart disease. Type II diabetes is characterized by a decreased glucose tolerance (the efficiency with which glucose is metabolized for energy) and increased insulin resistance (a reduced response to insulin resulting in a decreased ability to stimulate glucose uptake in the cells). Studies consistently show that endurance exercise training is associated with an improved glucose tolerance (if initially impaired) and insulin sensitivity (ACSM, 1998a).

FLEXIBILITY

Flexibility and Range of Motion

Flexibility is defined as the ability of a joint to move freely through its full range of motion. The range of motion is highly specific and varies from one joint to another. Many factors contribute to the range of motion at the joint, but the most important factor that influences the amount of movement possible at a joint is the length and extensibility of muscles and connective tissue (tendons and ligaments). To maintain good joint mobility, it is important to move each joint through its normal range of motion. When a joint is not used, the muscles and connective tissues shorten, reducing range of motion. This is especially true when the body repeatedly assumes a certain position for an extended period of time. For example, sitting in a chair places the hamstrings in a shortened position. For those who sit for many hours per day, the muscles adjust to that position and shorten, resulting in a reduced range of motion at the knee and hip.

Often, the importance of flexibility to good health is underestimated. Participating in a regular flexibility program prevents low back problems and contributes to good postural alignment. About 80% of Americans will experience low back pain at some point in their lives (Plowman, 1993). Low back pain is the second most common ailment in the United States, and the second most common reason for being absent from work. Although back pain can result from sudden traumatic injury, it is more often the long-term result of weak and inflexible muscles. Tight hamstrings, hip flexors, and lower back muscles along with weak trunk muscles all contribute to low back pain. Adequate flexibility is also critical for effective movement. Joints must be moved through their range of motion for normal locomotion and/or biomechanically correct movement. Due to a lack of flexibility, some older adults are unable to perform simple daily tasks such as bending forward or turning. Close observation of the body mechanics used by older adults to look behind themselves will illustrate this. Often, they will not turn their head or rotate their torso to look over their shoulder, but instead will step around 90 to 180° (Hoeger & Hoeger, 2000). This loss of flexibility may impact activities such as driving.

Flexibility decreases with age, with the greatest ranges of motion occurring in the second decade (ACSM, 1998). Substantial losses in flexibility occur relatively early in life, especially in movements that are not performed on a regular basis. A study by Einkauf, Gohdes, Jensen, and Jewell (1987) found that the greatest losses in back extension occurred between the ages of 30 and 50 years. These authors concluded that there are limited situations in which one must lean backward during normal daily activities. Roach and Miles (1991) compared the range of motion of the hip and knee in adults of all ages and found that the range of motion of these joints was related to age. The results of their study revealed that range of motion decreased as age increased.

Although flexibility has not been as widely studied as cardiorespiratory fitness and muscle strength in older adults, it appears that they can significantly improve range of motion with exercise (ACSM, 1998b; Hubley-Kozey, Wall, & Hogan, 1995; Morey et al., 1991). Lan, Lai, Chen, and Wong (1998) studied the effects of one year of Tai Chi in older adults. Low back flexibility improved by 11° in males and 9° in females. An added bonus was that the participants also experienced dramatic improvements in VO_2max and lower body strength.

Osteoarthritis

Osteoarthritis, the most common form of arthritis, is characterized by both degeneration of cartilage and new growth of bone around the joint. Because its prevalence increases with age, osteoarthritis is the leading cause of activity limitation among older adults, affecting more than half of those over age 65 (FIFARS, 2000; USDHHS, 1996).

Given the high prevalence of osteoarthritis among older people, it is important to determine whether persons with arthritis can safely participate in physical activity or if regular exercise will exacerbate the condition. In general, research on exercise with those who have osteoarthritis suggests that exercise does not worsen the disease (Nieman, 1999). This is an important consideration because people with arthritis have lower levels of cardiorespiratory fitness, weaker muscles, less joint flexibility, and are at higher risk for some chronic diseases including osteoporosis and coronary heart disease (Hoffman, 1993; Nieman, 1999). People with osteoarthritis can participate in an exercise program to improve their fitness level without detrimental effects on the joints.

Exercise does not cure or stop the progression of osteoarthritis. However, some studies have shown that regular exercise is beneficial as it relieves symptoms, improves function, reduces joint swelling, and raises the pain threshold (Ettinger, Burns, & Messier, 1997; Ettinger & Afable, 1994; Allegrante, Kovar, Mackenzie, Peterson, & Gutin, 1993; Fisher, Pendergast, Greshan, & Calkins, 1991; Fisher &

Pendergast, 1994; Minor, Hewett, Webel, Dreisinger, & Kay, 1988). Both aerobic and resistance training have been shown to improve symptoms associated with arthritis, but resistance training has been shown to be more economically efficient than aerobic training in improving physical function in older adults with osteoarthritis (Sevick et al., 2000).

BALANCE

Balance is the ability to maintain the body's position over its base of support, whether the base is stationary or moving (Spiraduso, 1995). Many different biological systems are important for maintaining balance including vision, the vestibular system (inner ear), the musculoskeletal system, and the somatosensory system. These systems all show decrements with aging, leading to decreases in balance and postural stability (Era & Heikkinen, 1985; Woollacott & Shumway-Cook, 1990).

Losing balance and falling during standing or locomotion is an ever-increasing problem in the elderly. It is estimated that, annually, falls are responsible for over 2 million injuries, 369,000 admissions to the hospital, and 9,000 deaths, at a cost of $8 billion per year (Rothschild & Leape, 2000). In the United States, one out of every three adults 65 years old or older falls each year (Sattin, 1992; Tinetti, Speechley, & Ginter, 1988). Reducing falls in the elderly is a major public health concern. Falls can be prevented by implementing a comprehensive program that includes all the major risk factors including sedentary lifestyle, cognitive status, postural hypotension, medication use, vision, and environmental hazards (ACSM, 1998a).

Exercise and Prevention of Falls

Exercise programs that include balance training, strength training, walking, and weight transfer should be part of a multifaceted intervention to reduce the risk of falling (ACSM, 1998a). Although more research needs to be completed to discern which type of exercise leads to improvement in balance, and the optimal frequency, intensity, and duration, a number of studies have shown that regular exercise has positive effects on balance in older adults.

Several studies have shown that participation in exercise programs reduces the number of falls compared to individuals who remain sedentary (MacRae, Feltner, & Reinsch, 1994; Province et al., 1995; Tinetti et al., 1994; Wolf et al., 1996). One 2-year study consisted of a home-based strength and balance exercise program for women 80 years and older. The exercise program was individually prescribed by a physical therapist during the first 2 months of the study. Compared to a sedentary control group, the women who complied with the program had a lower rate of falls (Campbell, Robertson, Norton, & Buchner, 1999). Older adults can reduce their chance of falls and injuries by participating in a program in their own homes.

Many studies on fall prevention have used balance tests to measure the effectiveness of their exercise intervention. Walking, dancing, Tai Chi, and resistance or strengthening exercises improved balance in the elderly (Jarnlo, 1991; Judge, Lindsey, Underwood, & Winsemius, 1993; Wolf et al., 1996). For example, older women who participated in 1 year of high-intensity strength training improved dynamic balance as measured by a timed backward, tandem walk (Nelson et al., 1994). During this same period, the inactive control subjects experienced a decrease in balance.

Because many studies have taken a multifaceted approach to fall prevention, that is, combining a program to reduce several risk factors simultaneously, there are many questions that remain to be answered. However, it appears reasonable to include exercise as a part of a comprehensive fall prevention program.

EXERCISE, DEPRESSION, AND COGNITIVE FUNCTION

Although depression is less common among older adults than those in younger age groups, 15% of people age 65 to 79, 21% of those 80 to 84, and 23% of those age 85 and older experience symptoms of severe depression (FIFARS, 2000). Rates are higher among those living in long-term care institutions, some reporting rates as high as 50% (Hogstel, 1995). The positive effects of exercise on depression have been well documented for years. Fox (1999) reviewed several hundred studies and over 20 reviews of research and concluded that sufficient evidence exists to document the effectiveness of exercise in the treatment of clinical depression. There is also good evidence that aerobic and resistance exercise enhances general mood states and weaker evidence that exercise can improve cognitive function in older adults (Fox, 1999).

In an 8-year longitudinal study of Finnish adults over age 65, more depressive symptoms were reported among those who had reduced their intensity of physical exercise during the study (Lampinen, Heikkinen, & Ruoppila, 2000). Other recent research, including studies that examined depression in relation to specific physical illnesses such as arthritis and cardiovascular disease, consistently found that exercise interventions had significant positive effects on depression (Barlow, Turner, & Wright, 2000; Christmas & Anderson, 2000; Paluska & Schwenk, 2000).

Rolland et al. (2000) studied the effects of a physical exercise program on several variables including cognitive function in patients with Alzheimer's disease and reported improvement in cognitive function following exercise. Although other studies found similar positive effects of exercise (Anstey & Smith, 1999), Anstey and Christensen (2000) concluded in a review article that results regarding the effect of physical activity on cognitive change were inconclusive. More research is needed to clarify the nature of the relationship between exercise and cognitive function.

SUMMARY

A great deal of research has been conducted to quantify the impact of exercise on older men and women. A vast majority of the research clearly indicates that regular exercise offers a wide range of benefits to older adults. Aerobic training and strength training may improve bone mineral density, glucose homeostasis, and the overall risk of falling. Strength training increases muscle mass and muscle strength. Aerobic training decreases high blood pressure and improves plasma lipid profiles. Flexibility training increases range of motion, making everyday movement easier. Balance training reduces the risk of falls. General positive effects of physical activity are noted in reducing the incidence of depression and improving cognitive function.

Perhaps the greatest contribution that regular exercise makes in older adults is an improvement in the quality of life. Those who exercise will be able to complete the activities of daily living more effectively, maintain the ability to participate in hobbies and social activities, and remain independent for a longer time that those who do not exercise.

A commonly asked question is "What is the best type of exercise?" Since each type of training has different benefits, the best recommendation for older adults who want to optimize their current and future health is to initiate a well-rounded physical activity program, one that includes aerobic, strength, flexibility, and balance training. It is beyond the scope of the book to include specific exercise programs, although resources for programs can be found in chapter 10.

REFERENCES

Allegrante, J. P., Kovar, P. A., Mackenzie, C. R., Peterson, M. G., & Gutin, P. A. (1993). A walking education program for patients with osteoarthritis of the knee: Theory and intervention strategies. *Health Education Quarterly, 20,* 63–80.

American College of Sports Medicine. (1995). Position stand on osteoporosis and exercise. *Medicine and Science in Sports and Exercise, 27,* i–vii.

American College of Sports Medicine. (1998a). Position stand on exercise and physical activity for older adults. *Medicine and Science in Sports and Exercise, 30,* 992–1008.

American College of Sports Medicine. (1998b). Position statement: The recommended quantity and quality for exercise for developing and maintaining cardiorespiratory and muscular fitness in healthy adults. *Medicine and Science in Sports and Exercise, 30,* 975–991.

Anderson, K. N. (1986). *Mosby's medical and nursing dictionary.* St. Louis: Mosby.

Anstey, K., & Christensen, H. (2000). Education, activity, health, blood pressure, and apolipoprotein E as predictors of cognitive change in old age: A review. *Gerontology, 46*(3), 163–177.

Anstey, K. J., & Smith, G. A. (1999). Interrelationships among biological markers of aging, health, activity, acculturation, and cognitive performance in late adulthood. *Psychological Aging, 14*(4), 605–618.

Barlow, J. H., Turner, A. P., & Wright, C. C. (2000). A randomized controlled study of the Arthritis Self-Management Programme in the UK. *Health Education Research, 15*(6), 665–680.

Bloomfield, S. A. (1997). Changes in musculoskeletal structure and function with prolonged bed rest. *Medicine and Science in Sports and Exercise, 29,* 197–206.

Booth, F. W., Weedem, S. H., & Tseng, B. S. (1994). Effect of aging on human skeletal muscle and motor function. *Medicine and Science in Sports and Exercise, 26,* 556–560.

Brooks, S. V., & Faulkner, J. A. (1994). Skeletal muscle weakness in old age: Underlying mechanisms. *Medicine and Science in Sports and Exercise, 26,* 432–439.

Campbell, A. J., Robertson, M. C., Norton, R. N., & Buchner, D. M. (1999). Falls prevention over 2 years: A randomized controlled trial in women 80 years and older. *Age Ageing, 6,* 513–518.

Campbell, W., Crim, M., Young, V., & Evans, W. (1994). Increased energy requirements and changes in body composition with resistance training in older adults. *American Journal of Clinical Nutrition, 60,* 167–175.

Chilibeck, P. D., Sale, D. G., & Webber, C. E. (1995). Exercise and bone mineral density. *Sports Medicine, 19,* 103–122.

Chow, R. K., Harrison, J. E., Brown, C. F., & Hajek, V. (1986). Physical fitness effect on bone mass in postmenopausal women. *Archives of Internal Medicine and Rehabilitation, 67,* 231–234.

Christmas, C., & Anderson, R. A. (2000). Exercise and older patients: Guidelines for the clinician. *Journal of the American Geriatrics Society, 48*(3), 318–324.

Cononie, C. C., Graves, J. E., Pollock, M. L., Philips, M. I., Sumners, C., & Hagberg, J. M. (1991). Effect of exercise training in blood pressure in 70- to 79-yr-old men. *Medicine and Science in Sports and Exercise, 23,* 505–511.

Dalsky, G. P., Stocke, K. S., Ehsani, A. A., Slatopolsky, E., Lee, W. C., & Birge, S. J. (1988). Weight-bearing exercise training and lumbar bone mineral content in postmenopausal women. *Annals of Internal Medicine, 108,* 824–828.

Doherty, T. J., Vandervoort, A. A., Taylor, A. W., & Brown, E. F. (1993). Effects of motor unit losses on strength in older men and women. *Journal of Applied Physiology, 74,* 868–874.

Dook, J. E., James, C., Hendersen, N. K., & Price, R. I. (1997). Exercise and bone mineral density in mature female athletes. *Medicine and Science in Sports and Exercise, 29,* 291–296.

Einkauf, D. K., Gohdes, M. L., Jensen, G. M., & Jewell, M. J. (1987). Changes in spinal mobility with increasing age in women. *Physical Therapy, 67,* 370–375.

Era, P., & Heikkinen, E. (1985). Postural sway during standing and unexpected disturbance of balance in random samples of men of different ages. *Journal of Gerontology, 40,* 287–295.

Ettinger Jr., W. H., & Afable, R. F. (1994). Physical disability from knee osteoarthritis: The role of exercise as an intervention. *Medicine and Science in Sports and Exercise, 26,* 1435–1440.

Ettinger, W. H., Burns, R., & Messier, S. P. (1997). A randomized trial comparing aerobic exercise and resistance exercise with a health education program in older adults with knee osteoarthritis: The fitness arthritis and seniors trial (FAST). *JAMA, 277,* 25–31.

Federal Interagency Forum on Aging Related Statistics. (2000). *Older Americans 2000: Key indicators of well-being.* Hyattsville, MD: Author.

Fiatarone, M. A., Marks, E. C., Ryan, N. D., Meredith, C. N., Lipsitz, L. A., & Evans, W. J. (1990). High-intensity strength training in nonagenarians. *JAMA, 263,* 3029–3034.

Fisher, N. M., & Pendergast, D. R. (1994). Effects if a muscle exercise program on exercise capacity in subjects with osteoarthritis. *Archives of Physical Medicine and Rehabilitation, 73,* 792–797.

Fisher, N. M., Pendergast, D. R., Gresham, G. E., & Calkins, E. (1991). Muscle rehabilitation: Its effect on muscular and functional performance of patients with knee osteoarthritis. *Archives of Physical Medicine and Rehabilitation, 72,* 367–374.

Fleg, J., O'Connor, F., Gerstenblith, G., Becker, L., Clulow, J., Schulman, S., & Lakatta, E. (1995). Impact of age on the cardiovascular response to dynamic upright exercise in healthy men and women. *Journal of Applied Physiology, 78,* 890–900.

Fox, K. R. (1999). The influence of physical activity on mental well-being. *Public Health and Nutrition, 2*(3A), 411–418.

Frontera, W. R., Meredith, C. N., O'Reilly, K. P., Knuttgen, H. G., & Evans, W. J. (1988). Strength conditioning in older men: Skeletal muscle hypertrophy and improved function. *Journal of Applied Physiology, 64,* 1038–1044.

Geographic profile of the aged (1993). *Statistics Bulletin, 74,* 2–9.

Haddock, B. L., Hopp, H. P., Mason, J. J., Blix, G., & Blair, S. N. (1998). Cardiorespiratory fitness and cardiovascular disease in postmenopausal women. *Medicine and Science in Sports and Exercise, 30,* 893–898.

Hagberg, J., Graves, J., Limacher, M., Woods, D., Cononie, C., Leggett, S., Gruber, J., & Pollock, M. (1989). Cardiovascular responses of 70- to 79-year-old men and women to exercise training. *Journal of Applied Physiology, 66,* 2589–2594.

Hagberg, J., Montain, S., Martin, W., & Ehsani, A. (1989). Effect of exercise training on 60- to 69-year-old persons with essential hypertension. *American Journal of Cardiology, 64,* 348–353.

Hakkinen, K., & Pakarinen, A. (1993). Muscle strength and serum testosterone. Cortisol and SHBG concentrations in middle-aged and elderly men and women. *Acta Physiologica Scandinavica, 148,* 199–207.

Hakkinen, K., & Pakarinen, A. (1995). Acute hormonal responses to heavy resistance exercise in men and women at different ages. *International Journal of Sports Medicine, 16,* 507–513.

Harries, U. J., & Bassey, E. J. (1990). Torque-velocity relationships for the knee extensors in women in their 3rd and 7th decades. *European Journal of Applied Physiology, 60,* 187–190.

Hartz, S. C. (1992). In S. C. Hartz, R. M. Russell, & I. A. Rosenberg (Eds.), *Nutrition in the Elderly: The Boston Nutritional Status Survey* (pp. 1–287). London: Smith Gordon.

Heath, G., Hagberg, J., Ehsani, A., & Holloszy, J. (1981). A physiological comparison of young and older endurance athletes. *Journal of Applied Physiology, 51,* 634–640.

Hersey, W., Graves, J., Pollock, M., Gingerish, R., Shireman, R., Heath, G., Spierto, F., McCole, S., & Hagberg, J. (1994). Endurance exercise training improves body composition and plasma insulin responses in 70- to 79-year-old men and women. *Metabolism, 43,* 847–854.

Hoeger, W. K., & Hoeger, S. A. (2000). *Lifetime physical fitness and wellness* (6th ed.). Engelwood, CO: Morton Publishing Company.

Hoffman, C., Rice, D., & Sung, H. Y. (1996). Persons with chronic conditions: Their prevalence and costs. *JAMA, 276,* 1473–1479.

Hoffman, D. F. (1993). Arthritis and exercise. *Primary Care, 20,* 895–910.

Hogstel, M. (1995). *Geropsychiatric nursing* (2nd ed.). St. Louis: C. V. Mosby.

Hubley-Kozey, C. L., Wall, J. C., & Hogan, D. B. (1995). Effects of a general exercise program on passive hip, knee, and ankle range of motion of older women. *Topics in Geriatric Rehabilitation, 10,* 33–44.

Hughes, J. R. (1984). Psychological effects of habitual aerobic exercise: A critical review. *Preventive Medicine, 13,* 66–78.

Hutchinson, T. M., Whalen, R. T., Cleek, T. M., Vogel, J. M., & Arnaud, S. B. (1995). Factors in daily physical activity related to calcaneal mineral density in men. *Medicine and Science in Sport and Exercise, 27,* 745–750.

Institute of Medicine, Division of Health Promotion and Disease Prevention (1990). *The second fifty years: Promoting health and preventing disability.* Washington, DC: National Academy Press.

Jackson, A. S., Beard, E. F., Wier, L. T., Ross, R. M., Stuteville, J. E., & Blair, S. N. (1995). Changes in aerobic power of men ages 25 to 70 yr. *Medicine and Science in Sports and Exercise, 27,* 113–120.

Jackson, A. S., Wier, L. T., Ayers, G. W., Beard, E. F., Stuteville, J. E., & Blair, S. N. (1996). Changes in aerobic power of women ages 20 to 64 yr. *Medicine and Science in Sports and Exercise, 28,* 884–891.

Jarnlo, G. B. (1991). Hip fracture patients: Background and function. *Scandinavian Journal of Rehabilitative Medicine, 24*(Suppl), 1–31.

Jette, A. M., & Branch, L. G. (1981). The Framingham disability study: II—Physical disability among the aging. *American Journal of Public Health, 71,* 1211–1216.

Judge, J. O., Lindsey, C., Underwood, M., & Winsemius, D. (1993). Balance improvements in older women: Effects of exercise training. *Physical Therapy, 73,* 254–265.

Kash, F. W., Boyer, J. L., Van Camp, S. P., Verity, L. S., & Wallace, J. P. (1990). The effect of physical activity on aerobic power in older men (a longitudinal study). *The Physician and Sports Medicine, 18,* 73–83.

Katzel, L., Bleeker, E., Colman, E., Rogus, E., Sorkin, J., & Goldberg, A. (1995). Effects of weight loss vs. aerobic training on risk factors for coronary heart disease in healthy, obese middle-aged and older men. *JAMA, 274,* 1915–1920.

Kirwan, J., Kohrt, J., Wojta, D., & Holloszy, J. (1993). Endurance exercise training reduces glucose-stimulated insulin levels in 60- to 70-year-old men and women. *Journal of Gerontology, 48,* M84–M90.

Klag, M. J., Whelton, P. K., & Appel, L. J. (1990). Effect of age on blood pressure treatment strategies. *Hypertension, 26,* 700–705.

Kohrt, W., Malley, M., Coggan, A., Spina, R., Ogawa, T., Ehsana, A., Bourey, R., Martin III, W., & Holloszy (1991). Effects of gender, age, and fitness level on response on VO₂max to training in 60- to 71-yr-olds. *Journal of Applied Physiology, 71,* 2004–2011.

Kohrt, W., Snead, D. B., Slatopolsky, E., & Birge, S. J. (1995). Additive effects of weight-bearing exercise and estrogen on bone mineral density in older women. *Journal of Bone Mineral Research, 20,* 1303–1311.

Kraemer, W. J., Fleck, S. J., Dziados, J. E., Harman, E., Marchitelli, L. J., Gordon, S. E., Mello, R., Frykman, P. N., Koziris, L. P., & Triplett, N. T. (1993). Changes in hormone concentrations following different heavy resistance training protocols in women. *Journal of Applied Physiology, 75,* 594–604.

Kraemer, W. J., Gordon, S. E., Fleck, S. J., Marchitelli, L. J., Mello, R., Dziados, J. E., Friedl, K., Harman, E., Maresh, C., & Fry, A. C. (1991). Endogenous anabolic hormones and growth factor responses to heavy resistance exercise in males and females. *International Journal of Sports Medicine, 12,* 228–235.

Lampinen, P., Heikkinen, R. L., & Ruoppila, I. (2000). Changes in intensity of physical exercise as predictors of depressive symptoms among older adults: An eight-year follow-up. *Preventive Medicine, 30*(5), 371–380.

Lan, C., Lai, J., Chen, S., & Wong, M. (1998). Twelve-month Tai Chi training in the elderly: Its effect on health fitness. *Medicine and Science in Sports and Exercise, 30,* 345–351.

Larsson, L. (1978). Morphological and functional characteristics of the aging skeletal muscle in man. *Acta Physiologica Scandinavica, 457*(Suppl), 1–36.

Larsson, L. (1982). Physical training effects on muscle morphology in sedentary males at different ages. *Medicine and Science in Sports and Exercise, 14,* 203–206.

Lee, E. J., Long, K. A., Risser, W. L., Poindexter, H. B. W., Gibbons, W. E., & Goldzieher, J. (1995). Variations on bone status of contralateral and regional sites in young athletic women. *Medicine and Science in Sports and Exercise, 27,* 1354–1361.

Lexell, J., Henriksson-Larsen, K., Winbald, B., & Sjostrom, M. (1983). Distribution of different fibers in human skeletal muscles: Effects of aging studies in whole muscle cross section. *Muscle and Nerve, 6,* 588–595.

Lexell, J., Taylor, C. C., & Sjostrom, M. (1988). What is the cause of aging atrophy? Total number, size, and proportion of different fiber types studied in whole vastus lateralis muscle from 15- to 83-year-old men. *Journal of Neurological Science, 84,* 275–294.

MacRae, P. G., Feltner, M. E., & Reinsch, S. (1994). A 1-year exercise program for older women: Effects on falls, injuries, and physical performance. *Journal of Aging and Physical Performance, 2,* 127–142.

McArdle, W. D., Katch, F. I., & Katch, V. L (1996). *Exercise physiology: Energy, nutrition and human performance* (4th ed.). Baltimore, MD: Williams & Wilkins.

Minor, M. A., Hewett, J. E., Webel, R. R., Dreisinger, T. E., & Kay, D. R. (1988). Exercise tolerance and disease-related measures in patients with rheumatoid and osteoarthritis. *Arthritis and Rheumatism, 15,* 905–911.

Morey, M. C., Cowper, P. A., Feussner, J. R., DiPasquale, R. C., Crowley, G. M., & Sullivan, R. J. (1991). Two-year trends in physical performance following supervised exercise among community dwelling old veterans. *Journal of the American Geriatric Society, 38,* 549–554.

Motoyama, M., Sunami, Y., Kinoshita, F., Kiyonaga, A., Tanaka, H., Shindo, M., Irie, T., Urata, H., Sasaki, J., & Arakawa, K. (1998). Blood pressure lowering effect of low intensity aerobic training in elderly hypertensive patients. *Medicine and Science in Sports and Exercise, 30,* 818–823.

National Center for Health Statistics (1997). *Health, United States, 1996–1997 and Injury chart book.* Hyattsville, MD: Author.

Nelson, M. E., Fiatarone, M. A., Morganti, C. M., Trice, I., Greenberg, R. A., & Evans. W. J. (1994). Effects of high-intensity strength training on multiple risk factors for osteoporotic fractures: A randomized trial. *JAMA, 272,* 1909–1914.

Nieman, D. C. (1999). *Exercise testing and prescription* (4th ed.). Mountain View, CA: Mayfield Publishing Company.

Ogawa, T., Spina, R., Martin III, W., Kohrt, W., Schecgtman, K., Holloszy, J., & Ehsani, A. (1992). Effects of aging, sex and physical training on cardiovascular responses to exercise. *Circulation, 86,* 494–503.

Paluska, S. A., & Schwenk, T. L. (2000). Physical activity and mental health: Current concepts. *Sports Medicine, 29*(3), 167–880.

Paterson, D. H., Cunningham, D. A., Koval, J. J., & St. Croix, C. M. (1999). Aerobic fitness in a population of independently living men and women aged 55 to 86 years. *Medicine and Science in Sports and Exercise, 31,* 1813–1820.

Plowman, S. A. (1993). Physical fitness and healthy low back function. *President's Council on Physical Fitness and Sports: Physical activity and fitness research digest, series 1, 3,* 3.

Province, M. A., Hadley, E. C., Hornbrook, M. C., Lipsitz, L. A., Miller, J. P., Mulrow, C. D., Ory, M. G., Sattin, R. W., Tinetti, M. E., & Wolf, S. L. (1995). The effects of exercise on falls in elderly patients: A preplanned meta-analysis of the FISCIT trials. *JAMA, 273,* 1341–1347.

Roach, K. E., & Miles, T. P. (1991). Normal hip and knee active range of motion: The relationship to age. *Physical Therapy, 70,* 656–665.

Rolland, Y., Rival, L., Pillard, F., Lafont, C., Rivere, D., Albarede, J., & Vellas, B. (2000). *Journal of Nutrition and Health in Aging, 4*(2), 109–113.

Ross, P. D. (1996). Osteoporosis: Frequency, consequences, and risk factors. *Archives of Internal Medicine, 156,* 1399–1411.

Rothschild, J. M., & Leape, L. L. (2000). AARP research: The nature and extent of medical injury in older patients—executive summary [online]. Available: Research.aarp.org/health/2000_17_injury_1.html.

Saltin, B. (1990). *Aging, health and exercise performance.* Provost Lecture Series, Muncie, IN: Ball State University.

Sattin, R. W. (1992). Falls among older persons: A public health perspective. *Annual Review of Public Health, 13,* 489–508.

Schwartz, R. W., Shuman, W., Larson, V., Cain, K., Fellingham, J., Beard, J., Kahn, S., Stratton, J., Cerqueira, M., & Abrass, I. (1991). The effect of intensive endurance exercise training on body fat distribution in young and older men. *Metabolism, 40,* 545–551.

Seals, D., Hagberg, J., Hurley, B., Ehsani, A., & Holloszy, J. (1984). Effects of endurance training on glucose tolerance and plasma lipid levels in older men and women. *JAMA, 252,* 645–649.

Sevick, M. A., Bradham, D. D., Muender, M., Chen, G. J., Enarson, C., Dailey, M., & Ettinger, W. H. (2000). Cost-effectiveness of aerobic and resistance exercise in seniors with knee osteoarthritis. *Medicine and Science in Sports and Exercise, 32,* 1534–1540.

Spiraduso, W. W. (1975). Reaction and movement time as a function of age and physical activity. *Journal of Gerontology, 30,* 435–439.

Spiraduso, W. W. (1995). *Physical dimensions of aging*. Champaign, IL: Human Kinetics.

Stratton. J., Levy, W., Cerqueira, M., Schwartz, R., & Abrass, I. (1994). Cardiovascular responses to exercise effects of aging and exercise training in healthy men. *Circulation, 89,* 1648–1655.

Tinetti, M. E., Baker, D. I., McAvay, G., Claus, E. B., Garrett, M., Gottschalk, M., Koch, M. L., Trainor, K., & Horwitz, R. I. (1994). A multifactorial intervention to reduce the risk of falling among elderly people living in the community. *New England Journal of Medicine, 331,* 821–827.

Tinetti, M. E., Doucette, J. T., & Claus, E. B. (1995). The contribution of predisposing and situational risk factors to serious fall injuries. *Journal of the American Geriatric Society, 43,* 1207–1213.

Tinetti, M. E., Speechley, M., & Ginter, S. F. (1988). Risk factors for falls among elderly persons living in the community. *New England Journal of Medicine, 319,* 1701–1707.

U.S. Department of Health and Human Services. Public Health Service. (1996). *Physical activity and health: A report of the Surgeon General.* Atlanta, GA: Author.

Vokonas, P. S., Kannel, W. B., & Cupples, L. A. (1988). Epidemiology and risk of hypertension in the elderly: The Framingham study. *Journal of Hypertension, 6*(Suppl. 1), S3–S9.

Warren, B. J., Nieman, D. C., Dotson, R. G., Adkins, C. H., O'Donnell, K. A., Haddock, B. L., & Butterworth, D. E. (1993). Cardiorespiratory responses to exercise training in septuagenarian women. *International Journal of Sports Medicine, 14,* 60–65.

Wiebe, C. G., Gledhill, N., Jamnki, V. K., & Ferguson, S. (1999). Exercise cardiac function in young through elderly endurance trained women. *Medicine and Science in Sports and Exercise, 31,* 684–691.

Wilcox, S. M., Himmelstein, D. U., & Woolhandler, S. (1994). Inappropriate drug prescribing for the community dwelling elderly. *JAMA, 278,* 292–296.

Wilmore, J. H., & Costill, D. L. (1994). *Physiology of sport and exercise.* Champaign, IL: Human Kinetics.

Wolf, S. L., Barnhart, H. X., Kutner, N. G., McNeely, C., Coogler, C., & Xu, T. (1996). Reducing frailty and falls in older persons: An investigation of Tai Chi and computerized balance training—Atlanta FISCIT Group: Frailty and injuries—cooperative studies of intervention techniques. *Journal of the American Geriatric Society, 44,* 489–497.

Wolinsky, F. D., Fitzgerald, J. F., & Stump, T. E. (1997). The effect of hip fracture on mortality, hospitalization, and functional status: A prospective study. *American Journal of Public Health, 87,* 398–403.

Woollacott, M. H., & Shumway-Cook, A. (1990). Changes in posture control across the life span: A systems approach. *Physical Therapy, 70,* 799–807.

Zernicke, R. F., Vailas, A. C., & Salem, G. J. (1990). Biomechanical response of bone to weightlessness. *Exercise and Sports Science Reviews, 18,* 167–192.

CHAPTER 2

The Challenges of Exercise in Older Adults

Carol Ewing Garber and Bryan J. Blissmer

> "Challenges are what make life interesting; overcoming them is what makes life meaningful."
>
> ~Joshua J. Marine

There are numerous challenges to assisting older adults to adopt and maintain a program of regular exercise. These difficulties are demonstrated on one hand by the very high prevalence of sedentary behavior among older adults, and on the other by the failure of extensive public health efforts to significantly increase their amount of physical activity (Federal Interagency Forum on Aging Related Statistics [FIFARS], 2000; United States Department of Health and Human Services [USDHHS], 1996; United States Department of Health and Human Services [USDHHS], 2000). Interventions to increase physical activity are complicated by the many health, cognitive, behavioral, cultural, social, economic, environmental, and other factors affecting physical activity behavior in older adults (Stewart et al., 1998; Elward, Wagner, & Larson, 1992;

Leaf & Reuben, 1996; Wilcox, Castro, King, Houseman, & Brownson, 2000; King et al., 2000; Eyler et al., 1999; King, Rejeski, & Buchner, 1998; Brownson et al., 2000; King, 1997; Mills et al., 1996; Resnick & Spellbring, 2000). In this chapter we will address some of these issues and challenges to increasing physical activity in the older adult and suggest solutions whenever possible.

MEDICAL AND HEALTH CONCERNS IN OLDER ADULTS

The health status of older adults is often compromised by acute and chronic illnesses and conditions, many of which affect the type, quantity, and quality of exercise that can be recommended, as well as the safety of unsupervised exercise (Larson, 1992; Shephard, 1990). Chronic illness and conditions are highly prevalent in older adults, and nearly 80% of adults over 70 years of age report having at least one chronic condition (National Center for Health Statistics, 2000; Kramarow, Lentzer, Rooks, Weeks, & Saydah, 1999). Among the most commonly reported chronic conditions include arthritis (afflicting nearly all), hypertension (33%), coronary heart disease (25%), diabetes mellitus (11%), respiratory diseases (11%), and stroke (9%). The proportion of older adults with chronic conditions is generally higher in black and Hispanic adults and other minority groups. Further complicating the ability to engage in physical activity are physical, visual, and auditory impairments affecting between 9 and 26% of older adults (FIFARS, 2000).

Screening for Exercise and Exercise Supervision: Current Recommendations

For older adults, most experts recommend screening for contraindications to exercise and obtaining clinical information relevant to developing the exercise prescription (American College of Sports Medicine [ACSM], 2000; Fletcher et al., 1995). Elders who are not medically stable, have an acute illness, or whose condition can be exacerbated by exercise should delay embarking on an exercise-training program until the condition has resolved or is under good control (ACSM, 2000; Fletcher et al., 1995). Any medical conditions where the risks of physical activity outweigh the benefits in the opinion of the attending physician and clinical exercise physiologist would preclude exercise in the older adult. The reader is referred to the exercise standards of the American Heart Association (Fletcher et al., 1995) and the *Guidelines for Exercise Testing and Prescription* by the American College of Sports Medicine (ACSM, 2000) for further details on screening prior to exercise, including the indications and contraindications to exercise.

A number of older adults with chronic illnesses and conditions may require increased levels of medical supervision to assure safety during exercise (ACSM, 2000; Fletcher et al., 1995). Indications for a medically based exercise program may include the following conditions, several of which are commonly encountered in the older adult (ACSM, 2000; Fletcher et al., 1995):

- Coronary heart disease
- Congestive heart failure
- Peripheral vascular disease
- Valvular heart disease
- Stroke
- Chronic obstructive pulmonary disease
- Chronic renal failure
- Diabetes mellitus
- Severe arthritis or rheumatoid disease
- Morbid obesity
- Moderate to severe orthopedic or neuromuscular limitations to exercise
- Moderate to severe cognitive impairment
- Mental illness

The Dilemma of Participant Screening and Supervision

Although public health officials recommend exercise for most adults (USDHHS, 1996), the issues of screening, exercise testing, and exercise supervision often present a dilemma for health professionals wishing to offer community and/or medically based programs for older adults. This is particularly true in our litigious society, where even exercise equipment, videos, and publications come with the warning, "See your doctor before using [this equipment, video, book, etc.]." These pervasive warnings send a message that exercise is dangerous and provide yet one more barrier to those interested in beginning an exercise program. In no group is exercise perceived as more dangerous than the older segment of our population.

How dangerous is exercise for the older adult? While often perceived otherwise, exercise training is fairly safe in persons without coronary heart disease, although the data do not include many older adults (Malinow, McGarry, & Kuehl, 1984; Vander, Franklin, & Rubenfire, 1982). In older adults, there are concerns about falling during exercise because many elders have significant problems with balance, agility, and impairments in muscular strength and flexibility (Tinetti, Liu, & Claus, 1993; Tinetti, Doucette, Claus, & Marottoli, 1995; Tinetti, Doucette, & Claus, 1995; ACSM, 1998). However, the risk of falling can be minimized by modification of the exercise program by using seated exercise or assistive devices, and thus the risk of falls becomes minimal.

Studies of the general population, including the elderly, have shown that the risk of cardiovascular events during exercise is increased by as much as 56 times in sedentary individuals, but this risk is reduced to 5 times the risk during rest in persons who exercise regularly (Siscovick, 1997; Siscovick, Weiss, Fletcher, & Lasky, 1984). Although the risk of cardiovascular events is acutely greater during exercise, both the acute and long-term risk of these events declines significantly with participation in regular exercise (Siscovick, 1997; Siscovick et al., 1984; USDHHS, 1996). The cause for concern about the safety of exercise comes primarily from the fact that the risks of exercise are substantially greater in persons with coronary artery disease, and it is difficult to accurately identify those at higher risk of cardiovascular events (Haskell, 1994; Haskell et al., 1994; Franklin, Bonzheim, Gordon, & Timmis, 1998; ACSM, 2000).

The issue of whether and how to screen older adults prior to embarking on an exercise regime presents the health professional with an ethical quandary: Will the safety of older adults be compromised? Although the risks of exercise are relatively low, it is clear that there are some individuals for whom this risk is elevated, leading several major organizations to recommend extensive screening, including comprehensive medical evaluation and exercise testing, of older adults prior to exercise (ACSM, 2000; Fletcher et al., 1995).

However, the cost and practicality of these procedures are a major obstacle to exercise from the viewpoint of both the potential participant and the health professional.

Further complicating matters, the utility of exercise testing in older adults has recently been questioned, with the argument posed that the risks of remaining sedentary far outweigh the risks of not testing (Gill, DiPietro, & Krumholz, 2000). Gill and colleagues (2000) suggest that exercise testing is of limited value in the older adult, and that the current recommendations for exercise testing are not applicable to most older adults who wish to exercise regularly. However, as the authors point out, there has not been enough research examining the efficacy of exercise (or other types of) testing, particularly in asymptomatic older adults, prior to starting an exercise program as a means of identifying persons at high risk of suffering a major cardiovascular event. It must be concluded that, in absence of definitive evidence to the contrary, pre-screening, including an exercise test, is recommended for most older adults and should be a part of all physical activity interventions if at all possible (ACSM, 2000; Fletcher et al., 1995). Refer to Table 2.1.

TABLE 2.1   Indications for Exercise Stress Testing Before Starting Exercise Training*

Condition
Post myocardial infarction
Suspected or known cardiovascular disease
Post revascularization (Coronary artery bypass surgery or percutaneous transluminal coronary angioplasty) • Patients with recurrent symptoms
Asymptomatic individuals: • Sedentary men > 40 years and women > 50 years • Patients at high risk for coronary heart disease

*Adapted from American College of Sports Medicine, 2000; Gibbons et al., 1997.

For those instances where extensive screening procedures are not practical, such as community-based interventions, the use of a screening instrument designed for use in older adults, such as the Physical Activity Readiness Questionnaire [PAR-Q] (Thomas, Reading, & Shephard, 1992) is suggested. The PAR-Q has been modified and evaluated for use in older adults (Cardinal, Esters, & Cardinal, 1996) and is reported to have 100% sensitivity and 80% specificity for the detection of contraindications to exercise (Shephard, 1988; Shephard, Cox, & Simper, 1981; Thomas et al., 1992). It has been administered to over 1 million people of all ages without serious cardiovascular sequelae (Cardinal et al., 1996; Shephard, 1988; Shephard et al., 1981), and has been recommended by the American College of Sports Medicine (2000) for pre-exercise screening. The revised version of the PAR-Q for use in older adults has an exclusion rate of approximately 48% (Thomas et al., 1992).

Should All Older Adults Participate in Medically-Supervised Exercise Interventions?

Given the pervasive health problems in older adults and the potential risks of exercise, should all seniors participate in medically supervised exercise programs? In an ideal world, the answer would be, "yes." There is no doubt that traditional, medically supervised exercise programs are effective and provide increased levels of safety for those who attend (USDHHS, 1995). This supervision can be provided at several levels and formats and generally involves medical personnel including clinical exercise physiologists, nurses, physical therapists, psychologists, dieticians, and other allied health professionals who work under the supervision of a physician. However, the costs of such programs are prohibitive and there are only a few indications for medically supervised programs that are covered by health insurance (if the participant has insurance). In addition, there are not enough medically based programs available for older adults, especially for those residing in rural or inner city locales.

If we are to reach a substantial portion of the older adult population we must provide exercise programs by a variety of delivery systems and in formats that involve medical supervision as needed. Incorporation of cognitive, behavioral, and motivational components using several theoretical models, including the Transtheoretical Model (Prochaska & DiClemente, 1983), can improve the efficacy of physical activity interventions, as is discussed later in this chapter and throughout this book. However, there is a real need for research on increasing and maintaining physical activity in older adults to guide health professionals in designing effective interventions for all segments of the elderly population. In the absence of these data, it is a challenge for the health professional to design and implement effective programs for the diverse population of older adults throughout our communities.

COMMUNITY AND HOME-BASED EXERCISE: A MODEL FOR THE FUTURE?

Providing exercise programs in or near the residences of older adults may overcome several obstacles to exercise and, therefore, may be an attractive alternative to traditional exercise programs. Home based and lifestyle exercise programs may overcome barriers to exercise such as accessibility, safety, time, and other factors discussed in more detail below. Studies of healthy and obese sedentary adults have shown that physical activity programs using a lifestyle approach result in similar improvements in coronary heart disease risk factors and adherence as more traditional structured programs (Dunn et al., 1999; Andersen et al., 1999). Lending support for the use of home and community-based interventions in older adults are studies evaluating the efficacy of home and community-based exercise in low- to moderate-risk patients with coronary artery disease (DeBusk et al., 1985; DeBusk et al., 1994; Miller, Haskell, Berra, & DeBusk, 1984; Sirvarajan et al., 1982; Fletcher et al., 1994; Haskell et al., 1994) and community-dwelling older adults (Stewart et al., 1998; Leaf & Reuben, 1996). These interventions have been effective and have not resulted in any untoward effects for the participants. Most of these studies, however, have included carefully screened subjects who have been supervised in community-based programs (Stewart et al., 1998; Leaf & Reuben, 1996) or by transtelephonic monitoring in the home (e.g., DeBusk et al., 1994; DeBusk et al., 1985). The safety of home and community-based exercise in a general population of older adults cannot be inferred from these studies, so the issues of screening and exercise testing still loom as a barrier for both exercise participants and health professionals who may recommend exercise for older adults.

CULTURAL, SOCIAL, ECONOMIC, AND OTHER FACTORS AFFECTING PHYSICAL ACTIVITY IN OLDER ADULTS

A number of social and economic factors can affect the physical activity levels of older adults, and these factors can challenge the health professionals designing interventions to increase physical activity in seniors. It is often those whose life circumstances and medical conditions are the most complicated who most need our intervention to increase physical activity: Physical inactivity is more prevalent in older adults of minority status, persons with lower income and educational levels, and those with arthritis and disabilities.

Social Isolation

A typical, yet unfortunate, facet of aging is increased solitude and social isolation resulting from causes such as deaths, retirement, and moving. This isolation is clearly related to conditions such as depression, however, it may also directly impact an individual's opportunities and motivation for exercise. As discussed later in this chapter, social support for exercise is an important determinant of exercise participation. The older adult who has limited social relations also has a limited opportunity to garner the beneficial effects of social support for physical activity.

Exercise can prove a valuable source of affiliation and interaction for older adults, while simultaneously providing more resources to expand their social interactions (McAuley, Marquez, Jerome, & Blissmer, 2000). A qualitative study of the motives underlying exercise participation in a group of older adults found that the participants exercised because they enjoyed the regular social contact and it made them feel better about themselves (Stead, Wimbush, Eadie, & Teer, 1997). The physiological changes resulting from participation in regular physical activity can enhance the energy and mobility levels of older adults, affording them further social engagement (Everard, Lach, Fisher, & Baum, 2000). As with many of the physical factors associated with old age, the key is to stop the downward spiral that comes from leading a sedentary lifestyle. In this instance, increased isolation can lead to increasingly sedentary behavior, which in turn limits the ability and opportunity for future social interaction. It is promising that increased physical activity can reverse the progression of the interaction between social isolation and physical decline, and this fact should be taken into consideration when designing programs for older adults. Incorporation of opportunities for social interaction can be an important component of a physical activity program for older adults.

Ethnicity

While we know that physical inactivity is more prevalent in older adults belonging to a minority group, little attention has been paid to identifying factors that promote or impede physical activity participation in these subpopulations of elders. This serious disparity in our knowledge comes at a time when the proportion of older adults belonging to ethnic and racial minority groups is growing rapidly. It is projected that by the year 2030, minorities will make up about 25% of the elder population (FIFARS, 2000).

Further complicating our ability to promote physical activity is the fact that one eighth of the older adult population is non-English speaking and 10% are foreign-born (FIFARS, 2000). Members of these populations often need health promotions that are tailored to be culturally relevant and in their own language. Literacy in their native tongue cannot be assumed, thus the issues of literacy and information delivery must be considered when designing appropriate interventions for these older adults.

Economic Issues Affecting Older Adults

Approximately 11% of older adults live in poverty, which affects ethnic minorities disproportionately. Twenty percent of Hispanic and nearly 25% of Black older Americans are impoverished, compared with 8% of whites (FIFARS, 2000). Being impoverished can greatly affect the access of older adults to resources for physical activity. For example, exercise programs, even public recreation programs, may be too costly or provided in locations that are inaccessible to a senior living in a low-income neighborhood. Safety concerns are also rampant in elders living in poverty, making many fearful of leaving their residence for any reason. Further, the challenges of poverty, including lack of nutritious food, can leave little energy for exercise.

Education and Literacy

Although only 18% of older adults have not completed high school, more than 70% of older adults have difficulty reading prose and about 68% have difficulty in locating and processing numeric information (Kirsch, Jungeblut, Jenkins, & Kolstad, 1993; FIFARS, 2000). Four out of five older adults struggle with filling out forms, reading and following directions, and using schedules. These data translate into the startling fact that a large proportion of older adults are functionally illiterate, that is, they do not have reading, writing, and computational skills adequate to meet the needs of everyday life situations. Although highly correlated with poverty, education, income, and former occupation, functional illiteracy exists in all segments of society and in all geographical areas (Kirsch et al., 1993). In spite of the widespread problem of illiteracy among older adults, there are wide gaps between the reading level of health promotion materials and the literacy skills of the target population (Weiss, Reed, & Kligman, 1995; Doak, Doak, & Root, 1995; Weiss & Coyne, 1997; Baker, Parker, Williams, Clark, & Nurss, 1997). Even if written materials are at a grade level appropriate for an elder with low literacy skills, factors such as the conceptual complexity, tone of the text, or visual layout of the passage may render the materials ineffective (Plimpton & Root, 1994). Thus, literacy of the target population is a vital consideration when designing a program for promoting physical activity in seniors, because if the information provided cannot be understood, then it has little possibility of affecting the behavior of the participant.

Gender Issues

The physical activity and exercise experiences among the current group of elderly are marked by vastly different socialization and practical experiences in men and women. Older adult males were encouraged to and often engaged in sports and physical activity throughout their youth, whereas the leisure of the older females in the United States rarely consisted of any strenuous physical activity, as that was considered to be "unladylike." The non-strenuous activity patterns evidenced throughout adulthood are maintained into old age, with epidemiological evidence indicating that older women exercise less than older males (Jones et al., 1998; USDHHS, 1996). The discrepancy between the activity levels of older males and females may in part be explained by their own perceptions of which activities are appropriate for males and females. A survey of older adults found that they considered a variety of physical activities to be more appropriate for men than women across the age spectrum (Stead et al., 1997). Thus, the socialization patterns established earlier in life appear to be salient into old age.

The problem of older women not exercising at the same level as older men is compounded by the demographics of aging. The proportion of females to males grows throughout old age, as more women survive than men and those older women are faced with a number of unique challenges. This inevitably leads to a growing number of older, widowed women. This may be their first opportunity to take time for themselves after spending a lifetime caring for their families, but these opportunities unfortunately coincide with a time when they have fewer financial resources, greater levels of illness and disability, and increasing social isolation. Having no previous experience with, or exposure to, regular exercise during their lifetimes, older women are unlikely to adopt such a lifestyle without some significant aid.

Those older women who are not widowed are often placed in the role of caregiver to an ailing husband, limiting their time and opportunities for social interaction, while at the same time sapping their energy levels and limiting their exercise opportunities (King & Brassington, 1997). A later chapter in this book is devoted to examining exercise interventions among caregivers, but those caregivers are primarily women who have special needs and concerns.

MOTIVATIONAL FACTORS

As discussed previously, the vast majority of older adults do not engage in enough physical activity to realize the numerous health benefits associated with exercise (Jones et al., 1998; USDHHS, 2000; USDHHS, 1996). In order to design effective interventions for older adults, an essential question remains to be addressed: "How do we get older adults to want to be more active?" That is, what factors underlie the motivation to be active on a regular basis? Moreover, once they become active, how can we help older adults maintain their program of regular physical activity? Over 50% of individuals who begin an exercise program will drop out within the first 6 months of the program (Dishman, 1988).

Psychological Determinants of Physical Activity in Older Adults

There have been a number of studies of the psychological factors related to exercise participation across the age spectrum, including the elderly. Although these studies of exercise in older adults have used a variety of psychological theories to explain and predict exercise behavior, all of the theories have, at their heart, some common psychological concepts. These include attitudes toward physical activity and exercise, social influences on exercise, barriers to exercise, and confidence in the ability to exercise. Without going into specific details on the role of these constructs within theories such as social cognitive theory, the theory of planned behavior, and the Transtheoretical Model (TTM), the following sections will briefly introduce each psychological construct and summarize the findings of its relationship with the physical activity behavior of older adults. For a more in-depth review of each of these theories and their utility in predicting and explaining exercise behavior the reader is directed to a number of excellent reviews (see Hausenblas, Carron, & Mack, 1997; McAuley & Blissmer, 2000 for reviews of planned behavior and social cognitive theory applications to exercise).

Attitudes toward Physical Activity

An important element in determining an individual's overall motivation for any behavior is their attitude about behavior (Fishbein &

Ajzen, 1975). Attitudes are beliefs that reflect the value or worth a person ascribes to that behavior (such as physical activity). A person's attitudes about, or their perception of the benefits (pros) of engaging in physical activity, are core components in a variety of psychological theories that have been used to explain physical activity behavior. Attitudes toward physical activity have been shown to be good predictors of a person's intentions to engage in physical activity as well as their actual physical activity behavior across the age spectrum (Godin, 1994; Hausenblas et al., 1997; Rhodes et al., 1999). That is, the more positive the attitude an older adult holds about physical activity, the more likely he/she is to both want to and actually engage in a program of regular physical activity (Gravelle, Pare, & Laurencelle, 1997; Gorely & Gordon, 1995). Attitudes about physical activity may be more important in determining whether a person starts to exercise rather than whether they stick with a program once they start. For example, Brenes, Strube, and Storandt (1998) found that physical activity attitudes were related to physical activity behavior during the first month of a structured physical activity program, but not in later months.

Recent research on attitudes toward physical activity has suggested that there may be two distinct aspects of these attitudes that may influence a person's motivation to participate: affective and evaluative attitudes. Evaluative attitudes are the values associated with physical activity, such as whether the person thinks it is useful and beneficial. Affective attitudes reflect how an individual actually feels about the behavior. For example, it is quite possible that an older adult may think that physical activity is good for him or her (i.e., positive evaluative attitudes), but, she/he may also think that exercise is boring, too hard, or painful (i.e., negative affective attitudes).

Some studies have suggested that it may be necessary for an older adult to have a positive evaluative attitude regarding physical activity (i.e., belief that physical activity is good), before s/he will begin a program of regular physical activity (Clark, 1999). Of concern, Clark (1999) found that older adults do not have adequate knowledge about the benefits of physical activity or how to set up a personal physical activity program. These data indicate a need to better educate adults about the benefits of physical activity and how to structure a proper program of regular exercise.

On the other hand, it is possible that no matter how good an older adult thinks physical activity is for them (evaluative attitude), they will be unlikely to start or continue an activity for which they hold negative affective attitudes (Emmons & Diener, 1986; Wankel, Mummery, Stephens, & Craig, 1994). For example, Stead and colleagues (1997) reported that older adults who were physically active did so, not for the health benefits, but rather for the enjoyment associated with the social interaction they received as part of exercising regularly.

Social Influences on Physical Activity

The social environment of an older adult can have a significant impact on their physical activity behavior. Social influences can operate at both a cultural and individual level. As a society we have formed expectations about "appropriate" behaviors for the elderly. Even as early as age 3, children appear to believe that the elderly are supposed to be less active than younger adults (Ostrow, Keeney, & Perry, 1986). Further research has shown that older adults recognize and have adopted these beliefs regarding the appropriateness of their own physical activity participation. A study of 62 adults asked them to indicate the appropriateness of engaging in a variety of physical activities that ranged from running in a marathon to bowling to ballet for men and women of different ages (Ostrow & Dzewaltowski, 1986). Across every activity, older adults reported that physical activities were less appropriate with increasing age. In addition, all of the activities were considered more appropriate for males than females. The existence of these social norms and their acceptance among the current cohort of older adults constitutes a powerful influence on whether or not an older adult exercises. Without appropriate role models, older adults may fail to even consider the idea that they can and should exercise throughout their life.

On an individual level we can examine the social influences within the framework of social support and examine the support that older adults receive regarding their levels of regular physical activity. Social support may be either instrumental, such as actually driving an older adult to a physical activity program, or it may be more emotional: simply encouraging activity and providing emotional support. Studies have shown that having a social network that is supportive of physical activity behavior is an important predictor of physical activity levels (e.g., Brenes, Strube, & Storandt, 1998; Courneya, Nigg, & Estabrooks, 1998; Courneya, Plotnikoff, Hotz, & Birkett, 2000; Eyler et al., 1999). However, it is important to note that social support is not necessarily positive, especially in the case of older adults (Chogahara, Cousins, & Wankel, 1998). Family and friends may exert negative influences through their benevolent efforts to protect and take care of older adults. The implicit message is that they are too old or frail to be physically active. Although well intentioned (can a Boy Scout helping an old woman across the street be anything less?), this type of social support intended to protect and ease the lives of the elderly may serve to facilitate their sedentary lifestyles and dependency.

The Role of the Physician in Social Support

A very important source of social support and influence among older adults are their physicians, because they are likely to see their physician several times each year (Woodwell, 1997). A major barrier for older adults is the belief that regular activity may be painful or cause injury, fears that a physician can help to assuage. However, statistics indicate that the majority of physicians fail to prescribe physical activity despite its many beneficial effects (Damush, Stewart, Mills, King, & Ritter, 1999; Lewis & Lynch, 1993; Washburn, Janney, & Caswell, 1990). There has been recognition of the importance of the physician in helping older adults to become more active, and some interventions have successfully increased the role of the physician in physical activity prescription. The Activity Counseling Trial (ACT) study documented the effectiveness of physician counseling for increasing activity levels in a variety of patients (Albright et al., 2000).

However, physicians experience many barriers to providing preventive care to their patients, including physical activity counseling, due to factors such as low interest level, skepticism about its effectiveness, uncertainty about how to do the counseling, as well as numerous barriers in the health care system (Woolf, Jonas, & Lawrence, 1996). Without the proper incentives, there is almost no likelihood that physicians will use their limited and valuable contact time to give comprehensive exercise prescriptions to their patients.

Social Support and Changing Times

Research supports the fact that social influences on physical activity behavior need to be carefully examined. Although the current cohort of older adults may have had particular socialization experiences, it is possible that future generations will not be subject to the ageist view that certain activities, such as physical activity, are not for the elderly. It is also important to recognize the powerful influence of individuals including friends, family, and physicians, while also acknowledging that their protective practices may actually be exerting a negative influence.

Barriers to Physical Activity

Despite the fact that many individuals hold positive attitudes regarding the health benefits of regular physical activity, and that most people would want older adults to be active and healthy, we know that most seniors fail to exercise regularly. Thus, a considerable amount of research has examined the reasons why people don't exercise. Barriers to exercise may be either external to the individual (environmental) or internal (personal). Whatever their focus, it is important to recognize that it is the perception of a barrier that is important, not necessarily the objective situation. For example, even though an older adult may have a mall in their neighborhood, if they feel that it is not accessible to them for whatever reason, they will not go there to walk, even if there is a special walking program offered for older adults

Many of the typical barriers to physical activity are similar among younger and older adults (Whaley & Ebbeck, 1997), however, there are several barriers that may take on special significance among older adults.

Among adults of all ages, the time required to exercise on a regular basis has typically been reported as the largest obstacle preventing individuals from exercising on a regular basis (Richter, Macera, Williams, & Koerber, 1993; Whaley & Ebbeck, 1997). Logic would seem to suggest that time would be a less significant barrier due to decreases in the demands on the time of the older adult. Because of reductions in work and child-rearing responsibilities, older adults typically are viewed as having more discretionary time than working adults. In reality, this is not always the case because individuals continue to work into old age, take on new responsibilities, and engage in caretaker roles. Just as with younger adults, it is necessary to examine each individual situation to determine the salient barriers that prevent the individual from exercising.

There are also financial barriers associated with physical activity because there is often some cost associated with exercising, such as YMCA or health club memberships or buying new shoes and workout clothes. As already mentioned, an alarming number of older adults live in poverty and often have less discretionary income to spend on exercise-related expenses such as walking shoes. It is important for practitioners to recognize these financial limitations when developing and suggesting programs for the elderly. There are numerous inexpensive forms of physical activity, not the least of which is a program of regular walking, which can be recommended as exercise for older adults.

Another major external barrier is accessibility to physical activity facilities or programs. This barrier is related to much that we have previously discussed in this chapter. Limitations in mobility, inability to travel to a workout center, lack of appropriate programs, safety concerns, and financial restrictions all play a role in limiting access to facilities. Even when physical activity facilities or classes are located close by, the perceptions of older adults may still be that they are inconvenient (Whaley & Ebbeck, 1997). From an environmental perspective, we can design our communities and buildings to facilitate regular activity (King et al., 2000), but that is typically in the realm of public policy. On a more personal level, a proper assessment is required before implementing an exercise program to determine what the older adults want and whether they will attend. These needs assessments can provide valuable insight into the preferences of older adults and ultimately increase program adherence.

Lack of social support and increased social isolation can be a barrier to regular physical activity participation. An older adult may rely on another individual for transportation to a physical activity facility. Research has also documented the beneficial effects of exercising with a "buddy" who can serve as additional motivation and provide emotional support (e.g., Wankel, 1984). Many older adults enjoy the social interaction involved with exercise participation, and approximately 33% of older adults report that they would rather exercise with others than alone (Wilcox, King, Brassington, & Ahn, 1999). Even those older adults who prefer to exercise outside of a formal program may require someone to teach them proper exercise techniques and help them develop a physical activity program if they have had little or no prior exercise experience.

Quite possibly the largest barrier to exercise participation in older adults is the fear that exercise will cause injury, pain, and discomfort or exacerbate existing conditions. These can be very significant, and often realistic, fears that require careful consideration. The typical older adult will spend several years of their late life with one or more disabling conditions that may limit their activity choices (Ferrucci et al., 1996). Beginning a program of exercise often has attendant pain and discomfort, especially when individuals start out too fast. Older adults need to be instructed that this mild pain is not a sign of their age or infirmity and that it should dissipate with modifications of their activity, and the activity will get easier as they continue to exercise. Compounding the problem is the assumption of many older adults that they have limited energy and that it should not be wasted on exercise. When older adults have responsibilities, such as being a caregiver, they may be operating with limited energy resources and feel that exercising will simply make them too tired to do what they have to do (King & Brassington, 1999). Proper counseling by the physician and a trained exercise professional can help decrease this barrier to exercise.

Self-Efficacy

Knowing that older adults will encounter most or all of these barriers to exercise does little on its own to explain their participation or lack of participation in physical activity. What is more important is their perception of their ability to exercise in the face of these barriers. These perceptions of their abilities, or self-confidence regarding exercise, have typically been examined within the framework of a psychological construct called self-efficacy.

Self-efficacy is an individual's belief in his or her capabilities to complete a course of action or behavior. It is the central construct in Bandura's (1986) social cognitive theory. Research has found self-efficacy to be an important predictor of whether an older adult will adopt an exercise program and continue to exercise after the completion of a supervised program (Hallam & Petosa, 1998; McAuley, Lox, & Duncan, 1993).

In line with the reported differences in exercise levels between men and women, males typically report greater exercise self-efficacy (confidence) than women (McAuley et al., 1999). These results may be explained by the fact that the most significant source of efficacy is an individual's past accomplishments (Bandura, 1997). Thus, older males are more likely to have greater exercise self-efficacy due to their previous positive exercise and sport experiences. Older women who have had fewer physical activity experiences have had less opportunity to develop self-confidence in their ability to exercise. However, it is important to note that when both older males and females are given an opportunity to exercise on a regular basis, they both become more confident in their ability to exercise (McAuley et al., 1999).

When examining an older adult's confidence in their ability to exercise in spite of the many barriers (barrier efficacy), people who have more confidence that they can overcome barriers to exercise actually exercise more (Brenes et al., 1998). There are also a number of studies using the framework of the TTM that document that higher levels of self-efficacy are associated with greater physical activity levels (e.g., Herrick, Stone, & Mettler, 1997; Gorely & Gordon, 1995). These studies clearly support the importance of older adults having a strong sense of confidence that they can overcome the many barriers to regular exercise.

Self-efficacy is a construct that predicts whether or not a person starts (adopts) an exercise program, and it also has been shown to increase when people engage in a program of exercise (see McAuley & Blissmer, 2000 for a review). This mutual relationship also exists with all of the other motivational factors we have previously discussed. For example, social support for exercise is an important predictor of exercise participation, and participating in a structured exercise program will place an older adult within a social network that obviously values exercise. The complexities of these relationships illustrate the need to examine the process of adoption and maintenance of exercise. Understanding why an individual chooses to be active, what factors change when they are active, and why they do or do not remain active is the real goal of exercise researchers and will ultimately have the greatest impact on the health of the elderly.

DYNAMIC NATURE OF EXERCISE

When attempting to understand and predict the exercise behavior of older adults, it is important to recognize that exercise behavior is a dynamic process. The reasons that individuals do or do not adopt an exercise program may be different than the reasons they do or do not continue an exercise program. Likewise, the barriers that face a beginning exerciser may be different than those facing a veteran exerciser. Researchers have begun to recognize that different approaches may be required to deal with individuals at various stages of readiness for exercise and at different points in their personal exercise histories (Dunn, Andersen, & Jakicic, 1998).

The model that has been adopted to attempt to explain and understand the process underlying exercise behavior has been the TTM (Nigg et al., 1999; Cardinal, 1997; Marcus & Simkin, 1994). At the heart of this model are the stages and processes of change, but the model also includes many of the components we previously described as important motivational determinants. Decisional balance measures capture the constructs of attitudes and barriers, self-efficacy is an important part of the TTM, and although not distinctly measured, the TTM recognizes the importance of social support in the processes of change that underlie behavioral change.

As the remainder of this book is dedicated to the TTM and its application to the exercise behavior of older adults, discussion of these constructs and their application to exercise behavior in older adults will be saved for later. The important thing to remember is the necessity of examining the motivational processes underlying exercise behavior during the different periods and stages of exercise behavior.

INTERVENTIONS

There are clearly a number of specific concerns that need to be addressed when developing programs to enhance the physical activity of adults. These factors include health, social, economic, cultural, physical, environmental, and safety concerns as well the motivational determinants of exercise and the dynamic nature of the exercise process. There have been a number of studies that have specifically attempted to intervene to increase the physical activity levels of older adults (for an excellent review see King, Rejeski, & Buchner, 1998). These interventions address many of the concerns presented in this chapter using a mix of theoretical and behavioral approaches. However, as reviewers have pointed out (King & Brassington, 1997; King et al., 1998), there remains a definite need to examine strategies based on our knowledge of the determinants of exercise in older adults and their effects on various subgroups of the elderly population including different gender, racial, and socioeconomic groups. There is also a need to assess the most effective and cost-efficient implementation methodology to effectively reach the largest population of elderly. Future approaches must also acknowledge the dynamic nature of exercise and respect the fact that different older adults may be at different stages in the exercise process.

REFERENCES

Albright, C. L., Cohen, S., Gibbons, L., Miller, S., Marcus, B., Sallis, J., Imai, K., Jernick, J., & Simons-Morton, D. G. (2000). Incorporating physical activity advice into primary care: Physician-delivered advice within the Activity Counseling Trial. *American Journal of Preventive Medicine, 18,* 225–234.

American College of Sports Medicine. (1998). ACSM Position stand on exercise and physical activity for older adults. *Medicine and Science in Sports and Exercise, 30*(6), 992–1008.

American College of Sports Medicine. (2000). *Guidelines for Exercise Testing and Exercise Prescription* (6th ed.). Philadelphia: Lippincott Williams and Williams: Author.

Andersen, R. E., Wadden, T. A., Bartlett, S. J., Zemael, B., Verde, T. J., & Franckowiak, S. C. (1999). Effects of lifestyle activity vs. structured aerobic exercise in obese women. *Journal of the American Medical Association, 281,* 2335–2340.

Baker, D. W., Parker, R. M., Williams, M. V., Clark, W. S., & Nurss, J. (1997). The relationship of patient reading ability to self-reported health and use of health services. *American Journal of Public Health, 87,* 1027–1030.

Bandura, A. (1986). *Social foundations of thought and action: A social cognitive theory.* Englewood Cliffs, NJ: Prentice Hall.

Bandura, A. (1997). *Self-efficacy: The exercise of control.* New York: W. H. Freeman and Company.

Brenes, G. A., Strube, M. J., & Storandt, M. (1998). Application of the theory of planned behavior to exercise among older adults. *Journal of Applied Social Psychology, 28,* 2274–2290.

Brownson, R. C., Eyler, A. A., King, A. C., Brown, D. R., Shyu, Y. L., & Sallis, J. F. (2000). Patterns and correlates of physical activity among U.S. women 40 years and older. *American Journal of Public Health, 90*(2), 264–270.

Cardinal, B. J. (1997). Construct validity of stages of change for exercise behavior. *American Journal of Health Promotion, 12*(1), 68–74.

Cardinal, B. J., Esters, J., & Cardinal, M. K. (1996). Evaluation of the revised physical activity readiness questionnaire in older adults. *Medicine and Science in Sports and Exercise, 28*(4), 468–472.

Chogahara, M., Cousins, S. O., & Wankel, L. M. (1998). Social influences on physical activity in older adults. *Journal of Aging & Physical Activity, 6,* 1–17.

Clark, D. O. (1999). Physical activity and its correlates among urban primary care patients aged 55 or older. *Journals of Gerontology: Series B, 54B,* S41–S48.

Courneya, K. S., Nigg, C. R., & Estabrooks, P. A. (1998). Relationships among the theory of planned behavior, stages of change, and exercise behavior in older persons over a three year period. *Psychology and Health, 13,* 355–367.

Courneya, K. S., Plotnikoff, R. C., Hotz, S. B., & Birkett, N. J. (2000). Social support and the theory of planned behavior in the exercise domain. *American Journal of Health Behavior, 24*(4), 300–308.

Damush, T. M., Stewart, A. L., Mills, K. M., King, A. C., & Ritter, P. L. (1999). Prevalence and correlates of physician recommendations to exercise among older adults. *Journals of Gerontology: Series A, Biological Sciences & Medical Sciences, 54*(8), M423–M427.

DeBusk, R. F., Haskell, W. L., Miller, N. H., Berra, C., Taylor, C. B., Berger, W. E., & Lew, H. (1985). Medically directed at home-rehabilitation soon after uncomplicated acute myocardial infarction: A new model for patient care. *American Journal of Cardiology, 55,* 251–257.

DeBusk, R. E., Houston-Miller, N., Superko, H. R., Dennis, C. A., Thoma, R. J., Lew, H. T., Berger, W. E., Heller, R. S., Rompf, J., & Gee, D. (1994). A case management system for coronary risk factor modification after acute myocardial infarction. *Annals of Internal Medicine, 120,* 721–729.

Dishman, R. K. (1988). *Exercise adherence: Its impact on public health.* Champaign, IL: Human Kinetics.

Doak, C. C., Doak, L. G., & Root, J. (1995). *Teaching patients with low literacy skills* (2nd ed.). Philadelphia: J. B. Lippincott.

Dunn, A. L., Andersen, R. E., & Jakicic, J. M. (1998). Lifestyle physical activity interventions. History, short- and long-term effects, and recommendations. *American Journal of Preventive Medicine, 15*(4), 398–412.

Dunn, A. L., Marcus, B. H., Kampert, J. B., Garcia, M. E., Kohl, H. W., & Blair, S. B. (1999). Comparison of lifestyle and structured interventions to increase physical activity and cardiorespiratory fitness: A randomized study. *Journal of the American Medical Association, 281,* 327–334.

Elward, K. S., Wagner, E. H., & Larson, E. B. (1992). Participation by sedentary elderly persons in an exercise promotion session. *Family Medicine, 24,* 607–612.

Emmons, R. A., & Diener, E. (1986). A goal-affect analysis of everyday situational choices. *Journal of Research in Personality, 20*(3), 309–326.

Everard, K. M., Lach, H. W., Fisher, E. B., & Baum, M. C. (2000). Relationship of activity and social support to the functional health of older adults. *Journal of Gerontology: Social Sciences, 55B,* S208–S212.

Eyler, A. A., Brownson, R. C., Donatelle, R. J., King, A. C., Brown, D., & Sallis, J. F. (1999). Physical activity social support and middle- and older-aged minority women: Results from a U.S. survey. *Social Science and Medicine, 49*(6), 781–789.

Federal Interagency Forum on Aging Related Statistics. (2000). *Older Americans 2000: Key indicators of well-being.* Hyattsville, MD: Author.

Ferrucci, L., Guralnik, J. M., Simonsick, E., Salive, M. E., Corti, C., & Langlois, J. (1996). Progressive versus catastrophic disability: A longitudinal view of the disablement process. *Journals of Gerontology Series A-Biological Sciences & Medical Sciences, 51*(3), M123–M130.

Fishbein, M., & Ajzen, I. (1975). *Belief, attitude, intention and behavior: An introduction to theory and research.* Reading, MA: Addison-Wesley.

Fletcher, G. F., Balady, G., Froelicher, V. F., Hartley, L. H., Haskell, W. L., & Pollock, M. L. (1995). Exercise standards: A statement for healthcare professionals from the American Heart Association. *Circulation, 91,* 580–615.

Fletcher, B. J., Dunbar, S. B., Flener, J. M., Jensen, B. E., Almon, L., Cotsonis, G., & Fletcher, G. F. (1994). Exercise testing and training in physically disabled men with clinical evidence of coronary heart disease. *American Journal of Cardiology, 73,* 170–174.

Franklin, B. A., Bonzheim, K., Gordon, S, & Timmis, O. C. (1998). Safety of medically supervised outpatient cardiac rehabilitation exercise therapy: A 16-year follow-up. *Chest, 114,* 902–906.

Gibbons, R. J., Balady, G. J., Beasley, J. W., Bricker, J. T., Duvemoy, W. F., Froelicher, V. F., Mark, D. B., Mawick, T. H., McCallister, B. D., Thompson, P. D., Jr., Winters, W. L., Yanowittz, F. G., Ritchie, J. L., Gibbons, R. J., Cetlin, M. D., Eagle, K. A., Gardener, T. J., Garson, A.,

Jr., Lewis, R. P., O'Rourke, R. A., & Ryan, T. J. (1997). ACC/AHS guidelines for exercise testing: A report of the American College of Cardiology/American Heart Association task force on practice guidelines (committee on exercise testing). *Journal of the American College of Cardiology, 30*(1), 260–315.

Gill, T. M., DiPietro, L., & Krumholz, H. M. (2000). Exercise stress testing for older persons starting an exercise program. *Journal of the American Medical Association, 284*(3), 342–349.

Godin, G. (1994). Theories of reasoned action and planned behavior: Usefulness for exercise promotion. *Medicine and Science in Sport and Exercise, 26*, 1391–1394.

Gorely, T., & Gordon, S. (1995). An examination of the transtheoretical model and exercise behavior in older adults. *Journal of Sport & Exercise Psychology, 17*, 312–324.

Gravelle, F., Pare, C., & Laurencelle, L. (1997). Attitude and enduring involvement of older adults in structured programs of physical activity. *Perceptual & Motor Skills, 85*, 67–71.

Hallam, J., & Petosa, R. (1998). A worksite intervention to enhance social cognitive theory constructs to promote exercise adherence. *American Journal of Health Promotion, 13*, 4–7.

Haskell, W. L. (1994). The efficacy and safety of exercise programs in cardiac rehabilitation. *Medicine and Science in Sports and Exercise, 26*, 815–882.

Haskell, W. L., Alderman, E. L., Fair, J. M., Maron, D. J., Mackey, S. F., Superko, H. R., Williams, P. T., Johnstone, I. M., Champagne, M. A., Krauss, R. M., et al. (1994). Effects of intensive multiple risk factor reduction on coronary atherosclerosis and clinical cardiac events in men and women with coronary artery disease. The Stanford Coronary Risk Intervention Project (SCRIP). *Circulation, 89*, 975–990.

Hausenblas, H. A., Carron, A. V., & Mack, D. E. (1997). Application of the theories of reasoned action and planned behavior to exercise behavior: A meta-analysis. *Journal of Sport & Exercise Psychology, 19*, 36–51.

Herrick, A. B., Stone, W. J., & Mettler, M. M. (1997). Stages of change, decisional balance, and self-efficacy across four behaviors in a worksite environment. *American Journal of Health Promotion, 12*, 49–56.

Jones, D. A., Ainsworth, B. E., Croft, J. B., Macera, C. A., Lloyd, E. E., & Yusuf, H. R. (1998). Moderate leisure-time physical activity: Who is meeting the public health recommendations? A national cross-sectional study. *Archives of Family Medicine, 7*, 285–289.

King, A. C., & Brassington, G. (1997). Enhancing physical and psychological functioning in older family caregivers: The role of regular physical activity. *Annals of Behavioral Medicine, 19*, 91–100.

King, A. C. (1997). Intervention strategies and determinants of physical activity and exercise behavior in adult and older adult men and women. *World Reviews of Nutrition & Diet, 82,* 148–158.

King, A. C., Castro, C., Wilcox, S., Eyler, A. A., Sallis, J. F., & Brownson, R. C. (2000). Personal and environmental factors associated with physical inactivity among different racial-ethnic groups of U.S. middle-aged and older-aged women. *Health Psychology, 19,* 354–364.

King, A. C., Rejeski, W. J., & Buchner, D. M. (1998). Physical activity interventions targeting older adults: A critical review and recommendations. *American Journal of Preventive Medicine, 15,* 316–333.

Kirsch, I. S., Jungeblut, A., Jenkins, L., & Kolstad, A. (1993). *Adult literacy in America: A first look at the results of the national adult literacy survey.* Washington, DC: National Center for Education Statistics, U.S. Department of Education, U.S. Government Printing Office.

Kramarow, E., Lentzner, H., Rooks, R., Weeks, J., & Saydah, S. (1999). *Health and aging chartbook: Health, United States, 1999.* Hyattsville, MD: National Center for Health Statistics.

Larson, E. B. (1992). Benefits of exercise for older adults. A review of existing evidence and current recommendations for the general population. *Clinics in Geriatric Medicine, 8*(1), 35–50.

Leaf, D. A., & Reuben, D. B. (1996). "Lifestyle" interventions for promoting physical activity: A kilocalorie expenditure-based home feasibility study. *American Journal of Medical Science, 312*(2), 68–75.

Lewis, B. S., & Lynch, W. D. (1993). The effect of physician advice on exercise behavior. *Preventive Medicine, 22,* 110–121.

Malinow, M. R., McGarry, D. K., & Kuehl, K. S. (1984). Is exercise testing indicated for asymptomatic active people. *Journal of Cardiac Rehabilitation, 4,* 376–379.

Marcus, B. H., & Simkin, L. R. (1994). The transtheoretical model: Applications to exercise behavior. *Medicine and Science in Sports and Exercise, 26*(11), 1400–1404.

McAuley, E., & Blissmer, B., (2000). Social cognitive determinants and consequences of physical activity. *Exercise and Sports Science Reviews, 28,* 85–88.

McAuley, E., Katula, J., Mihalko, S. L., Blissmer, B., Duncan, T. E., Pena, M., & Dunn, E. (1999). Mode of physical activity and self-efficacy in older adults: A latent growth curve analysis. *Journal of Gerontology: Psychological Series, 54B,* P283–P292.

McAuley, E., Lox, D. L., & Duncan, T. (1993). Long-term maintenance of exercise, self-efficacy, and physiological change in older adults. *Journal of Gerontology: Psychological Series, 48,* P218–P223.

McAuley, E., Marquez, D., Jerome, G., & Blissmer, B. (2000). Physical activity effects on social support: Generalized or specific? *The Gerontologist, 40,* A47.

Miller, N. H., Haskell, W. L., Berra, K., & DeBusk, R. F. (1984). Home versus group exercise training for increasing functional capacity after myocardial infarction. *Circulation, 70,* 645–649.

Mills, K. M., Stewart, A. L., King, A. C., Roitz, K., Sepsis, P. G., Ritter, P. L., & Bortz, W. M., 2nd (1996). Factors associated with enrollment of older adults into a physical activity promotion program. *Journal of Aging & Health, 8*(1), 96–113.

National Center for Health Statistics. (1999). *Health, United States, with health and aging chartbook.* Hyattsville, MD: Author.

Nigg, C. R., Burbank, P. M., Padula, C., Dufresne, R., Rossi, J. S., Velicer, W. F., Laforge, R. G., & Prochaska, J. O. (1999). Stages of change across ten health risk behaviors for older adults. *Gerontologist, 39,* 473–482.

Ostrow, A. C., & Dzewaltowski, D. A. (1986). Older adults' perceptions of physical activity participation based on age-role and sex-role appropriateness. *Research Quarterly for Exercise and Sport, 57,* 167–169.

Ostrow, A. C., Keeney, R. E., & Perry, S. A. (1986). The age grading of physical activity among children. *International Journal of Aging & Human Development, 24,* 101–111.

Plimpton, S., & Root, J. (1994). Materials and strategies that work in low literacy health communication. *Public Health Reports, 109,* 86–92.

Prochaska, J. O., & DiClemente, C. C. (1983). Stages and processes of self-change of smoking: Toward an integrative model of change. *Consultations in Clinical Psychology, 51*(3), 390–395.

Resnick, B., & Spellbring, A. M. (2000). Understanding what motivates older adults to exercise. *Journal of Gerontological Nursing, 26*(3), 34–42.

Rhodes, R. E., Martin, A. D., Taunton, J. E., Rhodes, E. C., Donnelly, M., & Elliot, J. (1999). Factors associated with exercise adherence among older adults: An individual perspective. *Sports Medicine, 28,* 397–411.

Richter, D. L., Macera, C. A., Williams, H., & Koerber, M. (1993). Disincentives to participate in planned exercise activities among older adults. *Health Values, 17,* 51–55.

Shephard, R. J. (1988). Canadian Home Fitness Test and screening alternatives. *Sports Medicine, 5,* 185–195.

Shephard, R. J. (1990). The scientific basis for prescribing exercise for the very old. *Journal of the American Geriatrics Society, 38,* 62–70.

Shephard, R. J., Cox, M. H., & Simper, K. (1981). An analysis of "PAR-Q" responses in an office population. *Canadian Journal of Public Health, 72,* 37–40.

Sirvarajan, E. S., Bruce, R. A., Linskog, B. D., Almes, M. J., Belanger, L., & Green, B. (1982). Treadmill responses to an early exercise program after myocardial infarction: A randomized study. *Circulation, 65,* 1420–1428.

Siscovick, D. S. (1997). Exercise and its role in sudden cardiac death. *Cardiology Clinics, 15*(3), 467–472.

Siscovick, D. S., Weiss, N. S., Fletcher, R. H., & Lasky, T. (1984). The incidence of primary cardiac arrest during vigorous exercise. *New England Journal of Medicine, 311,* 874–877.

Stead, M., Wimbush, E., Eadie, D., & Teer, P. (1997). A qualitative study of older people's perceptions of aging and exercise: The implications for health promotion. *The Health Education Journal, 56,* 3–16.

Stewart, A. L., Mills, K. M., Sepsis, P. G., King, A. C., McLellan, B. Y., Roitz, K., & Ritter, P. L. (1998). Evaluation of CHAMPS, a physical activity promotion program for older adults. *Annals of Behavioral Medicine, 19*(4), 353–361.

Thomas, S., Reading, J., & Shephard, R. J. (1992). Revision of the physical activity readiness questionnaire (PAR-Q). *Canadian Journal of Sport Sciences, 17,* 338–345.

Tinetti, M. E., Doucette, J. T., & Claus, E. B. (1995). The contribution of predisposing and situational risk factors to serious fall injuries. *Journal of the American Geriatric Society, 43*(11), 1207–1213.

Tinetti, M. E., Doucette, J., Claus, E., & Marottoli, R. (1995). Risk factors for serious injury during falls by older persons in the community. *Journal of the American Geriatric Society, 43*(11), 1214–1221.

Tinetti, M. E., Liu, W. L., & Claus, E. B. (1993). Predictors and prognosis of inability to get up after falls among elderly persons. *Journal of the American Medical Association, 269,* 65–70.

U.S. Department of Health and Human Services. Public Health Service. Agency for Health Care Policy and Research. National Heart, Blood and Lung Institute (1995). *Clinical practice guideline number 17: Cardiac rehabilitation.* (AHCPHR Publication number 96-0672). Rockville, MD: Author.

U.S. Department of Health and Human Services. Public Health Service. (1996). *Physical activity and health: A report of the Surgeon General.* Atlanta, GA: Author.

U.S. Department of Health and Human Services. Public Health Service. (2000). *Healthy people 2010* (2nd ed.) *With understanding and improving health and objectives for improving health* (2 vols.). Washington, DC: U.S. Government Printing Office: Author.

Vander, L., Franklin, B., & Rubenfire, M. (1982). Cardiovascular complications of recreational physical activity. *Physician and Sports Medicine, 10,* 89–94.

Wankel, L. M. (1984). Decision-making and social support structures for increasing exercise adherence. *Journal of Cardiac Rehabilitation, 4,* 124–128.

Wankel, L. M., Mummery, W. K., Stephens, T., & Craig, C. L. (1994). Prediction of physical activity intention from psychological variables: Results from the Campbell's survey of wellbeing. *Journal of Sport and Exercise Psychology, 16,* 56—69.

Washburn, R. A., Janney, C. A., & Caswell, C. (1990). Physicians recommendation influences walking for exercise in older people. *Medicine and Science in Sports and Exercise, 22,* 546.

Weiss, B. D., & Coyne, C. (1997). Communicating with patients who cannot read. *New England Journal of Medicine, 337*(4), 272–274.

Weiss, B. D., Reed, R. L., & Kligman, E. W. (1995). Literacy skills and communication methods of low-income older persons. *Patient Education and Counseling, 25,* 109–119.

Whaley, D. E., & Ebbeck, V. (1997). Older adults constraints to participation in structured exercise classes. *Journal of Aging & Physical Activity, 5,* 190–212.

Wilcox, S., Castro, C., King, A. C., Housemann, R., & Brownson, R. C. (2000). Determinants of leisure time physical activity in rural compared with urban older and ethnically diverse women in the United States. *Journal of Epidemiology and Community Health, 54*(9), 667–672.

Wilcox, S., King, A. C., Brassington, G., & Ahn, D. (1999). Physical activity preferences of middle-aged and older adults: A community analysis. *Journal of Aging & Physical Activity, 7,* 386–399.

Woodwell, D. A. (1997). *National ambulatory medical care survey: 1996 summary. Advanced data from vital and health statistics.* Hyattsville, MD: National Center for Health Statistics.

Woolf, S. H., Jonas, S., & Lawrence, R. S. (1996). Introduction. In S. H. Woolf, S. Jonas, & R. S. Lawrence (Eds.), *Health promotion and disease prevention in clinical practice.* Philadelphia: Williams and Wilkins.

CHAPTER 3

Overview of the Transtheoretical Model

Gary J. Burkholder and Claudio C. Nigg

> "Without change, something sleeps inside us, and seldom awakens. The sleeper must awaken."
>
> ~Frank Herbert

As the public emphasis on healthy living increases, more and more people seek ways to improve their health. Individuals are living longer and preservation of activity and health into older age is becoming increasingly important. Exercise, proper diet, and stress management have been identified as key to preserving health in older age (Perry, 1995). Most individuals intuitively know that some change is necessary, but in reality, making the changes necessary for a healthier lifestyle, such as quitting smoking, moderating fat intake, or protecting oneself against HIV/AIDS infection is typically easier said than done.

For some, change may be easy; for many, however, the attainment of such goals seems nearly impossible. For example, consider smoking, a behavior that has been the focus of public health campaigns for many years. Some may recognize the need to quit smoking but do not feel that the "time is right." Others may not even be thinking about quitting. There are those who have been successful at quitting but at some point started smoking again. These people are all changers, however, each is at a different level of readiness to change. Thus, the goal for the health professional is to find a behavior change approach that can be designed for an individual depending upon where he or she is in terms of intending to change. The person who has been thinking about quitting smoking for some time will most likely respond to a different approach than someone who has never even considered quitting.

But shouldn't knowledge of risk be enough? Why, given the evidence of the long-term impact on health, do some people continue to engage is risky and problematic behaviors? National dietary recommendations include increasing fruit, vegetable, and fiber consumption and decreasing total dietary fat, yet the consumption of dietary fiber, fruits, and vegetables is currently lower, and fat intake is higher than recommended levels (Block, 1993; Public Health Service, 1988). More people than ever are classified as overweight or obese (U.S. Department of Health and Human Services [USDHHS], 2000). Evidence overwhelmingly supports inclusion of exercise in one's daily routine to prevent cardiovascular disease (Powell, Thompson, Caspersen, & Kendrick, 1987; USDHHS, 2000), yet many Americans (about 30%) report not exercising regularly (Stephens & Casperson, 1993; USDHHS, 1996). Millions of young adults, primarily between the ages of 15 and 29, contract at least one sexually transmitted disease (STD) (Centers for Disease Control and Prevention, 1991), yet interventions have had little effect on condom use (Catania et al., 1994). Interestingly, even impact on a single behavior can have positive health implications for other problem behaviors. Unger (1996) found that those who quit smoking also tended to adjust other health behaviors, including increasing exercise and decreasing alcohol use.

Researchers and health professionals generally agree that finding effective ways to reduce health risk is an important priority. It is also recognized that improving knowledge alone does not result in behavior change. Additionally, in the case of smoking, traditional interventions target individuals who are ready to quit, but are not as effective with the majority of smokers who are not considering quitting (Velicer & DiClemente, 1993). Finding the correct approach to use with clients presenting unique circumstances can be challenging. How does the practitioner, considering the physical and psychological needs of the client, help him or her to adopt healthier lifestyle choices?

The purpose of this chapter is to present an overview of the Transtheoretical Model of Behavior Change (TTM) (Prochaska & DiClemente, 1983) by summarizing and synthesizing some of the research pertaining to this model. The TTM is revolutionary in that it can be used to assess the "readiness" of an individual to change and then to tailor an intervention program unique to that individual. Applications of the TTM, originally used to understand the process of smoking cessation (Prochaska, DiClemente, Velicer, & Rossi, 1993; Prochaska & DiClemente, 1983), have rapidly expanded to include a number of other health behaviors, including weight loss (Laforge, Velicer, Richmond, & Owen, 1999), reduced exposure to sun to lower risk of skin cancer (Rossi, 1989), dietary fat reduction (Kristal, Glanz, Curry, & Patterson, 1999; Laforge, Velicer, Richmond, & Owen, 1999); safer sex (Grimley, Prochaska, & Prochaska, 1997; Harlow et al., 1999; Prochaska, Redding, Harlow, Rossi, & Velicer, 1994); exercise adoption (Bark & Nicholas, 1990; Marcus, Banspach, Lefebvre, Rossi, & Carlton, 1992; Marcus, Eaton, Rossi, & Harlow, 1994); and mammography screenings (Rakowski, Fulton, & Feldman, 1993).

This chapter will include the historical origins of the TTM, explanations of the major constructs in the model, and some strengths and limitations of the model. The next chapter will survey in more detail the variety of applications of the model; remaining chapters will examine specific application of the TTM to increasing exercise in older adults.

HISTORICAL ORIGINS OF THE TRANSTHEORETICAL MODEL

Kurt Lewin has generally been given credit for establishing the foundation for our current understanding of health behavior change. Lewin (1951) and Lewin, Dembo, Festinger, and Sears (1944) proposed that people exist in positively, negatively, or neutrally valued spaces, and that forces work to move people to spaces of positive value and less tension. For example, disease would exist in negatively valued space for the individual; the person would be moved to seek remedies for the disease in order to remove it and thus move toward a positively valued space of lower tension and stress. An individual's behavior depends upon two factors: (a) The value placed on a given outcome by the individual (or, in other words, the "pull" the individual feels toward a particular outcome; an individual will be pulled toward the possibility of future health) and (b) the individual's estimate of the probability that a given action would result in that outcome (the "push" of the action: Lewin et al., 1944). The process an individual uses in estimating the outcome of his or her disease became the basis of several decision-making models, including the performance behavior model of Tolman (1955) and Atkinson's (1957) achievement motivation theory.

The Health Belief Model (HBM) (Rosenstock, 1974) is one of the earliest theories of health behavior change. This theoretical perspective was initially conceived in the 1950s to address a growing public health concern that few people at risk for disease were taking advantage of community health programs geared toward early diagnosis. There was a practical need for public health officials to increase awareness of diseases such as tuberculosis, for which screenings might result in early detection. Not only did applied researchers need to address the problem of who was and was not taking advantage of the low-cost or free screenings, but scientists also needed to persuade a largely asymptomatic population of the inherent risk of disease. Using Lewin's Value Expectancy theory, Rosenstock (1974) translated the abstract concept of *valence* into a series of statements applicable to a public health interest. These statements concerned perceived susceptibility ("I can get this disease"), perceived severity ("This disease has the capacity to interfere with my life") of the disease, and perceived benefits of taking action ("If I go to a tuberculosis screening, I can find out early if I test positive").

Decision-making research and the increased focus on public health were important to the development of the TTM. The TTM is the result of accumulating wisdom in the public health tradition. It is used to evaluate where an individual is relative to changing a problematic behavior. The individual stage is strongly related to the manner in which a person rates the benefits of the behavior relative to the costs of the behavior. This relative rating of costs and benefits comes directly from the decision-making theory of Janis and Mann (1977); however, when one examines the history of behavior change and public health and the extent to which the TTM has been tested, it is clear that the model is grounded in a rich public health research tradition.

THE TRANSTHEORETICAL MODEL

Development of the TTM has its roots in the areas of therapy evaluation and smoking cessation. Prochaska (1979), in his research into how people change in the context of therapy as well as those who self-change, identified the *processes of change* variable in his analysis of 18 principle therapy systems. In his search for an eclectic system of psychotherapy that would "rein in" the proliferation of therapy systems during the 1960s and 1970s, the five processes of consciousness-raising, catharsis, commitment, conditional stimuli, and contingency management were identified as being common to the systems analyzed. Further research (Prochaska & DiClemente, 1982, 1983, 1984) indicated that there were 10 basic processes used in the client-therapist context that helped both to attain the therapeutic goal behavior change. Although people changing their behavior were found to use over 100 techniques to help them (Prochaska, Velicer, DiClemente, & Fava, 1988), the techniques used were found to be substantive components of these ten processes. Further investigation revealed that individuals who change with or without the benefit of therapy use similar processes of change (Prochaska & DiClemente, 1982; Prochaska & DiClemente, 1984).

From a retrospective pilot study of smokers who had successfully quit, DiClemente and Prochaska (1982) discovered that successful quitters had used a variety of processes, and different processes were emphasized depending upon where the individual was in the process of change. It was found that, generally, people described the use of specific processes based on whether they were just thinking about quitting smoking, were actively preparing to quit, had actually made an attempt to quit, or quit but were struggling to find ways to keep themselves smoke-free. Initially, research in smoking cessation indicated that there were five primary stages. However, mathematical analysis indicated four stages, and for a time, the 4-stage model of behavior change was used. Cumulative research in the TTM has supported the existence of a 5-stage model of behavior change (DiClemente et al., 1991; Prochaska & DiClemente, 1992).

What follows is a general description of the core constructs of the TTM as they are used in contemporary research and intervention. These constructs are: (a) five principle *stages of change*— precontemplation, contemplation, preparation, action, and maintenance; (b) ten *processes of change* (the processes therapists and self-changers use to facilitate behavior change; (c) *decisional balance*, a relative weighting of benefits of the behavior (pros) to costs of the behavior (cons); and (d) *self-efficacy* for behavior change. Figure 3.1 shows a general model relating the core TTM constructs; each predictor construct has an important relationship to stages of change.

The Stages of Change

Individuals changing behavior move through a series of five stages (a sixth stage, *termination*, is sometimes used and will be discussed here (DiClemente & Prochaska, 1982; Prochaska, Norcross, & DiClemente, 1994). Figure 3.2 shows a visual display of the stages.

1. *Precontemplation.* The individual has no intention to change his or her behavior in the foreseeable future (empirically defined as within the next six months). The behavior is not necessarily seen as high risk and, if it is, there is no feeling of need to change the behavior. In fact, many in this stage may see not their own behavior but that of others as the problem. For example, a precontemplator might say, "My parents have smoked all their lives, they are still alive and healthy, and society just doesn't accept the right of people to smoke if they want to."

2. *Contemplation.* This stage is characterized by an intention to change behavior in the foreseeable future (*within the next six months*). This individual will have begun to examine the consequences of his or her behavior. He or she is most likely beginning to ask questions about the short-term and long-term effects the behavior is/will be having on his or her life.

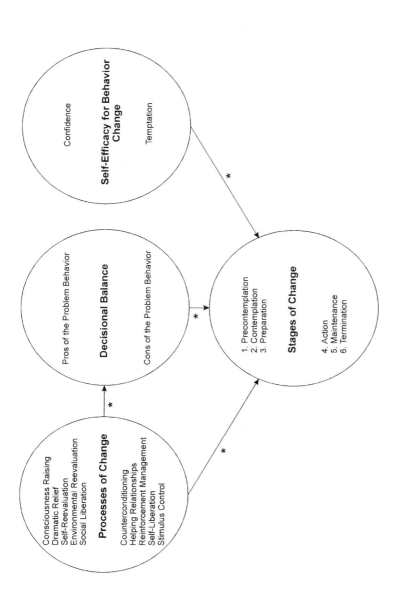

FIGURE 3.1 The Transtheoretical Model of behavior change.

*Different relationships exists for the different stage transitions. More research is needed for development of stage-specific models.

Precontemplation → Contemplation → Preparation → Action → Maintenance → Termination

FIGURE 3.2   The stages of change.

3.   *Preparation.* An individual is intending to take action to change his/her behavior in the near future (usually defined as *within the next month*). This individual is most likely beginning to think about strategies that could be used to help change the behavior.

4.   *Action.* A person in the *action* stage has already made the behavior change, but for less than six months. The criterion for entrance into the action stage is typically set at a level that represents a significant reduction in risk for disease. In some behaviors, this criterion is relatively straightforward (for example, the cessation of smoking). For other behaviors, such as the reduction of dietary fat, the criterion must be based on epidemiological studies providing information on risks associated with the particular behavior. An individual in this stage is at highest risk for relapse as the benefits of the new healthy behavior are not apparent immediately.

5.   *Maintenance.* In this stage the individual has maintained the healthy behavior for an extended period of time (typically defined as a period of *at least six months or longer*). This person will start to realize the benefits of the behavior. There is still some risk of relapse, so the individual must attend to temptations to resume the problem behavior.

6.   *Termination.* The final stage, termination, is characterized by no temptation to resume the habit and 100% self-efficacy for the healthy behavior. Termination has been defined as starting *after five years* of changing the behavior (Prochaska & Velicer, 1997). For some behaviors such as exercise or fruit and vegetable consumption (adoption behaviors), it is unclear if a point in time exists at which a person can be defined as being in termination.

The items used to assess stages are straightforward and involve temporal aspects of the behavior change (i.e., where the person is in relation to change quantified in specific time frames). The behavior in question should be defined carefully such that frequency, duration, and intensity, as well as the criteria for what is considered "taking action" for exercise, are included in the behavioral definition. An example of a stage of change instrument for exercise is provided in chapter 5.

Movement through the six stages of change does not have to be linear. In fact, many people who change their behavior find that they slip back into engaging in the problem behavior (i.e., a person resumes smoking or stops exercising). This is called relapse. The most common path for individuals changing behavior is one in which they advance and regress (relapse) through the stages of change ("spiral model of change": Prochaska, Norcross, & DiClemente, 1994). A person might move into the preparation phase, but then relapse to contemplation, and that same person, once having attained maintenance, may relapse to the preparation stage. The longer the time in maintenance, however, the less likely a person is to relapse (to resume the unhealthy behavior).

Ten Processes of Change

The ten processes can be grouped into two categories. *Experiential processes* are those in which individuals obtain information based on their own experiences. *Behavioral processes* are those in which information is generated from the environment (i.e., outside of the individual). A brief summary of the processes (Burbank, Padula, & Nigg, 2000) is provided in Table 3.1.

Experiential

1. *Consciousness-raising.* A person utilizing this process of change would be interested in obtaining information about the current behavior in order to better understand the impact the behavior has on self and others. The goal is to increase awareness of the consequences of the problem behavior. For example, someone who is trying (or thinking of trying) to lower dietary fat intake might begin reading materials that provide education on the long-term effects of higher fat diets.

TABLE 3.1   The Processes of Change

Process	Definition
Experiential	
Consciousness Raising	Efforts by the individual to seek new information and to gain understanding and feedback about the problem behavior.
Dramatic Relief	Affective aspects of change, often involving intense emotional experiences related to the problem behavior.
Self-Reevaluation	Emotional and cognitive reappraisal of values by the individual regarding the problem behavior.
Environmental Reevaluation	Consideration and assessment by the individual of how the problem affects the physical and social environments.
Social Liberation	Awareness, availability, and acceptance by the individual of alternative, problem-free lifestyles in society.
Behavioral	
Counterconditioning	Substitution of alternative behaviors for problem behavior.
Helping Relationships	Trusting, accepting, and using the support of caring others during attempts to change the problem behavior.
Reinforcement Management	Changing the contingencies that control or maintain the problem behavior.
Self-Liberation	The individual's choice and commitment to change the problem behavior, including the belief that one can change.
Stimulus Control	Control of situations and other causes that trigger the problem behavior.

2.   *Dramatic Relief.* This process represents a type of catharsis in which the individual moves closer to change through direct emotional response to the behavior he or she is trying to change. For example, and individual who is trying to increase his or her level of exercise might find that a colleague had a heart attack because of being unfit. This emotional experience may help move the individual closer to adopting a regular exercise routine.

3.   *Self-reevaluation.* Using this process, the individual seeks change through cognitive or emotional appraisal of the impact of the behavior on him- or herself. For example, the person who smokes might begin to reflect on the ways that such behavior affects his or her life and how life might be different without the problem behavior.

4. *Environmental reevaluation.* This is similar to self-reevaluation. In environmental reevaluation, however, the individual begins to assess his or her impact on the surrounding environment. In the case of a smoker, that assessment might include consideration of the impact of secondhand smoke on family members.

5. *Social liberation.* Social liberation involves the recognition that societal norms are moving to promote a healthier lifestyle that is free of the effects of the problem behavior. There are many examples of this in our culture—the increasing number of laws restricting the places where people can smoke, or the nationwide advertising campaigns targeting drivers who operate vehicles while intoxicated. In both cases, social norms are favoring lifestyles without the effects of these problem behaviors. An individual using this process of change would come to understand the reasons for and benefits of changing to behaviors normative to society and how this relates to his or her own behavior.

Behavioral

6. *Counterconditioning.* A person using this process of change would actively seek ways to substitute healthier behaviors for the current problem behavior. A person who is attempting to quit drinking alcohol, for example, might seek a number of behaviors to substitute for drinking. This might include such actions as calling an Alcoholics Anonymous (AA) member when the urge to drink happens, or to have a cup of coffee instead of alcohol. Someone who smokes might replace cigarettes with candy, or take several very deep breaths. In this process, the individual changes his or her response to the urge to engage in the problem behavior.

7. *Helping relationships.* Helping relationships involve the support of friends or loved ones during the process of change. Such people in the life of one he or she is changing behavior can act as a source of support for the behavior change. Social support can come from a number of other sources, including a family doctor, spiritual leader, or therapist.

8. *Reinforcement management.* Someone using reinforcement management will seek ways to continually reinforce positive behaviors and decrease problem behaviors. This typically would take the form

of some kind of reward system. For example, an individual who wants to quit smoking might place a certain amount of money in a jar for every cigarette avoided. For some, behavior change may be self-rewarding, such as in the case of a person who engages in exercise and is rewarded with lower blood pressure readings.

9. *Self-liberation.* Self-liberation comes from making the definite commitment to change. This process benefits from the extent to which the commitment is made to others. For example, many people who quit smoking make the decision to do so and then relate this information to a close friend or family member. In this way, the act of making a public commitment serves as a reinforcement for abstinence from the problem behavior.

10. *Stimulus control.* This process is similar to counterconditioning, except that now the environment, rather than the thoughts or actions of the individual, is altered to provide cues for positive, healthier behaviors. A person who wants to begin a regular exercise program might hang pictures of athletes in the living space or place an exercise machine in a frequently visited part of the house. Such environmental cues are used to remind the person of the commitment to the process of behavior change.

Decisional Balance

The decision-making theory of Janis and Mann (1977) formed the basis for decisional balance. They evaluated the extent to which people rated costs of a behavior relative to benefits. The Janis and Mann model indicated four cost factors (losses for self, losses for others, disapproval from self, and disapproval from others) and four benefit factors (gains for self, gains for others, approval from self, and approval from others). However, Velicer, DiClemente, Prochaska, and Brandenburg (1985), in a study of smoking cessation, found only two stable factors—one relating to the benefits of the behavior (pros) and costs of engaging in the behavior (cons). This two-factor model, referred to as *decisional balance,* has since been replicated for at least 12 other behaviors including exercise (Prochaska, Velicer, DiClemente, & Fava, 1994).

Generally a client is asked to assess his or her level of agreement with a series of statements. Some of these statements will reflect positive aspects (pros) of a behavior, as well as negative aspects (cons) of a behavior (a decisional balance instrument used for exercise behavior is given in chapter 5). Research has indicated that the degree to which a person rates the pros of a behavior higher than the cons is strongly related to stage of readiness for change.

Self-Efficacy for Behavior Change

Self-efficacy for behavior change, derived from the general self-efficacy theory of Bandura (1977, 1982), generally refers to the degree to which a person feels he or she can be successful at engaging in or resisting a behavior in a variety of contexts. This construct was operationalized for the TTM using two components (Prochaska, Redding, & Evers, 1996)—confidence and temptation. Confidence refers to the level to which a person feels he or she can respond to situational demands without relapsing. A smoker might have a certain level of confidence that he or she can resist smoking when under work stress. Temptation represents the urge to involve oneself in the risky behavior in the context of stressful situations. An example of this would be physical cravings experienced by a person withdrawing from substances. A sample exercise self-efficacy scale is presented in chapter 5.

RELATIONSHIPS AMONG TTM CONSTRUCTS

Figure 3.3 provides a pictorial display of how processes, stage, decisional balance, and self-efficacy are related in an ideal situation in which the individual progresses linearly and successfully through each of the stages. It should be noted that the processes may be variable with specific behaviors, and that the relationships indicated represent a general synthesis based on a number of discussions of processes (Prochaska, DiClemente, & Norcross, 1992; Prochaska, Norcross, & DiClemente, 1994; Prochaska, Redding, & Evers, 1996). For example, some of the processes may be more appropriate for specific problem behaviors, or fewer processes may be used in behavior change (Prochaska, Redding, & Evers, 1996).

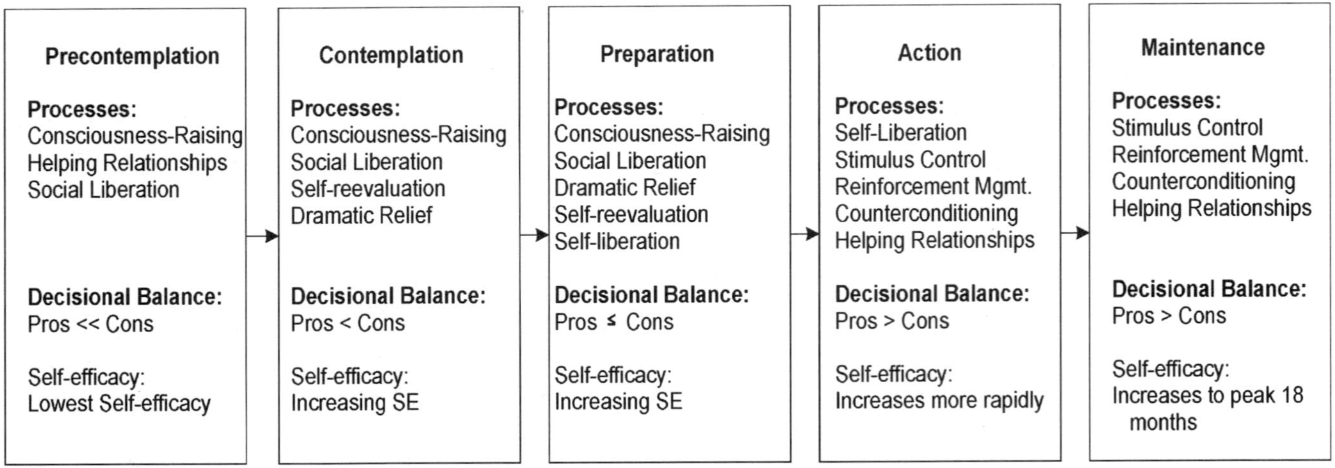

Precontemplation

Processes:
Consciousness-Raising
Helping Relationships
Social Liberation

Decisional Balance:
Pros << Cons

Self-efficacy:
Lowest Self-efficacy

Contemplation

Processes:
Consciousness-Raising
Social Liberation
Self-reevaluation
Dramatic Relief

Decisional Balance:
Pros < Cons

Self-efficacy:
Increasing SE

Preparation

Processes:
Consciousness-Raising
Social Liberation
Dramatic Relief
Self-reevaluation
Self-liberation

Decisional Balance:
Pros ≤ Cons

Self-efficacy:
Increasing SE

Action

Processes:
Self-Liberation
Stimulus Control
Reinforcement Mgmt.
Counterconditioning
Helping Relationships

Decisional Balance:
Pros > Cons

Self-efficacy:
Increases more rapidly

Maintenance

Processes:
Stimulus Control
Reinforcement Mgmt.
Counterconditioning
Helping Relationships

Decisional Balance:
Pros > Cons

Self-efficacy:
Increases to peak 18 months

FIGURE 3.3 Relationship between stages of change, processes of change, and decisional balance.

Processes and Stages of Change

Prochaska and DiClemente (1983) found a relationship between a person's stage and specific processes used in that stage. This relationship is very important as it forms the basis of using staging models to tailor unique, individual-specific interventions.

1. *Precontemplation.* A person in this stage utilizes all processes less than people who are in any other stage. A person in this stage would be characterized as being resistant and in denial that there is a problem. This person may appear to be rationalizing his or her behavior and might appear to be blaming his behavior on the insensitivity of others. People in precontemplation may benefit most from receiving general information about the problem behavior (consciousness-raising), the unconditional encouragement from close friends and family (helping relationships), and receiving more information about problem behaviors (social liberation), which happens frequently in the context of social norms (for example, establishment of no-smoking sections helps to increase the awareness of the ills of smoking).

2. *Contemplation.* Those in the contemplation stage are more likely to use consciousness-raising, self-reevaluation, and dramatic relief to progress to the preparation stage. Thus, awareness techniques that help the client to become more deeply aware of the ways in which the problem behavior affects one's life and helping him or her to understand how the problem behavior is really conflicting with that person's basic life values would be most beneficial to someone in the contemplation stage of change. Additionally, informing others about the contemplation of changing a problem behavior maximizes encouragement from others. Social liberation is also important for continuing to recognize the ways in which social pressure is applied to change the problem behavior.

3. *Preparation.* In this stage helping the person to continue self-reevaluation and continuing to offer support are the best strategies for helping in the behavior change process. The client is ready to make the change (recalling that, by definition, preparation occurs when someone intends to change his or her behavior in the next 30 days). The moment of self-liberation is at hand! This would also

be the time to begin to engage the client in thought and discussion of techniques associated with the behavioral processes, such as reinforcement management, which will be useful once action has been taken.

4. *Action.* In this stage self-liberation, stimulus control, reinforcement management, and counterconditioning are the processes used most. The latter three are the behavioral processes. Types of strategies used include altering the environments to reinforce positive behaviors, the use of contracts or other public demonstrations of commitment to change, and reward systems for continued successful performance.

5. *Maintenance.* In this stage the person has been successful at change for at least six months. The temptations will still exist but typically will become weaker and less frequent as the time over which behavior change has been successful increases. During this time the continuing self-reevaluation and redefinition by the individual of life without the problem behavior and the continuing reliance on helping relationships are valuable in helping the person to achieve the commitment of the specific behavior change. The need for processes of stimulus control, counterconditioning, and reinforcement management should decrease as the length of maintenance increases and the individual creates a life without the problem behavior.

Decisional Balance and Stage of Change

The rating of pros relative to cons is most prevalent in the earlier stages of change (precontemplation, contemplation, and preparation). In the precontemplation stage, the individual would tend to rate the benefits of the unhealthy behavior as far exceeding the costs. As progress through the stages occurs, this relationship changes such that the benefits of the problem behavior receive less weight and the costs of the problem behavior are weighted more strongly in the action and maintenance stages. In the preparation stage, the person tends to rate pros and cons equally. However, the pros for a healthy behavior increase across the stages and the cons decrease with the crossover (the decisional balance point at which pros = cons). Decisional balance does not generally predict progress in the action and maintenance stages (Prochaska, DiClemente, & Norcross, 1992). Empirical evidence for several problem behaviors (Prochaska, Velicer, Rossi, et al., 1994) indicated this classical crossover pattern. Therefore, the evidence suggests that *decreasing pros and increasing cons of a particular unhealthy behavior* would be a practical goal in moving people through the early stages of change (Prochaska, Redding, & Evers, 1996).

Self-Efficacy and Stages of Change

Self-efficacy (confidence) was found to increase as forward progress was made through the stages of change; less research has been done on temptations. It was interesting that temptations did not level off until 3 years after smoking had been stopped (DiClemente, Prochaska, & Gilbertini, 1985), and that self-efficacy actually peaked at 18 months after the behavior had been changed. This implies that self-efficacy seems to be important as the health behavior comes under one's control. Over time, temptations may play an increasingly important role in maintaining the health behavior for life.

EVALUATION OF THE TTM

Assumptions

There are several assumptions underlying the TTM, some of which are discussed in Prochaska, Redding, and Evers (1996). These include: (a) multiple theoretical perspectives are required to account for the number of ways people change their behavior, both in and out of the context of therapy; (b) changing behavior happens in steps and, except in rare cases, does not happen instantly. Development in the TTM indicates that the process of change begins well before the actual adoption of the health behavior. In fact, as noted earlier, the change process is best described as a "spiral of change" that includes advancements and relapses in behavior; (c) change in health behavior of the population will rarely happen on its own—change requires the use of materials tailored to specific individuals unique to their stage of change. Although many of the traditional behavior change programs, such as quitting smoking or ceasing alcohol use, assume that the individual is at the preparation stage, this is seldom the case.

Another important assumption is that health behavior is primarily under the control of the individual. The model does not explicitly include socioeconomic or cultural influences that have been demonstrated to have an impact on behavior. For example, Caron et al. (2000) found that the interaction of neighborhood-level factors such as poverty and educational level, family-level factors such as a measure of income to needs, and individual-level factors is important in explaining change in physical activity.

Strengths of the TTM

There are several aspects of the TTM that make it particularly useful in the public health domain.

1. *Tailored interventions.* A behavior change program can be uniquely tailored to an individual. As noted at the beginning of this chapter, different people are going to be at different levels of readiness to change their behavior. Some will not even be thinking about change, and others may have changed their behavior but are searching for ways to make maintenance of the new behavior easier. Health practitioners, in theory, can quickly assess where a client is in terms of the process of change, and then be able to counsel a client on specific techniques for progress toward higher stages. The varied processes of change can also be tailored to what works best with the client. Velicer, Norman, Fava, and Prochaska (1999) submitted the TTM to a rigorous test of several predictions based on stage of change, and the majority of the predictions were confirmed, indicating strong statistical support for a tailored stage-of-change model. Additionally, public health issues, such as cigarette smoking, alcohol use, drug use, and compliance with medication regimes can be approached on a population level through public interventions that can reach large numbers of people quickly with individualized attention.

2. *It works even if your willpower is low.* The old adage, "it takes willpower" to change has been rendered false. The willpower hypothesis suggests that people who engage in risky health behaviors need

to have willpower in order to succeed. However, the TTM offers an explanation and a means to behavior change that depends less upon willpower than it does on the scientific application of appropriate processes that can nudge the change process along, regardless of what stage a person is currently in. It is also clear that smoking cessation, for example, is not a one-time event, but rather represents a process that is cyclic and dynamic (Cohen et al., 1989).

3. *Broad scope.* The TTM has been shown to be applicable to a wide variety of health behaviors. Research is suggesting that such an integrated model of behavior change does very well at explaining change encompassing a variety of problem behaviors, many of which are public health concerns. Application of the model represents an effective means of effecting behavior change.

4. *Usefulness to practitioners.* The TTM, a model that represents an extremely powerful approach to behavior change, is clear enough to be used by virtually any type of practitioner as well as by researchers. More testing of the model is needed to find ways to more easily and accurately match intervention to stages. However, as the model is validated for each behavior, doctors, nurses, social workers, psychologists, and other health care professionals will, in the future, have access to the model in their offices. The TTM has the capacity to combine clinical and public health interventions to maximize success in problem behavior change (Prochaska, 1996).

5. *Success compared with other interventions.* There have been few studies in which the TTM has been compared to other interventions. Prochaska, DiClemente, Velicer, and Rossi (1993) conducted an experiment with smokers who were randomly assigned either a standardized self-help manual, individualized manuals matched to stage, interactive expert system reports (a computer-generated report matching stage of change to written materials; detailed description of the expert system is provided in Velicer, Rossi, Ruggiero, & Prochaska, 1994), or personalized counselor calls plus individualized manuals. The results indicated that those assigned to the interactive expert system showed the best quit rates at all follow-ups. Rossi (1994) found that stage-matched interventions produce two to three times more change than action-oriented programs, and that participation rates in stage-matched programs were as high as 80% compared with 1 to 5% participation in action programs. While it is unclear if these success rates could be attained in interventions with other problem

behaviors, the results do suggest that, at least for smoking, stage-matched interventions outperform the best self-help programs. The results should be encouraging to researchers interested in doing similar comparison studies with other problem health behaviors.

Limitations of the TTM

Although the TTM is a powerful model for behavior change, some limitations have been noted.

1. *Is behavior change best represented as a stage model?* Joseph, Breslin, and Skinner (1999) critiqued the stage construct and the question was raised as to whether stage models are most appropriate for behavior change. The researchers noted that the change in the number of stages, the number of processes, and the items used to evaluate both stages and processes have changed since the original conception of the TTM, although more recent work has settled on the use of a five-stage and 10-process model of change. This suggested the need for more work on the nature of the stages and whether the current interventions are best matched to the individual stage of readiness to change.

Hedeker, Mermelstein, and Weeks (1999) provided evidence to suggest that even the thresholds of change (the transitions between stages) could be uniquely described apart from the stages they separate. These researchers discovered a contemplation threshold (the transition from precontemplation to contemplation) and an action threshold (the transition from preparation to action). It was found that self-efficacy has a stronger effect at the action threshold. This provided empirical support for additional stages to which interventions could be tailored. In the case of thresholds, a specific, tailored program might urge the individual into the next stage.

The five-stage TTM model has demonstrated usefulness in a number of behaviors. However, it is possible that behavior change can be described by additional stages that might differ based on health domain. Given that there is evidence for more stages, and that, as noted in the description of processes, there are some discrepancies in the literature as to the processes most appropriate for each stage, additional research into the impact of process in specific health domains is required.

2. *Application of the TTM.* Joseph et al. (1999) noted in their critique of the TTM that nearly half of the applications to content areas outside of smoking and alcohol addiction adapted constructs without critical analysis. For example, some researchers have changed the wording of existing staging algorithm scales to fit the particular health behavior of interest. While this is a first step in determining the usefulness of the TTM in a new behavior, scientific rigor is required to test the reliability (how well the scale works in multiple samples) and validity (does the scale actually measure stage of change for the behavior in question, and are the processes valid for the particular stage of change) of the adapted scales. Milstein, Lockaby, Fogarty, Cohen, and Cotton (1998) provided support for the TTM processes using qualitative interview data from 45 urban women. It was found that women mentioned at least one of the processes in their descriptions of how they changed their high-risk behavior. Such studies increase confidence in the utility of the processes for specific health behaviors. While the model has been showing some very positive results, practitioners and researchers need to be aware of the limits of the model's application to a behavioral domain that has not been thoroughly tested.

3. *Relapse.* More research is needed on predictors of relapse behavior. This area has been understudied relative to other dimensions of the TTM. Velicer, DiClemente, Rossi, and Prochaska (1990) found three dimensions of relapse in cigarette smokers: (a) negative/affective (involving negative emotional states and inadequate motivation; (b) positive/social (involving positive emotional states in social situations; and (c) habit/addictive (reflecting the physical cravings associated with smoking cessation). Fitzgerald and Prochaska (1990) found that chronic relapsers underuse helping relationships and stimulus control. Lower self-efficacy has been implicated in other studies (e.g., Sullum, Clark, & King, 2000, exercise). It would be useful to undertake qualitative research to better understand the mechanisms involved in relapse behavior. Additionally, it is plausible that some of the reasons for relapse vary from behavior to behavior, necessitating careful study of this dimension in other content areas for which the TTM has been useful.

Although the mechanism of relapse still needs research, this has minimal impact on the application of the TTM to intervention. The person who relapses has merely reverted to an earlier stage. Although knowledge of the reasons for the relapse would improve tailoring of the behavior change program, the processes of change and their associated techniques should be appropriate to the new stage of change. For example, if a person who has been successful at quitting smoking for some time relapses to the contemplation stage, contemplation stage interventions would be appropriate, along with a discussion and preparation for situations that facilitated the relapse. Therefore, a clearer understanding of relapse would provide additional direction to clinicians working with clients who revert to problem behaviors.

4. *Complete model testing.* There need to be more studies that examine the model in its entirety. Many researchers have investigated specific components, such as the relationship between decisional balance and stage of change, but few have incorporated all constructs (specifically, the relation of processes of change to stages of change). This is extremely important for application of the processes of change to other health behavior areas. The TTM can be considered to still be in the theory development stage as many studies are undertaken to understand how it operates in a variety of health-related contexts. As more information is collected and model testing that includes processes, decisional balance, stages of change, and self efficacy are tested, the precision of the model's predictive ability should improve.

5. *Congruence of philosophical perspectives.* Prochaska, DiClemente, and Norcross (1992) noted an objection raised by others with the TTM concerning its combination of a number of therapeutic systems that are philosophically incompatible. The processes of change represent a combination of behavior and experiential processes that are integrated into a model that is essentially a model of decision making (cognitive). For example, the philosophic position of the behaviorist who uses stimulus control techniques is incompatible with that of the cognitive theorist interested in decision making.

Analysis of the theoretical positions indicated that, although a number of cognitive, emotional, and behavioral constructs were critical to the models, all are essentially cognitive models. The TTM is one of the few models that incorporates both cognitive and behavioral strategies to elicit behavior change. It is acknowledged that different techniques are appropriate at different stages along the change continuum. The TTM endorses the different approaches (hence, "transtheoretical") and does not rely on one specific approach. Thus, individuals may use a number of philosophically different approaches that result in the desired behavior change. There is also the position, of course, that regardless of the degree of congruence between theory and philosophy, the optimal outcome is whatever works for the client. If an individual responds more quickly through behavioral techniques, then these should be used to assist the client in the process toward maximizing health.

6.   There has been much research done with the TTM in a variety of areas, however, there are some populations that have been, in general, underserved in research on the model. Burbank, Padula, and Nigg (2000) noted in their description of the application of the TTM to physical exercise that few of the studies involved older adults, a population that is becoming increasing large. Using another example, much of the work in the HIV/AIDS content area is with college samples, or combinations of college and community samples. There is a need for the model to be tested, in its entirety, in more diverse communities of men and women. For example, Lauby et al. (1998) in a sample of 4,036 women recruited from high-risk communities, found patterns of stage prediction by TTM mediators consistent with those in other studies. These types of studies are necessary to ensure that the model can be adapted to a variety of populations, particularly those representing higher risk (e.g., women, adolescents, older adults, African Americans, and Hispanics).

SUMMARY

The TTM offers an exciting opportunity for researchers and clinicians working in the area of behavior change. The potential applications of the model make it a viable approach to meeting the objectives established by the federal government for healthier behavior. Understanding an individual's stage of readiness for change and the processes of change most effective for that stage allows the opportunity to provide interventions tailored specifically to that person that will be most effective in facilitating progress toward permanent behavior change. The model constructs have been described, as well as their interrelationships. Some of the assumptions, strengths, and limitations have been discussed. It is important to appreciate the power of the model as well as the time and resources required to scientifically explore its application to various health domains.

In the next chapter, results of research using the TTM with a variety of health behaviors is described and summarized.

REFERENCES

Atkinson, J. W. (1957). Motivational determinants of risk taking behavior. *Psychological Review, 64,* 359–372.

Bandura, A. (1977). Self-efficacy: Toward a unifying theory of behavioral change. *Psychological Review, 84,* 191–215.

Bandura, A. (1982). Self-efficacy mechanism in human agency. *American Psychologist, 37,* 122–147.

Bark, C. R., & Nicholas, P. R. (1990). Physical activity in older adults: The stages of change. *Journal of Applied Gerontology, 9,* 216–223.

Block, G. (1993). Dietary guidelines and the results of food consumption surveys. *American Journal of Clinical Nutrition, 53,* 356s–357s.

Burbank, P. M., Padula, C. A., & Nigg, C. R. (2000). Changing health behavior of older adults. *Journal of Gerontological Nursing, 26,* 26–33.

Caron, C., Burkholder, G. J., Kirtania, U., Keith, N., Garber, C., & Lasater, T. (2000, November). *Using GIS in public health: A multilevel analysis of SES in health.* Presented at the American Public Health Association National Conference, Boston, MA.

Catania, J. A., Coates, T. J., Golden, E., Dolcini, M. M., Peterson, J., Kegeles, S., Siegel, D., & Fullilove, M. T. (1994). Correlates of condom use among Black, Hispanic, and White heterosexuals in San Francisco: The AMEN longitudinal survey. *AIDS Education and Prevention, 6,* 12–26.

Centers for Disease Control and Prevention. (1991). *Division of STD/HIV Prevention Annual Report.* U.S. Department of Health and Human Services, Atlanta, GA.

Cohen, S., Lichtenstein, E., Prochaska, J. O., Rossi, J. S., Gritz, E. R., Carr, C. R., Orleans, C. T., Schoenbach, V. J., Biener, L., Abrams, D., DiClemente, C. C., Curry, S., Marlatt, G. A., Cummings, K. M., Emont, S. L., Giovino, G., & Ossip-Klein, D. (1989). Debunking myths about self-quitting: Evidence from 10 prospective studies on persons who attempt to quit smoking by themselves. *American Psychologist, 44,* 1355–1365.

DiClemente, C. C., & Prochaska, J. O. (1982). Self-change and therapy change of smoking behavior: A comparison of processes of change in cessation and maintenance. *Addictive Behaviors, 7,* 133–142.

DiClemente, C. C., Prochaska, J. O., Fairhurst, S. K., Velicer, W. F., Velasquez, M. M., & Rossi, J. S. (1991). The process of smoking cessation: An analysis of precontemplation, contemplation, and preparation stages of change. *Journal of Consulting and Clinical Psychology, 59,* 295–304.

DiClemente, C. C., Prochaska, J. O., & Gilbertini, M. (1985). Self-efficacy and the stages of self-change of smoking. *Cognitive Therapy and Research, 9,* 181–200.

Fitzgerald, T. E., & Prochaska, J. O. (1990). Nonprogressing profiles in smoking cessation: What keeps people refractory to self-change? *Journal of Substance Abuse, 2,* 87–105.

Grimley, D. M., Prochaska, G. E., & Prochaska, J. O. (1997). Condom use adoption and continuation: A transtheoretical approach. *Heath Education Research: Theory and Practice, 12,* 61–75.

Harlow, L. L., Prochaska, J. O., Redding, C. A., Rossi, J. S., Velicer, W. F., Snow, M. G., Schnell, D., Galavotti, C., O'Reilley, K., & Rhodes, R. (1999). Stages of condom use in a high HIV-risk sample. *Psychology and Health, 14,* 143–157.

Hedeker, D., Mermelstein, R. J., & Weeks, K. A. (1999). The thresholds of change model: An approach to analyzing stages of change data. *Annals of Behavioral Medicine, 21,* 61–70.

Janis, I. L., & Mann, L. (1977). *Decision making: A psychological analysis of conflict, choice, and commitment.* New York: Free Press.

Joseph, J., Breslin, C., & Skinner, H. (1999). Critical perspectives on the transtheoretical model and stages of change. In J. A. Tucker, D. M. Donovan, & G. A. Marlatt (Eds.), *Changing addictive behavior: Bridging clinical and public health strategies* (pp. 160–190). New York: Guilford Press.

Kristal, A. R., Glanz, K., Curry, S. J., & Patterson, R. E. (1999). How can stages of change be best used in dietary interventions? *Journal of the American Dietetic Association, 99,* 679–684.

Laforge, R., Velicer, W., Richmond, R., & Owen, N. (1999). Stage distributions for five health behaviors in the U.S. and Australia. *Preventive Medicine, 28,* 61–74.

Lauby, J. L., Semaan, S., Cohen, A., Leviton, L., Gielen, A., Pulley, L. V., Walls, C., & O'Campo, P. (1998). Self-efficacy, decisional balance and stages of change for condom use among women at risk for HIV infection. *Health Education Research: Theory and Practice, 13,* 343–356.

Lewin, K. (1951). The nature of field theory. In M. H. Marx (Ed.), *Psychological theory.* New York: MacMillan.

Lewin, K., Dembo, T., Festinger, L., & Sears, P. S. (1944). Level of aspiration. In J. Hunt (Ed.), *Personality and the behavior disorders: A handbook based on experimental and clinical research* (pp. 333–378). New York: Ronald Press.

Marcus, B. H., Banspach, S. W., Lefebvre, R. C., Rossi, J. S., & Carlton, R. A. (1992). Using the stages of change model to increase the adoption of physical activity among community participants. *American Journal of Health Promotion, 6,* 424–429.

Marcus, B. H., Eaton, C. A., Rossi, J. S., & Harlow, L. L. (1994). Self-efficacy, decision making, and stages of change: An integrative model of physical exercise. *Journal of Applied Social Psychology, 24,* 489–508.

Milstein, B., Lockaby, T., Fogarty, L., Cohen, A., & Cotton, D. (1998). Processes of change in the adoption of consistent condom use. *Journal of Health Psychology, 3,* 349–368.

Perry, D. (1995). Researching the aging well process. *American Behavioral Scientist, 39,* 152–171.

Powell, K., Thompson, P., Caspersen, C., & Kendrick, J. (1987). Physical activity and the incidence of coronary heart disease. *Annual Review of Public Health, 8,* 253–287.

Prochaska, J. O. (1979). *Systems of psychotherapy: A transtheoretical analysis.* Homewood, IL: Dorsey Press.

Prochaska, J. O. (1996). A stage paradigm for integrating clinical and public health approaches to smoking cessation. *Addictive Behaviors, 21,* 721–732.

Prochaska, J. O., & DiClemente, C. C. (1982). Transtheoretical therapy: Toward a more integrative model of change. *Psychotherapy: Theory, Research, and Practice, 19,* 276–288.

Prochaska, J. O., & DiClemente, C. C. (1983). Stages and processes of self-change in smoking: Towards an integrative model of change. *Journal of Consulting and Clinical Psychology, 51,* 390–395.

Prochaska, J. O., & DiClemente, C. C. (1984). *The transtheoretical approach: Crossing traditional boundaries of change.* Homewood, IL: Dorsey Press.

Prochaska, J. O., & DiClemente, C. C. (1992). Stages of change in the modification of problem behaviors. In M. Hersen, R. M. Eisler, & P. M. Miller (Eds.), *Progress in behavior modification* (pp. 184–214). Sycamore, IL: Sycamore Press.

Prochaska, J. O., & DiClemente, C. C. (1994). *The transtheoretical approach: Crossing traditional boundaries of therapy.* Malabar, FL: Krieger Publishing.

Prochaska, J. O., DiClemente, C. C., & Norcross, J. C. (1992). In search of how people change: Applications to Addictive Behaviors. *American Psychologist, 9,* 1102–1114.

Prochaska, J. O., DiClemente, C. C., Velicer, W. F., & Rossi, J. S. (1993). Standardized, individualized, interactive and personalized self-help programs for smoking cessation. *Health Psychology, 12,* 399–405.

Prochaska, J. O., Norcross, J. C., & DiClemente, C. C. (1994). *Changing for good.* New York: William Morrow and Company, Inc.

Prochaska, J. O., Redding, C. A., & Evers, K. E. (1996). The transtheoretical model and stages of change. In K. Glanz, F. Marcus Lewis, & B. K. Rimer (Eds.), *Health behavior and health education: Theory, research, and practice* (pp. 60–84). San Francisco: Jossey-Bass.

Prochaska, J. O., Redding, C. A., Harlow, L. L., Rossi, J. S., & Velicer, W. F. (1994). The transtheoretical model of change and HIV prevention: A review. *Health Education Quarterly, 21,* 471–486.

Prochaska, J. O., & Velicer, W. F. (1997). The transtheoretical model of behavior change. *American Journal of Health Promotion, 12,* 38–48.

Prochaska, J. O., Velicer, W. F., DiClemente, C. C., & Fava, J. S. (1988). Measuring processes of change: Applications to the cessation of smoking. *Journal of Consulting and Clinical Psychology, 56,* 520–528.

Prochaska, J. O., Velicer, W. F., Rossi, J. S., Goldstein, M. G., Marcus, B. H., Rokowski, W., Fiore, C., Harlow, L. L., Redding, C. A., Rosenbloom, D., & Rossi, S. R. (1994). Stages of change and decisional balance for 12 problem behaviors. *Health Psychology, 13,* 39–46.

Rakowski, W., Fulton, J. P., & Feldman, J. P. (1993). Women's decisions about mammography: A replication of the relationship between stages of adoption and decisional balance. *Health Psychology, 12,* 209–214.

Rosenstock, I. M. (1974). Historical origins of the health belief model. In J. H. Becker (Ed.), *The health belief model and personal health behavior* (pp. 1–8). Thorofare, NJ: Charles B. Slack.

Rossi, J. (1989). The hazards of sunlight: A report on the consensus development conference on sunlight, ultraviolet radiation, and the skin. *Health Psychology, 11,* 4–6.

Rossi, J. (1994). *Stages and processes of behavior change: Applications to the cessation of smoking.* Paper presented at the 18th Annual Conference of the New England High Blood Pressure Council, Worcester, MA.

Stephens, T., & Casperson, C. J. (1993). The demography of physical activity. In C. Bouchard, R. J. Shephard, & T. Stephens (Eds.), *Physical activity, fitness and health: Consensus statement* (pp. 204–213). Champaign, IL: Human Kinetics.

Sullum, J., Clark, M. M., & King, T. K. (2000). Predictors of exercise relapse in a college population. *Journal of American College Health, 48,* 175–180.

Tolman, E. C. (1955). Principles of performance. *Psychological Review, 62,* 315–326.

Unger, J. B. (1996). Stages of change of smoking cessation: Relationships with other health behaviors. *American Journal of Preventive Medicine, 12,* 134–138.

U.S. Department of Health and Human Services. Public Health Service. (1988). *The Surgeon General's report on nutrition and health.* DHHS (PHS) Publication No 88-50210.

U.S. Department of Health and Human Services. (1996). Centers for Disease Control and Prevention, National Center for Chronic Disease Prevention and Health Promotion. *Physical activity and health: A report of the Surgeon General.* Atlanta, GA: Author.

U.S. Department of Health and Human Services. (2000, January). *Healthy People 2010 (Conference Edition, in Two Volumes).* Washington, DC: Author.

Velicer, W. F., & DiClemente, C. C. (1993). Understanding and intervening with the total population of smokers. *Tobacco Control, 2,* 95–96.

Velicer, W. F., DiClemente, C. C., Prochaska, J. O., & Brandenburg, N. (1985). A decisional balance measure for assessing and predicting smoking status. *Journal of Personality and Social Psychology, 48,* 1279–1289.

Velicer, W. F., DiClemente, C. C., Rossi, J. S., & Prochaska, J. O. (1990). Relapse situations and self-efficacy: An integrative model. *Addictive Behaviors, 15,* 271–283.

Velicer, W. F., Norman, G. J., Fava, J. L., & Prochaska, J. O. (1999). Testing 40 predictions from the transtheoretical model. *Addictive Behaviors, 24,* 455–469.

Velicer, W. F., Rossi, J. S., Ruggiero, L., & Prochaska, J. O. (1994). Minimal interventions appropriate for an entire population of smokers. In R. Richmond (Ed.), *Intervention for smokers: An international perspective* (pp. 69–92). Baltimore, MD: Williams & Wilkins.

CHAPTER 4

Application of the Transtheoretical Model to Several Problem Behaviors

Gary J. Burkholder and Kerry A. Evers

> "The daily habits of people have a great deal more to do with what makes them sick and when they die than all influences of medicine"
>
> ~Lester Breslow, M.D.

The U.S. Department of Health and Human Services [USDHHS] (2000) has established a number of national public health goals including: (1) increased quality and years of healthy life, and (2) the elimination of health disparities based on ethnicity, sexual orientation, income, and education. These objectives require social scientists to develop and test models of behavior change, as well as interventions based on those models. The previous chapter provided a general description of the Transtheoretical Model of Behavior Change (TTM) (Prochaska & DiClemente, 1983), a model that has shown promise for its application to a number of problem health behaviors. In that chapter, a detailed discussion of TTM constructs (stage of change, processes of change, decisional balance, and self-efficacy) was provided. These are briefly reviewed here.

TRANSTHEORETICAL MODEL CONSTRUCTS

Stage of Change

An individual can generally be classified into one of five *stages of change*. In *precontemplation*, the individual is not thinking about changing his or her behavior. A person in the *contemplation* stage is considering the possibility of changing the problem behavior, operationally defined as within the next six months. The changer in the *preparation* stage intends to change the problem behavior within the next 30 days. At the point of *action*, the individual has made the commitment to change and has ceased the problem behavior. After six months of successful change, the person is considered in the *maintenance* stage and is working toward resisting the temptation to revert back to the old behavior.

Processes of Change

There are 10 processes of change shown to be consistent across a number of different therapy systems and across several problem behaviors (Prochaska & DiClemente, 1984; Prochaska & DiClemente, 1982). These processes are: (a) *consciousness raising* (efforts by the individual to seek new information and to gain understanding and feedback about the problem behavior); (b) *dramatic relief* (affective aspects of change, often involving intense emotional experiences related to the problem behavior); (c) *self-reevaluation* (emotional and cognitive reappraisal of values by the individual regarding the problem behavior); (d) *environmental reevaluation* (consideration and assessment by the individual of how the problem affects the physical and social environments); (e) *social liberation* (awareness, availability, and acceptance by the individual of alternative, problem-free lifestyles in society); (f) *counterconditioning* (substitution of alternative behaviors for problem behavior); (g) *helping relationships* (trusting, accepting, and using the support of caring others during attempts to change the problem behavior); (h) *reinforcement management* (changing the contingencies that control or maintain the problem behavior); (i) *self-liberation* (the individual's choice and commitment to change the problem behavior, including the belief that one can change); and (j) *stimulus control* (control of situations and other causes that trigger the problem behavior).

Decisional Balance and Self-Efficacy

Decisional balance is the result of weighing the pros and cons of a given behavior. At a certain point in the progression of change, the pros of changing the behavior will exceed the cons, generally before the individual takes action. Self-efficacy assesses the extent to which a person feels confident that he or she can maintain the behavior change in a number of different situations. In the TTM, self-efficacy has two components—*confidence* that the person can maintain behavior change and *temptations* for reengaging in the problem behavior.

The purpose of this chapter is to provide an overview and evaluate the application of the TTM to a number of problem behaviors. These behaviors include: (a) smoking cessation and acquisition; (b) HIV/AIDS risk (safer sex and condom use); (c) alcohol and drug cessation; (d) diet and weight control; (e) stress management; (f) sun exposure; (g) screening behavior (mammography and pap tests); (h) medication compliance; and (i) health care provider behavior. Application of the TTM to other behaviors will be briefly reviewed. Exercise will not be summarized here, as the succeeding chapters will provide an in-depth review of the state of the research in this area. Research summarized in this chapter should provide the reader with the strengths as well as the limitations of the current state of research as it has been applied to these problem behaviors.

RESEARCH REVIEW STRATEGIES

Empirical research is the accepted procedure in social science for testing hypotheses generated from theory. Research is " . . . a formal, systematic, and rigorous process of inquiry used to generate and test the concepts and propositions that comprise middle-range theories . . . " (Fawcett, 1999, p. 8). This definition allows for multiple forms of inquiry [for example, empirical (quantitative and/or qualitative investigation), historical, etc.]. Theory development is a process that begins with a basic description of constructs, continues with the exploration of relationships among constructs (correlations), and then tests those relationships in experimental designs. An important goal for social science is determining the causes of behavior. Practitioners and researchers seek answers to the question, "What causes people to change their behavior" (to quit smoking, begin regular exercise, etc.)?

The determination of cause and effect in the social sciences is usually a tricky proposition. The classic method is to conduct an experiment in which every variable that could be a potential explanation for the result is controlled. One hopes that, with such rigorous procedure, any change can be attributed to the one variable that is manipulated. Unfortunately, behavior is multivariate in nature. That is, there are many individual and contextual factors operating simultaneously in the behavior change process, and one usually cannot know with certainty which factor (if any) was primarily responsible for the change. Another option methodologists have of making at least tentative causal statements is by conducting studies that are longitudinal (i.e., behavior is measured for the same individual on several successive occasions). In this way, the researcher can see which factors are changing as the behavior of interest changes. The use of longitudinal analysis methods does not yield a definitive cause-and-effect statement; however, one can be more certain that human behavior and individual and contextual factors changing together are probably related to each other. This change can, in turn, lend support to the plausibility of behavior change theories.

Theory development can be evaluated by examining its progress through three phases of research: *descriptive, explanatory,* and *predictive.* First, there should be adequate *descriptive* studies that yield operational definitions of constructs considered essential to the behavior change theory. This would include quantitative studies (for example, examining the structure of scales used to measure behavior) as well as qualitative studies (for example, those that include interviews, focus groups, and other forms of direct inquiry to assess the meaning of the constructs). One would also expect to see extensive work on reliability (are the similar results found across studies using the same individuals?) and validity (are the scales measuring what they are supposed to, and could those scales be used to measure the behavior of the population at large?) of the measures (for example, in the case of the TTM, stage of change, decisional balance, processes of change, and self-efficacy). Evidence of further theoretical and empirical development would include correlation studies examining the relationships among constructs. For theory in the *explanatory* phase of development, one would expect to see studies that examine the nature of the relationship between processes and stage of change, or between pros and cons (decisional balance) and stage of change. Tests of the full model with all constructs, studies including experimental designs, intervention studies, and analyses based on longitudinal data analysis would all advance theory development to the *predictive* phase in which the isolation of causal mechanisms is important.

Chapter Organization

One goal of this chapter is the evaluation of TTM theory development. The chapter has been organized in such a way as to minimize confusion and to achieve a maximum level of usefulness for readers who may be interested in specific applications of the TTM. For each problem behavior, the following information is provided. First, an extensive review of the research using the TTM for the behavior is summarized. While an attempt has been made to include as much of the research as possible, it is impossible and impractical to guarantee that every study has been documented. However, the studies mentioned should provide the reader with a knowledge foundation related to application of the TTM to the specific behavior. For each behavior, the review of the research will be organized as much as possible by construct: stage of change (generally, the first step in applying the TTM to a new behavior is to define a valid and reliable criterion for action stage of change); processes of change; decisional balance; and self-efficacy. In some cases there will be some overlap, as several research studies include information on all model constructs.

Where available, interventions using the TTM as the theoretical framework will be described.

The large numbers of references and extensive analyses may be potentially confusing. Therefore, a summary following the literature review includes highlights from the detailed analysis with a minimum number of references. The review will hopefully provide the reader with a sense of the "breadth" of the research, defined as the extent to which a model has been tested in a variety of different populations (Barnum, 1990). One of the goals of social science is to investigate the "universals" of human behavior, and breadth is one means by which success of the TTM in behavior change in a variety of populations can be ascertained. Brief tables are also included, which provide quick snapshots of the published research for the problem behavior domain using key words and phrases (see Tables 4.1 through 4.11).

After the review of selected problem behaviors has been completed, summarizing remarks are provided to help integrate the findings across behaviors. One of the questions of model utility concerns scope. If the model is useful across the behaviors considered in this chapter, then it is likely that the TTM could be applied to other behaviors of interest that have not yet been thoroughly researched. While a large number of behaviors have been considered here, this list is not exhaustive. For example, there may be studies ongoing that are not yet reflected in the literature. It is important that researchers as well as practitioners understand the questions that have been answered and those that remain unanswered about the TTM.

SMOKING

Review of the Research

Cigarette smoking is the single most preventable cause of disease and death in the United States, however the number of deaths due to tobacco use each year is about 430,000, and 36% of adolescents in 1997 smoked compared to only 24% of the adult population. While the percentage of adult smokers has appeared to level off, that for adolescents is steadily increasing (USDHHS, 2000). It is clear that behavior change models showing potential for success

TABLE 4.1   Key References for TTM Overview/History (Presented in Order of Year of Publication)

Author(s) and Year	Brief Description of the Article
Prochaska, J. O. (1979)	Development of processes of change in psychotherapy.
Prochaska & DiClemente (1982)	Stage of change and processes of change in transtheoretical therapy.
Prochaska & DiClemente (1984)	Analysis of transtheoretical therapy.
Prochaska, DiClemente, & Norcross (1992)	Review of empirical support for the transtheoretical model.
Prochaska, Velicer, Rossi, Goldstein, et al. (1994)	Stage of change and decisional balance comparisons across 12 different behaviors.
Prochaska (1994)	Pros and cons mathematically related to stage movement.
Prochaska, Redding, & Evers (1997)	Easy-to-read explanation of the TTM, assumptions, constructs, applications.
Nigg et al. (1999)	Stage of change for 10 problem behaviors in older adults.
Joseph, Breslin, & Skinner (1999)	Excellent critical theoretical and empirical analysis of the TTM.
Burbank, Padula, & Nigg (2000)	Overview of the model with application to older adults.

in helping people to quit smoking will have a positive impact on public health.

1. *Stage of change.* The problem behavior first and most extensively studied using the TTM is smoking cessation. In the earliest study of smokers, DiClemente and Prochaska (1982) found that certain processes of change were used depending upon stage of change of smokers. In a study of approximately 900 volunteers, the 10 processes of change, self-efficacy, and decisional balance were

TABLE 4.2   Key References for TTM Applications to Smoking Cessation and Acquisition (Presented in Order of Year of Publication)

Author(s) and Year	Brief Description of the Article
DiClemente & Prochaska (1982)	Empirical comparison of self-changing and therapy-changing smokers.
DiClemente, Prochaska, & Gilbertini (1985)	Classic article on relationship between stage of change and self-efficacy.
Velicer, DiClemente, Prochaska, & Brandenburg (1985)	Classic article on development of the 2-factor decisional balance scale.
Prochaska, DiClemente, Velicer, Ginpil, & Norcross (1985)	Predictors of movement through stages of change for self-changing smokers.
Prochaska, Velicer, DiClemente, & Fava (1998)	Empirical development of processes of change.
Prochaska, Velicer, Guadagnoli, & Rossi (1991)	Longitudinal evidence for all constructs of the TTM.
Velicer, Hughes, Fava, Prochaska, & DiClemente (1995)	Subtype within stage of change analyses.
Velicer, Fava, Prochaska, et al. (1995)	Validation of stage of change distribution among various populations.
Martin, Velicer, & Fava (1996)	Longitudinal model supporting TTM predictions on stage movement.2
Dijkstra, DeVries, & Bakker (1996)	Decisional balance, self-efficacy, and stage of change in Dutch population.
Pallonen, Prochaska, Velicer, & Prokhorov (1998)	Stages of cessation and acquisition of smoking behavior in adolescents.
Velicer, Norman, Fava, & Prochaska (1999)	Extensive empirical testing of predictions from the TTM.

TABLE 4.2   *(continued)*

Author(s) and Year	Brief Description of the Article
Expert Systems	
Prochaska, DiClemente, Velicer, & Rossi (1993)	Description of expert systems.
Velicer, Prochaska, Bellis, et al. (1993)	Detail of expert system and potential applications.
Pallonen et al. (1998)	Expert system application to teenage smokers.

found to be the most important predictors of smoking status (Prochaska, DiClemente, Velicer, Ginpil, & Norcross, 1985). For smoking cessation, the universally accepted definition of action is quitting smoking. The stage of change variable has been widely validated for smoking cessation in both national [e.g., see Velicer, Fava, et al. (1995) for a comparison of two randomly drawn samples in Rhode Island and California, and a third sample from several work sites in different geographic locations] and international [e.g., see Pallonen, Fava, Salonen, and Prochaska (1992) in a study of Finnish men; Keller, Nigg, Jaekle, Baum, & Basler (1999) in a German sample] populations. A continuous-measure version of the stages of change has been validated as an alternative to the 5-item categorical scale (University of Rhode Island Change Assessment Scale—URICAS: McConnaughy, Prochaska, & Velicer, 1983).

The stage-of-change variable has also demonstrated adequate reliability (Donovan, Jones, Holman, & Corti, 1998, in a sample of Australian smokers; Morera et al., 1998). Some studies have reproduced subtypes within stages of change. For example, Fava, Rossi, Redding, Ding, and Prochaska (1994) found that those in precontemplation could be further classified based on whether or not they have made previous quit attempts, two groups that would probably respond maximally to different processes of change. Longitudinal analyses have provided support for the predicted movement through stages. Martin, Velicer, and Fava (1996) found evidence to support the nonlinearity of movement through stages, the probability for

TABLE 4.3   Key References for TTM Applications to Safer Sex (Presented in Order of Year of Publication)

Author(s) and Year	Brief Description of the Article
Prochaska, Redding, Harlow, Rossi, & Velicer (1994)	Comprehensive review of TTM and HIV prevention.
Grimley, Prochaska, Velicer, & Prochaska (1995)	Condom use and contraceptive staging.
Galavotti et al. (1995)	Stage of change, decisional balance, self-efficacy for condom use.
Bowen & Trotter (1995)	Stage of change for condom use among drug users.
Grimley et al. (1996)	Decisional balance and self-efficacy cross-validation for condom use.
Lauby et al. (1998)	Self-efficacy, decisional balance, and stage of change for condom use in high-risk women.
Milstein, Lockaby, Fogarty, Cohen, & Cotton (1998)	Qualitative (interview) support for processes of change applied to safer sex.
Evers, Harlow, Redding, & LaForge (1998)	Longitudinal support for stage movement and stability applied to condom use.
Redding & Rossi (1999)	Gender differences in situational self-efficacy for safer sex.
Harlow et al. (1999)	Staging of high-risk women for condom use.

forward movement being greater than the probability for backward movement through the stages, and the higher probably of moving into a subsequent stage of change rather than jumping ahead.

2. *Decisional balance.* Velicer, DiClemente, Prochaska, and Brandenburg (1985) developed a two-factor Decisional Balance measure derived from the Janis and Mann (1977) eight-factor model of decision making. This measure, pros of smoking and cons of smoking, have formed the basis for the decisional balance scale used across

TABLE 4.4 Key References for TTM Applications to Alcohol and Drug Cessation and Acquisition (Presented in Order of Year of Publication)

Author(s) and Year	Brief Description of the Article
DiClemente & Hughes (1990)	Stages of change in outpatient alcoholic treatment clients.
Migneault, Pallonen, & Velicer (1997)	Decisional balance and stage of change for adolescent drinking behavior.
Snow, Prochaska, & Rossi (1994)	Processes of change for clients in Alcoholics Anonymous.
Carney & Kivlahan (1995)	4-group staging of substance abuse clients.
Miller & Tonigan (1996)	Validation of the SOCRATES.
Werch (1997)	Stages of acquisition and cessation in adolescent drinking; STARS intervention.
Migneault, Velicer, Prochaska, & Stevenson (1999)	Decisional balance for college student drinking.

a number other problem behaviors. The consistent relationship between pros and cons and stage of change for smoking (the increase in pros and decrease in cons until the crossover point in the preparation stage, at which time pros outweigh cons of smoking) has been shown to be consistent across studies and thus continues to receive empirical support (see Etter & Perneger, 1999; Jaekle, Keller, Baum, & Basler, 1999; Keller, Nigg, Jaekle, Baum, & Basler, 1999; Norman, Velicer, Fava, & Prochaska, 1998), but this finding is not universal (see Lafferty, Heaney, & Chen, 1999, for a study of Asian males living in the United States who did not demonstrate the expected relationship between pros and cons in earlier stages of change).

3. *Processes of change.* Early research also validated the 10-factor processes of change scales for smoking cessation and identified two higher-order factors, *experiential* and *behavioral* (Prochaska, Velicer, DiClemente, & Fava, 1998). Rossi, Prochaska, and DiClemente

TABLE 4.5   Key References for TTM Applications to Diet/Weight Control (Presented in Order of Year of Publication)

Author(s) and Year	Brief Description of the Article
Clark, Abrams, Niaura, Eaton, & Rossi (1991)	Weight control and self-efficacy.
Prochaska, Norcross, Fowler, Follick, & Abrams (1992)	Processes and stages of change in a work site weight control program.
Greene, Rossi, Reed, Willey, & Prochaska (1994)	Stages of change for reducing dietary fat to 30% of energy or less.
Glanz et al. (1994)	Stages of change related to dietary fat and fiber.
Brug, Glanz, & Kok (1997)	Self-efficacy and stage of change related to fruit and vegetable consumption.
Glanz, Kristal, Tilley, & Hirst (1998)	Stages of change in a group of male auto workers.
Hargreaves et al. (1999)	Stage of change in dietary fat among African American women.
Kristal, Glanz, Curry, & Patterson (1999)	Excellent review of stage of change algorithms and suggested applications to diet.

(1988) found evidence that heavy and light smokers could be distinguished based on processes of change. Using dynamic typology, a type of longitudinal cluster analysis that identified certain groups of changers across time (for example, those who stayed in a given stage for the duration of the study and those who progressed into further stages), support was found for the relationship between processes of change and stage of change (Norman, Velicer, Fava, & Prochaska, 1998; Prochaska, Velicer, Guadagnoli, & Rossi, 1991). Norman et al. (1998) showed that processes of change could predict stage of change (for example, those who initially were in precontemplation and showed forward progress over the 2-year study tended to increase use of social support, dramatic relief, self-reevaluation,

TABLE 4.6   Key References for TTM Applications to Stress Management (Presented in Order of Year of Publication)

Author(s) and Year	Brief Description of the Article
Norman, Fava, et al., 1997	Development of confidence measure.
Fava, Norman, Levesque, et al., 1998	Development of decisional balance measure.
Fava, Norman, Redding, et al., 1998	Development of process of change measure.
Johnson, Norman, & Fava, 1998	Exploration of maintenance stage and relapse.
Robbins et al., 1998	Stages of change across three samples.
Velicer, Prochaska, Fava, Norman, & Redding, 1998	Review of TTM applied to smoking cessation and stress management.
Evers, Evans, Fava, & Prochaska, 2000	Development and validation measures.
Riley, Toth, & Fava, 2000	Application to women at risk for, or infected with, HIV.
Evers & Padula, 2001	Description of an intervention trail.

and self-liberation). Other analyses continue to refine the relationship between processes of change and stage of change. Perz, DiClemente, and Carbonari (1996) found that certain processes are maximally used in different stages (for example, it was discovered that social liberation reaches its highest level of use in the precontemplation stage). In another analysis, Velicer, Hughes, Fava, Prochaska, and DiClemente (1995) found multiple subtypes distinguishable by the use of particular processes of change within the precontemplation, contemplation, preparation, and action stages. These studies suggest the possibility for more precise tailoring of information to the person undergoing behavior change to maximize success. The processes of change appear to be used similarly between men and women (O'Connor, Carbonari, & DiClemente, 1996), and they ap-

TABLE 4.7 Key References for TTM Applications to Sun Exposure (Presented in Order of Year of Publication)

Author(s) and Year	Brief Description of the Article
Rossi, Blais, & Weinstock, 1994	Interventions conducted on the beaches.
Rossi, Blais, Redding, & Weinstock, 1995	Application of TTM and implications for interventions.
Maddock et al., 1998	Measure development for sun protection behaviors among adolescents.
Redding, Prochaska, Pallonen, et al., 1999	Interventions for smoking, diet, and sun for adolescents.
Weinstock, Rossi, Redding, Maddock, & Cottrill, 2000	Stage of change among beachgoers.

pear to be stable (i.e., the 10-process structure is consistent) for other ethnic groups [e.g., see Gottlieb, Galavotti, McCuan, & McAlister (1990) for an analysis of processes of change with a sample of Mexican Americans].

4. *Self-efficacy.* DiClemente, Prochaska, and Gilbertini (1985) provided the foundational work in understanding the important relationship between self-efficacy (confidence and temptation) and stage of change. Self-efficacy was found to steadily increase across the stages of change, while temptations decreased markedly as one moved through the stages of change into maintenance. Other studies have continued to support the predicted relationship between stages of change and self-efficacy (see Dijkstra, DeVries, & Bakker, 1996; Prochaska, Velicer, Guadagnoli, & Rossi, 1991).

5. *TTM across populations.* Studies with a variety of populations have supported the general structure of the TTM and, in some cases, point to differences by ethnicity or other discriminating factors. In a sample of predominantly white 7th graders, there were substantially more relapsers and fewer maintainers than found in adult populations (Pallonen, Murray, Schmid, Pirie, & Luepker, 1990). They also

TABLE 4.8 Key References for TTM Applications to Screening (Mammography and Cervical Cancer; Presented in Order of Year of Publication)

Author(s) and Year	Brief Description of the Article
Earp et al., 1995	Intervention for mammography screening with older black women.
Kelaher et al., 1999	Cervical cancer screening.
Lipkus, Rimer, & Strigo, 1996	Objective and subjective risk and stages of change.
Mah & Bryant, 1997	Effect of past mammography behavior and intention.
Pearlman et al., 1997	Decisional balance over a 1-year period.
Pearlman, Rakowski, Ehrich, & Clark, 1996	Race and ethnicity affect mammography.
Rakowski, Andersen, et al., 1997	Decisional balance construct.
Rakowski, Clark, et al., 1997	Single decisional balance measure for mammography and pap testing.
Rakowski, Dube, et al., 1992	Decisional balance measure.
Rakowski, Fulton, & Feldman, 1993	Replicated previous findings for stages of change and decisional balance.

noted that young teen smokers tend to cycle faster through the stages. Pallonen et al. (1994) found that use of stage-tailored manuals accelerated the smoking cessation process in a group of middle-aged Finnish men. Prokhorov et al. (1995) found similar stage of change distributions for Russian and U.S. students in vocational schools. Dijkstra, DeVries, and Bakker (1996) found similar patterns in pros and cons, self-efficacy, and stage of change in the Dutch population and in U.S. studies. Stage of change patterns among rural black male adults were similar to those found in other studies (Schorling, 1995). However, some ethnic differences have been noted. Ahijevych and Parsely (1999) found that African American women smoked

TABLE 4.9   Key References for TTM Applications to Medication Compliance (Presented in Order of Year of Publication)

Author(s) and Year	Brief Description of the Article
Johnson, Grimley, & Prochaska, 1998b	Process of change measure.
Johnson, 1998	Application to oral contraceptive adherence.
Johnson, Grimley, & Prochaska, 1998a	Prediction of adherence.
Willey, 1999	Methods for improving medication adherence.
Emmett & Ferguson, 1999	Stage and decisional balance for oral contraceptive pill use.

TABLE 4.10   Key References for TTM Applications to Health Care Provider (Presented in Order of Year of Publication)

Author(s) and Year	Brief Description of the Article
Pololi & Potter, 1996	Teaching internal medicine residents behavioral counseling skills for multiple risk factor modification.
Berger & Grimley, 1997	Pharmacists' readiness for rendering pharmaceutical care.
Cassidy, 1999	Facilitating behavior change in patients with chronic illness.
Taylor, Berger, Anderson-Harper, & Grimley, 2000	Pharmacists' readiness to assess consumers' over-the-counter product selections.

fewer cigarettes and consistently rated cons of smoking higher that white women. Development of a four-factor pros and cons scale for pregnant women (general pros, pregnancy-related pros, cons related to disapproval from others, and health-related cons) indicated that, although the general structure of pros and cons seems to apply, more of the variance may be explained if decisional balance scales

TABLE 4.11   Key References for TTM Applications to Other Behaviors (Alphabetical by Behavior)

Author(s) and Year	Behavior	Brief Description of the Article
Keefe et al., 2000	Arthritis	Stages of change for patients with persistent arthritis pain.
Levesque, Gelles, & Velicer, 2000	Batterer treatment	Measure of batterers' readiness to end their violence.
Humphreys, Thompson, & Miner, 1998	Breastfeeding	Assessment of women's intention to breast-feed.
Kloeblen, Thompson, & Miner, 1999	Breastfeeding	Breast-feeding intention among low-income women.
Levy, 1997	Bulimia	Application of the TTM to bulimia.
Treasure et al., 1999	Bulimia	Effect of stages of change on outcome of treatment for bulimia.
Nolan et al., 1999	CPR	Assessed readiness to perform CPR.
O'Neil, Bristow, & Brennan, 1999	Financial Behavior	TTM and financial behavior among New York residents.
Levesque, Prochaska, & Prochaska, 1999	Organizational Change	University's readiness for integrated service delivery.
Prochaska, 2000	Organizational Change	Family service agencies readiness to adopt time-limited therapy.
Prochaska, Prochaska, & Levesque, in press	Organizational Change	Application of the TTM to organizational change.
Kerns, Rosenberg, Jaminson, Caudill, & Haythornthwaite, 1997	Pain Management	Readiness to adopt a self-management of chronic pain.

(continued)

TABLE 4.11   *(continued)*

Author(s) and Year	Behavior	Brief Description of the Article
Jensen, Nielson, Romano, Hill, & Turner, 2000	Pain Management	Further evaluation of the pain stages of change questionnaire.
McConnaughy, Prochaska, & Velicer (1983)	Psychotherapy	Stage of change of clients in psychotherapy.
Prochaska (1991)	Psychotherapy	Stage of change applied to treating phobias.
Prochaska, Rossi, & Wilcox (1991)	Psychotherapy	Stage of change in psychotherapy.
Brogan, Prochaska, & Prochaska, 1999	Therapy Termination	TTM measures as predictors of termination of clients entering psychotherapy.

are tailored to the unique situation of the population in question (Bane, Ruggiero, Dryfoos, & Rossi, 1999).

6. *Interventions.* There have been a number of intervention studies done to assess the effectiveness of the TTM as compared to other programs of smoking cessation. Prochaska, DiClemente, Velicer, and Rossi (1993) reported on an intervention in which smokers were randomly assigned by stage of change to four conditions: (1) use of individualized self-help manuals, (2) use of manuals generated from the stage of change model, (3) use of tailored expert system computer feedback in addition to the manuals, and (4) use of four counselor calls in addition to expert system feedback and manuals. Those using the expert system feedback were found to have higher quit rates across all time points than those in the other interventions. In an expert system, the computer determines stage of change, and based on the person's decisional balance, self-efficacy score, and his or her relative use of the processes of change, a report designed to guide the individual in the behavior change process is generated that is unique to the individual and his or her stage of change.

Ruggiero, Redding, Rossi, and Prochaska (1997) ascertained the acceptability of the expert system with a culturally diverse group of pregnant smokers, and its utility for high school students has been demonstrated (Pallonen, Velicer, et al., 1998; in this study, however, there was no difference in quit rates between those using the system based on stage of change and a program adapted for use by the computer not employing stage of change). The importance of matching stages to intervention has not found universal support, however. In an experiment in which participants were randomly assigned to a matched tailored intervention or an action-only-oriented tailored approached, Quinlan and McCaul (2000) showed that more of those who received action-oriented materials attempted to quit smoking, regardless of participants' stage of change.

Summary

Application of the TTM to smoking cessation has been extensive. The research has established the utility of a stage-based model of smoking behavior change. A number of different populations have been used to test the model including white, African American, Asian American, and Mexican-American, as well as populations from countries outside of the United States including Germany, Switzerland, Finland, and Australia. There have been attempts to validate various constructs in the model for men, women, pregnant women, and middle and high school students. Only the studies with Finnish men were specifically targeted toward middle-aged or older adults, indicating the need to target more research to older adults. While research with adolescents and smoking cessation is impressive (Pallonen, Prochaska, Velicer, & Prokhorov, 1998; Pallonen, Velicer, et al., 1998), more intensive work with this population would be important, given that teenage smoking has, in recent years, become the target of public health awareness.

The good news is that while research support is not universal for the applicability of the TTM to smoking cessation, the preponderance of the evidence suggests that the model has scientific merit. Applications of the model using expert computer systems are demonstrating increased participation rates and increased success for quitting of all smokers, not just those that have decided to stop smoking.

The success of the smoking cessation model is exciting as an exemplar for other problem behaviors.

Review of the literature suggests the TTM is a well-established theory, at least as it is applied to smoking cessation. The fact that the 10 processes of change, the 5 stages of change, the 2-factor decisional balance construct, and self-efficacy have been verified in a number of populations, and that the relationships predicted by the TTM have consistently been replicated across studies, indicates that the scales have good external validity. The initial work on these TTM constructs, derived initially from a study of smokers who quit, has established the research tradition for application of the TTM to other problem behaviors.

SAFER SEX: CONDOM USE FOR HIV/AIDS PREVENTION

Review of the Research

HIV/AIDS continues to be a public health crisis. Seventy percent of the AIDS cases worldwide are the result of heterosexual transmission, with transmission among men having sex with men accounting for only 15% of the cases (Mann, Tarantola, & Netter, 1992). Women, particularly adolescent females, are at disproportionately higher risk for Human Immunodeficiency Virus (HIV) infection from heterosexual transmission, and women represented the fastest growing group infected with HIV in 1997 (Centers for Disease Control [CDC], 1997) with a 6% increase in the prevalence of HIV infection among women since 1988. Adolescents, Blacks, and Hispanics are also at highest risk for HIV infection (CDC, 1999). The TTM has been viewed as one means of understanding why some people do not modify their sexual risk for HIV infection despite the enormity of the problem worldwide. There has been some application of the TTM to the HIV/AIDS health domain, but this area has not been researched as extensively as has smoking cessation.

1. *Stage of change.* For condom use, the generally accepted criterion for entry into the action stage of change is the use of condoms at every sexual encounter. Several studies have found differences in

condom use between main and casual partners (more use with casual partners), and that people could be staged on intention to use condoms [Anderson, Cheney, Faruque, & Long (1996) in a study of intravenous drug users (IDUs); Galavotti et al., 1995; Grimley, Prochaska, & Prochaska, 1993; Grimley, Prochaska, Velicer, & Prochaska, 1995; Harlow et al., 1999; O'Reilly & Higgins, 1991; Rhodes & Malotte, 1996, in a study of IDUs and crack users; Stark et al., 1998, in a multicity sample of primarily African American women). Generally, these studies have shown that men and women are approximately equally distributed in each of the stages of change. Evers, Harlow, Redding, and LaForge (1998) found, in a longitudinal study, that precontemplation and maintenance were the most stable stages (the highest percentage of women in these stages at baseline were still in these stages 1 year later; without intervention, women in precontemplation probably remain at that stage), and the model indicated high rates of relapse in consistent condom use. Some ethnic differences with respect to safer sex and condom use have been noted. White participants were more likely to be in the action stage than blacks, and Hispanics were more likely to be in contemplation than blacks (Bowen & Trotter, 1995).

2. *Decisional balance.* Redding, Rossi, Velicer, and Prochaska (1989) developed a two-factor Decisional Balance scale for four safer sex dimensions (pros and cons of safer sex, discussion about safer sex, condom use, and partner selectivity). The relationship of pros and cons of safer sex to stage of change mirrored the relationship found in smoking cessation, a result also supported by Lauby et al. (1998) in their study of at-risk women. One study indicated that the cons of safer sex did not decrease significantly by stage of change, a pattern that was noted to be more characteristic of adoption rather than cessation of behaviors (Galavotti et al., 1995).

3. *Processes of change.* Redding and Rossi (1993) validated a processes of safer sex adoption scale that nearly replicated the 10 processes of change scale used in smoking cessation research (with the exception of one new process, interpersonal systems control; this was renamed Assertiveness for Condom Use: Grimley, Prochaska, & Prochaska, 1997), providing evidence for a generalization of the TTM to safer sex behavior. Milstein, Lockaby, Fogarty, Cohen, and Cotton (1998) found support for the processes of change in a qualita-

tive study of women at risk for HIV. Each woman interviewed in their study mentioned at least one of the 10 processes of change.

4. *Self-efficacy.* Decisional balance and self-efficacy measures developed in research on a high-risk sample (Galavotti et al., 1995) were successfully replicated in a sample consisting primarily of college women (Grimley et al., 1996). Redding and Rossi (1999) developed a situational self-efficacy scale for safer sex that included subscales reflecting sexual situations in which there was confidence in resisting unsafe sex and/or temptation to engage in that same behavior. Their analyses revealed no significant differences among men and women on these scales (with the exception of temptation for unsafe sex on which males scored higher), and the results were validated in an independent sample. The self-efficacy scales were able to discriminate stage of change as predicted by the TTM. Other studies have validated the importance of self-efficacy to stage of change (see Lauby et al., 1998, in a sample of women at high risk for HIV; Montoya, 1997, in a population of female crack cocaine users; Stark et al., 1998, in a study of inner-city women, primarily African American, at risk for HIV).

Summary

Much of the early work in the application of the TTM to safer sex used college samples. However, over time, the number of populations to which the TTM model for safer sex and condom use behavior change has been applied has increased to include men and women as well as drug users at high risk for HIV. Research with injection drug users and with women at risk for HIV infection has generally resulted in findings consistent with those predicted by the TTM. There has been less TTM research with other higher-risk populations, most notable gay men, African Americans, and Hispanics, probably given the higher levels of interest in the AIDS Risk Reduction Model (Catania, Kegeles, & Coates, 1990) developed specifically for use with gay men. Given that these groups are identified as most at risk for HIV infection, TTM more research is needed within these populations using the TTM. Although some regions in Africa have the highest rates of HIV infection, TTM studies were not identified outside of the United States.

Application of the TTM to safer sex and condom use is still primarily in its descriptive and explanatory phases. Some longitudinal analysis has been done as well as research establishing predictive success of processes of change, decisional balance, and self-efficacy for stage of change. No published intervention studies that clearly used the TTM to target specific materials based on stage of change were found. However, one study currently in progress is using the expert system to tailor materials to women at high risk for HIV (Redding et al., 2001)

Some issues still remain to be addressed. There are a number of studies that have shown the importance of cultural factors on condom use and safer sex (see Diaz, 1998 for a discussion of a psychocultural model of HIV risk for Latino gay men), yet the TTM does not explicitly consider how differing constructions of sexuality and gender affect behavior change. Application of the TTM to minority cultural groups requires more extensive research and instrument validation than has occurred thus far. The previously mentioned situational self-efficacy scale study by Redding and Rossi (1999) indicates that self-efficacy is variable depending upon sexual situation; this concept needs to be extended and validated in other populations. It is clear that there is much descriptive and explanatory work to be done for this application of the TTM, including more studies establishing longitudinal (over time) support for model constructs.

ALCOHOL AND DRUG DEPENDENCE

Review of the Research

There has been some research on TTM applications to alcohol and drug dependence, and only a few studies have attempted to replicate the TTM analyses done with smoking cessation. This is in spite of literature recommending specific ways of applying the model to substance addiction (see Peteet, Brenner, Curtiss, Ferrigno, & Kauffman, 1998). Substance abuse is associated with violence, injury, and HIV infection, and is a problem among adolescents, 23% of whom reported using substances in 1997 compared to 6% of the adults reporting drug use and 16% reporting binge drinking (USDHHS, 2000).

1. *Stages of change.* Migneault, Pallonen, and Vellicer (1997) found that for adolescents, a nine-stage acquisition and cessation of drinking scale adequately explained the stages of change. When dealing with adolescents it is important to understand the stages describing intention to *adopt* problem behaviors. Other staging algorithms have been proposed. Edens and Willoughby (1999) found two clusters of changers—preparation/action (those in this cluster were more likely to complete treatment) and precontemplation. In another study Rollnick, Heather, Gold, and Hall (1992) found a factor structure indicating three distinct stages—precontemplation, contemplation, and action. Other studies support the existence of a four-stage structure (precontemplation, contemplation, ambivalent, and participation, Carney & Kivlahan, 1995; DiClemente & Hughes, 1990). In an analysis by stage of change for patients admitting to an outpatient alcohol treatment program, DiClemente and Hughes (1990) found that five clusters emerged:

1. Precontemplation—those who did not intend to change and resisted admitting that their drinking might be problematic
2. Ambivalent—those with above average scores for alcohol use in all four stages, suggesting a group ambivalent about changing
3. Participation—those who seemed to be invested in changing their behavior
4. Uninvolved or Discouraged—those who appeared disinterested in change; it was hypothesized that these people may have given up on the change process
5. Contemplation—those who were serious about changing but not yet ready to make the commitment

A replication of the study found four stages (all except uninvolved/discouraged, Carney & Kivlahan, 1995). One observes from these studies that the stages of change for alcohol cessation may be different than the classical smoking cessation stages of change. Although the stages are consistent theoretically with those predicted by the TTM, research with alcohol dependence clarifies the importance of careful adaptation of the stages of change variable to other problem behaviors.

2. *Processes of change.* One study on the processes of change indicated that a relationship exists between use of behavioral processes of change and increased involvement in Alcoholics Anonymous (Snow, Prochaska, & Rossi, 1994). Rossi (1992a) found confirmation for the two hierarchical factors—experiential and behavioral—and the processes of change for alcohol, cocaine, and heroin addiction.

3. *Decisional balance.* Decisional balance was replicated in two studies of alcohol use with adolescents (Migneault, Pallonen, & Velicer, 1997; Migneault, Velicer, Prochaska, & Stevenson, 1999).

There have been few studies for TTM research in drug abuse, such as with heroin and cocaine. Rossi, Rosembloom, Monti, et al. (1993) found in a study of current and former cocaine users that stage of change, decisional balance, processes of change, and self-efficacy (confidence and temptation) were structurally identical to those used in the smoking cessation model, providing support for use of the model with cocaine addicts. Tejero, Trujols, Hernandez, de los Cobos, and Casas (1997) found that it was primarily behavioral processes of change that discriminated drug users by stage of change.

SUMMARY

It appears that TTM research in alcohol and drug dependence is in its initial, exploratory stages. More research is needed to determine whether the five original stages—precontemplation, contemplation, preparation, action, and maintenance—are the best means of staging alcohol cessation. The Stages of Change Readiness and Treatment Eagerness Scale (SOCRATES) described three basic motivational readiness-for-change processes—*recognition* of a drinking problem, *ambivalence* toward the extent of the problem, and *taking steps* to reduce or completely stop drinking (Isenhart, 1994; Miller & Tonigan, 1996)—that are similar to the classic stages of change. Stage of change based on alcohol acquisition has been also tested with adolescents (Kelley, Denny, & Young, 1999; Werch, 1997). There is much room for research at all levels of theory development, specifically descriptive studies that would provide information allowing for potential consensus by scientists and practitioners on staging for alcohol and drug-addicted individuals.

DIET AND WEIGHT MANAGEMENT

Review of the Research

Costs associated with obesity were estimated to be nearly $100 billion in 1995 (USDHHS, 2000). National dietary recommendations include increasing fruit, vegetable, and fiber consumption and decreasing total dietary fat consumption (USDHHS, 1991), yet the consumption of dietary fiber, fruits and vegetables is currently lower, and fat intake is higher than recommended levels (Public Health Service, 1988; World Cancer Research Fund, 1997). The number of people classified as overweight or obese continues to rise (USDHHS, 2000). More people than ever are classified as overweight or obese. Dietary behavior continues to be a public health concern, particularly as the population ages and risk for cancer and cardiovascular disease increase.

1. *Stage of change.* Reaching a consensus on the definition of "action" for this behavior has been difficult. If one asks the question, "Have you reduced your consumption of high-fat foods," around 65% of the population will be in either action or maintenance (Prochaska, 1992). Generally, people should consume no more than 30% of their total calories from fats (Kristal, Shattuck, & Henry, 1990). However, if one were to ask the average consumer, "Do you intend to reduce dietary fat consumption to no more than 30% of total calories from fats in the next 6 months," he or she would most likely not know how much of their total intake is from fats.

Curry, Kristal, and Bowen (1992) were one of the first groups of diet researchers to show how people could be staged according to the TTM model of behavior change. Theirs is an algorithm that includes measures of perceived overall fat content of diet, length of time following a low fat diet, success in following a low fat diet, and intentions to change diet. A similar staging algorithm was used by Glanz et al. (1994). Greene, Rossi, Reed, Willey, and Prochaska (1994) used an algorithm that included intention to avoid high fat foods, a behavioral measure (food frequency questionnaire) used to compute percent of energy intake from fat, and an instrument used to assess dietary behaviors. Hargreaves et al. (1999) used a similar algorithm for stage assignment of African American women. Rossi et al. (1993) compared four different algorithms for staging individuals on fat intake (limiting dietary fat intake, constantly avoiding high fat foods, eating a low fat diet, and eating a diet of which fat is 30% of the calories or less). Similar results were obtained using all 4 algorithms, although the first, limiting dietary fat, had the fewest in the maintenance stage, and levels of dietary fat decreased with increasing stage of change; decisional balance across the stages was generally as predicted for all four algorithms. What is consistent across algorithms is the strong relationship between dietary fat and stage of change (Kristal, Glanz, Curry, & Patterson, 1999).

2. *Other model constructs.* Brug, Glanz, and Kok (1997) found that *self-efficacy* predicted stage of change for increasing intake of fruits and vegetables as would be predicted from the TTM. Research on the processes of change has generally shown that the 10 TTM processes of change are also valid for diet (Bowen, Meishcke, & Tomoyasu, 1994; Rossi, 1992a; Rossi & Rossi, 1993).

Some work has also been accomplished specifically around weight control. In reviews of multiple behaviors, researchers have found stage of change and decisional balance for weight control to be consistent with TTM constructs in other behaviors studied (Nigg et al., 1999; Prochaska, Velicer, Rossi, Goldstein, et al., 1994). Prochaska, Norcross, Fowler, Follick, and Abrams (1992) found, in a work-site based weight control study, that participants used more action-related change processes compared to change processes they used during the 10-week period preceding the intervention. Additionally, self-efficacy increased as predicted by the TTM and was further validated as a predictor of stage of change [also see Clark, Abrams, Niaura, Eaton, & Rossi (1991) for a more detailed treatment of the importance of self-efficacy to weight loss].

3. *Interventions.* One intervention study was found that tailored feedback materials based on stage of dietary fat change, albeit in a limited fashion. Greene and Rossi (1998) used stages of change to classify individuals at baseline and provided them with a stage-tailored; feedback report more of those receiving the initial feedback progressed to the action stage at the end of 18 months.

Summary

The "correct" means of staging dietary behaviors has been a source of research effort, and there still is not one standardized algorithm accepted by all researchers. The stage of change variable has been tested in a variety of populations, including clinical, university, community, African American, and work sites. However, there have been relatively few studies testing the applicability of the four core measures of the TTM in a single study. More research on stage of change, processes of change, decisional balance, and self-efficacy is needed in order to broaden our understanding of the relationship among the four constructs. For example, is the classical relationship between pros and cons across stages of change maintained in different populations? This would be a fruitful area for further research. Research is still in the descriptive and explanatory phases; there clearly is a need for further descriptive inquiry into dietary behavior.

The question of the correct staging algorithm remains unanswered. However, Kristal et al. (1999) suggested that the best measure of diet is self-rated diet, because it provides information on what people think they are eating. Thus, the stage of change variable can be used as a means of intervening in dietary change rather than being a proxy for dietary fat intake. Given this, individuals can be provided with tailored information for stage of readiness to eat a reduced fat diet based on their self-rated dietary behaviors. The study by Kristal et al. (1999), which includes several of the leading names in dietary research, should provide motivation for intervention studies that include tailored materials based on stage of change. Even though the majority of people tend to be classified into action and maintenance, tailoring can be targeted toward preventing relapse to less healthy eating behaviors.

STRESS MANAGEMENT

Review of the Research

Stress is an important behavioral risk factor for cancer and other chronic diseases. The 1985 U.S. National Health Institute Survey found that 30% of employed workers reported that exposure to mental stress was the work condition that most endangered their health (Shilling & Brackbill, 1987). In a national survey by the Northwestern Mutual Life Insurance Company (1991) with 28,000 workers in 215 organizations, it was found that stress was a predominant problem associated with employee burnout, acute and chronic health problems, and poor work performance. The costs of unmanaged stress can be considerable not only for individuals and their families, but for employers, health care systems, and government.

There have been several studies conducted that apply the TTM to the area of stress management (for a review, see Velicer, Prochaska, Fava, Norman, & Redding, 1998). The primary focus of these studies has been to examine the feasibility of applying the TTM to this area and developing and validating measures of the key TTM constructs. These studies have been conducted with a variety of populations including college students, work site samples, random digit dialing samples, and women who are infected with HIV (see Velicer et al., 1998; Riley, Toth, & Fava, 2000).

1. *Stage of change.* The development of staging as applied to stress management has involved seven separate samples. Current studies use two different definitions of stress management in the staging algorithm. The first asks if the individual "consistently practices stress management in daily life" (Robbins et al., 1998). The second approach focuses more on "effectively managing stress" (Evers, Evans, Fava, & Prochaska, 2000). In both formats, examples of typical stress management behaviors and activities are provided to assist individuals in accurately assessing their own stress management levels. The stage of change construct in these samples has proved robust across the different validating samples and a general picture of the overall stage distribution has emerged. Stage distributions have varied depending on the population, with anywhere from 58 to 75% of adults indicating that they are in action or maintenance stages of change for stress management. Different examinations of the staging questions have, at times, allowed individuals to indicate that they currently have no stress in their lives, which changes the stage distribution significantly.

2. *Processes of change.* There has also been initial measurement work conducted on the 10 processes of change for stress management (Fava et al., 1998; Evers et al., 2000). These instruments are modeled on the 10 traditional processes of change originally developed for smoking cessation (Prochaska, Velicer, et al., 1988). One study of a 30-item version of this measure found that it demonstrated good psychometric properties (Fava et al., 1998). Significant differences

were found for eight of the processes across the stages. In a second study, separate principal components analysis and confirmatory factor analysis were conducted, each in one half of the sample. All models showed adequate fit (CFI range .76 to .91, AASR range .05 to .067; Evers et al., 2000). Both studies also found differential process usage by stage, which was consistent with previously conducted research in smoking cessation. It was found that precontemplators use the processes the least, and process use increases with advancement through the stages of change (Evers et al., 2000; Fava et al., 1998). Specifically in a college population, environmental reevaluation, self-reevaluation, counterconditioning, helping relationships, and self-liberation were all found to differ significantly across the stages (Evers et al., 2000).

3. *Decisional balance.* Analyses of different versions of decisional balance have examined and supported the dimensions, reliability, and validity of the pros and cons of stress management with three different samples (Fava et al., 1998; Evers et al., 2000). In one series of studies, a principal components analysis was conducted in a sample of university students, and a confirmatory factor analysis using structural equation modeling was performed on a sample of parents of 9th-graders (Velicer et al., 1998). Both of these analyses supported the two-factor decisional balance construct. Other studies examining the external validity of similar assessments have found significant difference across the stages of change for both pros and cons (Evers et al., 2000). Graphs of the standardized score values of the pros and cons across the stages of change show the most dramatic shift in attitude occurring during the transition between the precontemplation and contemplation stages. During this time, the pros increase one full standard deviation, which is similar to findings in other areas of behavior change (Prochaska et al., 1994).

4. *Self-efficacy.* A 20-item scale assessing situational confidence (self-efficacy) for managing stress has also been developed and tested in two separate samples (Norman et al., 1997; Evers et al., 2000). Significant differences by stage of change were found for self-efficacy. There were also significant correlations between the confidence measure and a short behavioral index (Johnson, Norman, & Fava, 1998) of stress management, further establishing validity for the measure. In a separate population, situational confidence was devel-

oped and confirmed, and showed significant differences between the stages of change (Evers et al, 2000).

The various measures of TTM constructs as applied to stress management have been applied in other distinct populations. Riley et al. (2000) administered the measures of stage of change, decisional balance, and situational confidence to a population of women at risk for, or infected with, HIV. Results found that the majority of the HIV-positive women, and all of the women at risk for HIV were in the later stages of change (preparation, action, and maintenance). Women in the later stages of change reported significantly more situational confidence to manage stress than those women in earlier stages of change. Although the sample for this study was small ($N=19$), it represents an important application of the TTM measures as applied to stress management in a unique population.

5. *Interventions.* Clinical trials of interventions based on the TTM focusing on stress management have begun. One study in progress involves an interactive, individualized intervention for stress management based on the TTM, and impact of the intervention is being examined (Evers & Padula, 2001). This randomized clinical trial includes a TTM-based expert system as well as a manual. The feasibility of recruiting 70% of an at-risk population into a randomized clinical trial has been shown. Individuals in the intervention group indicated high acceptability of the materials, including more than 50% indicating they thought the materials were easy to read, use, and that they would recommend them to a friend. In addition, 64% indicated that they used the materials more than once (Evers & Padula, 2001).

Summary

Development of a stress management model of the TTM is in its early stages. The initial research is favorable for extending the TTM constructs into this important area for research. The research thus far supports the existence of five distinct stages, ten processes of change, and a two-factor decisional balance (pros and cons) model. Self-efficacy also appears to be important in predicting stage of change. Interventions are beginning to test the utility of the TTM in helping individuals to better manage stress in their lives. Attempts have been made to validate this model with different populations, including women, college students, and individuals in work sites. Review of the research indicates that this application is in its descriptive and explanatory phases of development; further research with other populations is needed to further establish the validity of the TTM in stress management.

SUN EXPOSURE

Sun exposure is one of the most important avoidable causes of skin cancer that accounts for approximately 1,000,000 cancers per year in the United States (Miller & Weinstock, 1994). The application of the TTM to sun risk behaviors has included both measurement development studies (Maddock et al., 1998) and intervention studies conducted with a variety of populations (Redding et al., 1999; Weinstock, Rossi, Redding, Maddock, & Cottrill, 2000).

1. *Stage of change.* Several studies have developed and validated TTM measures as applied to sun protective behaviors, including staging algorithms (Maddock et al., 1998; Rossi, Blais, Redding, & Weinstock, 1995). Staging algorithms focus on general sun protection based on intentions and behaviors for protecting oneself from the sun consistently by: (1) avoiding sun exposure; (2) covering up with clothing/hats; and (3) using SPF 15 sunscreens. An algorithm for stage of change focuses on protection by using SPF 15 sunscreens alone. Both measures have been well developed across more than 10 different study populations, including participants in self-help smoking cessation and work site health promotion programs, sun bathers on beaches, HMO members, and random telephone survey participants (Rossi et al., 1995). Rossi et al. (1995) reported in the same study that the vast majority of individuals are in the precontemplation stage for both reducing unprotected sun exposure and increasing sunscreen use.

Measures of decisional balance and situational self-efficacy have also been developed. Research has shown that they have good internal consistency and show similar patterns across the stages when compared to other behaviors (Maddock et al., 1998; Prochaska, Velicer, Rossi, Goldstein, et al., 1994). Development of the situational self-efficacy (confidence) measure found two subscales; sunscreen use and sun avoidance (Maddock et al., 1998). Early work on the processes of change has found a similar hierarchical structure to that found in other behaviors (Maddock et al., 1998; Rossi, 1992a).

2. *Interventions.* An intervention research project aimed at delivering skin cancer prevention and health promotion efforts directly to sunbathers at Rhode Island beaches contacted a total of 1,016 beachgoers during the course of the study (Rossi, Blais, & Weinstock, 1994). The project aided in the development of measurement models and questionnaires based on the TTM. In addition, interventions were developed and tested the feasibility of using the beach of an intervention site. Seven interventions were developed and tested: an educational pamphlet, distribution of free sunscreen samples, a sun sensitivity assessment and feedback, a sun scanner intervention, an educational and dramatic videotape, a skin microtopography (a plastic impression of the skin in the crow's feet area near the eye), and an ultraviolet and polarized light instant photography. This study demonstrated the feasibility of conducting interventions on the beach, and provided data on interventions provided and barriers to implementations of such interventions.

An intervention aimed at increasing adolescents' sun protective behaviors has also been developed. Redding et al. (1999) provides a description of the "Health Information Highway" program, which is a high school intervention research project that uses both multimedia expert computer systems and complementary school curriculum components to decrease smoking, increase sun protective behaviors, and decrease dietary fat consumption among high school students. Aspects of the program are based on the TTM. Baseline recruitment included 4,983 ninth graders, which represented a 90% recruitment rate. Adolescents enrolled in the program were followed throughout the 2-year intervention period and for 2 years afterward.

Another large intervention study recruited a representative sample of 2,324 beachgoers in southeastern New England (Weinstock et al., 2000; Weinstock & Rossi, 1998). Recruitment on the beach enrolled 83% of those approached about the research. Analyses of the baseline sample of this randomized controlled intervention study have been published. Individuals were placed into stages of change based on general readiness to consistently engage in protective behaviors and for sunscreen use with SPF of 15 or above. Analyses included stage of change for sun protective behaviors by demographic information including age, gender, and degree of sun sensitivity. Individuals who were in the precontemplation stage, who were not adequately protecting themselves from sun exposure, were more likely to be younger adults, male, lower socioeconomic status, and lower sun sensitivity. In addition, they were less likely to have personal knowledge of someone with skin cancer, family histories of melanoma, and were more likely to be tanning booth users. Smoking status, exercise status, personal history of skin cancer, and the presence of large moles were not related to stages of change.

Summary

The initial research examining the application of the TTM to the area of sun protective behaviors, although early in its development, is favorable. Research has supported the constructs of the TTM applied to this area, including the staging of two separate behaviors: a general sun protective index and use SPF 15 sunscreens. Many intervention studies have been conducted with a variety of populations. In addition to studying the impact of these interventions on sun protective behaviors, they have also shown the ability to recruit individuals into intervention programs in nontraditional settings such as on the beach.

SCREENING BEHAVIORS

Mammography

Colorectal, breast, and cervical cancers are expected to take the lives of over 100,000 Americans in 2000. Early detection through screening tests can significantly reduce morbidity and mortality associated with these cancers. The TTM has been applied to several different types of screening behaviors. The first of these is mammography. Several studies have applied the TTM to this behavior with a variety of populations including a work site sample (Rakowski et al., 1992), women in selected census tracts (Rakowski, Fulton, & Feldman, 1993), and random samples of women from an HMO in southeastern New England (Rakowski et al., 1996). The populations tended to be women ages 50 to 75 years of age.

1. *Stage of change.* The majority of the research in this area has focused on the stage of change and decisional balance measures (Rakowski, Fulton, & Feldman, 1993; Rakowski et al., 1996). Different research studies have conceptualized the stages of change as related to mammography in different ways. The traditional five stages of change, precontemplation, contemplation, preparation, action, and maintenance are represented. However, other stages are also incorporated into research design. Risk, defined as having been screened in the distant past but not intending to be screened in the future, and relapse risk, defined as having had regular screenings but no longer planning to continue are two such stages. In addition, studies have defined the stages as screeners (women who have had a mammogram in the past 24 months and plan to have another in 24 months); intenders (women who have not had a mammogram in the past 24 months but intent to in the next 24 months); and nonparticipants (women who have not had a mammogram in the past 24 months, nor intend to in the next 24 months, Mah & Bryant, 1997).

2. *Decisional balance.* Several studies have focused on the development and validation of the decisional balance measures for mammography use. Development and validation of the pros and cons of mammography were conducted on a sample of 142 women recruited from three work sites (Rakowski et al., 1992). Measures of the pros and cons were developed using principal components analysis, and were found to be associated with the stage of change for mammography adoption. A study conducted by Rakowski, Anderson, et al. (1997) allowed for further examination of the decisional balance measures. A total of 8,914 women ages 50 to 80 from 40 primarily rural communities in Washington state participated in research that confirmed previous measures. In addition, this research allowed for the testing of the measures in a different geographic region and had a sample large enough to conduct analysis in both a developmental and confirmatory sample. The structure of the pros and cons were confirmed and an analysis of variance confirmed the associations between readiness to obtain screening and opinions about mammography previously found.

Longitudinal studies of decisional balance have also been conducted. Women ages 50 to 74 (N = 1,144) participated in a longitudinal telephone study examining women's decision making about mammography over a 1-year period (Pearlman et al., 1997). Results showed that individuals who shifted to a less favorable view of mammography over the course of the study tended to be smokers and had not had a recent clinical breast examination and pap test. Change was also related to four dimensions of a woman's information environment. Those who rated opinions of physicians as somewhat or not important, felt that they lacked enough people in their social network with whom they could discuss health concerns, and who reported that at least one family member or friend discouraged them from having a mammogram were less likely to express favorable attitudes about mammography. In addition, those who consistently communicated the value of mammography to others expressed more favorable views of screening.

3. *Other predictors of stage of change.* Several studies have examined the impact of other variables on stage of change for mammography use. In a study examining the relationship of objective and subjective risk of breast cancer and the TTM as applied to mammography screening, significant relationships were found (Lipkus, Rimer, & Strigo, 1996). Women with objective and subjective risk were associated with being in a later stage of change for mammography. Another study found that race was an important factor to include when applying the TTM to mammography use (Pearlman, Rakowski, Ehrich, & Clark, 1996). By looking at data from the 1990 National Health Interview Survey, analyses of stage of change for mammography was stratified by three groups: blacks, Hispanics, and non-Hispanic whites. Results found that race is an important influencing factor for mammography use. Although it was found that those who reported less pap smear testing, breast self-examination, and clinical breast exams were less likely to have mammograms, the magnitude of the associations were different among the different racial groups.

Interventions based on the TTM have been developed to increase mammography screening. The North Carolina Breast Cancer Screening Program was developed to increase the rate of mammography screening by 20% in 3 years among older black women in five rural counties in the state (Earp, Altpeter, Mayne, Viadro, & O'Malley, 1995). The theoretical foundations of the program include the TTM, the Health Belief Model, the social ecological perspective, and the PRECEDE model of health promotion.

Cervical Cancer

The other screening behavior to which the TTM has been applied is cervical cancer screening—pap tests. One such study was conducted in Queensland, Australia, with Australian South Sea Islanders, Chinese, German, Greek, and Moslem women (Kelaher et al., 1999). This study conducted focus groups and structured interviews. During these, participants were classified into one of the stages of change, and were assessed on their knowledge of screenings, sources of information, and benefits and barriers. Participants were classified into one of six stages of change, which were modifications of the criteria developed for mammography. These included the traditional stages of precontemplation, contemplation, action, and maintenance. In addition, individuals who had no intention of being screened but had been screened in the distant past were classified into relapse, and individuals who had regular pap tests but no longer plan to continue having them were placed into the relapse risk stage. Knowledge and decisional balance scores supported classification into each stage of change. Analyses found that women in the earlier stages of change were more likely to express a preference for service delivery in their own language and by a female, while women in the action and maintenance stages were more likely to have had their last pap test by a female physician. Intention was found to be an important part of the stage construct in that women who indicated they intended to be screened in the future were more likely to have positive decisional balance scores and higher knowledge scores than others.

Screening for Multiple Cancers

Two studies have examined multiple-cancer screening behavior. The first assessed stage of change for colorectal, breast, and cervical cancer screening and explored the covariation of different screening behaviors (Driskell, Evers, Johnson, Johnson, & Prochaska, 2001).

A second study examined mammography screening and pap tests (described above) together (Rakowski, Clark, et al., 1997). A single index of recency and decisional balance for both screening behaviors was examined with baseline and one-year follow-up surveys with an HMO sample of 1,605 women ages 40 to 74. Results showed the ability to combine measures of decisional balance for both mammography and pap testing.

Summary

There have been a variety of studies of the TTM in the area of screening behavior, mainly mammography and pap tests. In the area of mammography, the stages of change have been examined extensively, and several different sets of stages have been identified by different studies. Decisional balance has also been examined and studies have found results across the stages as would be predicted from other behavioral areas. Other predictors of stage of change have also been examined, including objective and subjective risk of breast cancer, and race. The second screening behavior, pap tests, has mainly been examined in terms of stages of change, which were modified from the stages developed in mammography. One study, which examined both screening behaviors together, found a single index of decisional balance to be valid.

MEDICATION COMPLIANCE

The TTM has been applied to the area of medication adherence in a variety of different medications including oral contraceptive pills (Johnson, 1998; Johnson, Grimley, & Prochaska, 1998a, 1998b; Emmett & Ferguson, 1999), and antihypertensive drug therapy (Willey, 1999), where publications have provided descriptions of intervention strategies (Willey, 1999).

Adherence to oral contraceptive pill use has been examined using the TTM in a variety of studies. The development and validation of reliable measures of the TTM as applied to this behavior have occurred in two independent samples (Johnson, 1998; Johnson et al., 1998a). Decisional balance and self-efficacy have been found to vary systematically across the stages as expected based on the application of the TTM to other behaviors (Johnson, 1998). In addition, measures of the processes of change have also been developed and validated (Johnson et al., 1998a). Independent multivariate analyses of variance revealed that women in different stages of change differed significantly on process use in that women in post-action stages emphasized behavioral processes, whereas early stage individuals emphasized the experiential processes.

Another study examined oral contraceptive (OC) pill use among 94 women who completed an anonymous questionnaire (Emmett & Ferguson, 1999). Stage of change from the TTM was used as a framework for this research, with an additional stage (deciding not to act) from the precautionary adoption process added. The study examined decision making, including decisional balance, knowledge, perceived risk, and stage of change. Results showed differences between the stages on positive and negative aspects, perceived risks, and subjective knowledge of OC use.

Research studies have compared the predictive ability of the constructs of the TTM to demographics and sexual history characteristics (Johnson et al., 1998b). In two independent samples, demographic and sexual history variables did not add significantly to the prediction of adherence based on the TTM. Within both samples, the TTM variables accounted for a significant proportion of the variance in adherence.

Summary

Studies of the TTM applied to medication compliance have mainly focused on the area of oral contraceptive use. The decisional balance, confidence, and processes of change measures have been developed and validated in two separate samples. The Stages in this behavior have also been examined. The constructs of the TTM were found to account for a significant proportion of variance of compliance when compared to sexual history and demographics.

HEALTH CARE PROVIDER

The TTM has also been applied to changing behaviors among health care providers. Publications have often outlined how the TTM can be applied to changing health care provider behavior by providing programs and interventions that they can implement in their own practice. One such publication (Cassidy, 1999) outlines how nurse practitioners can use the TTM to facilitate behavior change with patients with chronic illness in an effort to facilitate behaviors such as exercising and self-monitoring and stop behaviors such as smoking. Pololi and Potter (1996) designed a program to teach internal medicine residents behavioral counseling skills for multiple risk factor modification. This program used small group discussions, negotiation skills, and physician-patient communication, and was based on the TTM. Application of the program with 18 residents found that the program increased ability to modify patient behavior during videotaped interviews. In addition, it found that that program increased both residents' self-efficacy and performance of behavioral counseling.

The TTM has also been applied to pharmacists' behavior in a variety of research projects. Berger and Grimley (1997) examined the pharmacists' readiness for rendering pharmaceutical care utilizing the TTM. Analysis of data collected at the 1996 American Public Health Association (APHA) Annual Meeting and Exposition helped identify and measure factors that facilitate and barriers to rendering pharmaceutical care, as well as the strength of these factors in each stage of readiness. The vast majority of pharmacists were not ready to take action within six months. Findings also showed that individuals in administrative positions were more likely to engage in behavior that leads to submitting documentation for compensation. As predicted based on research in other areas, the cons of engaging in a behavior tended to be more salient for individuals in the precontemplation and contemplation stages.

In another study pharmacists' readiness to adopt a proposed new standard for assessing consumers' over-the-counter product selections were examined (Taylor, Berger, Anderson-Harper, & Grimley, 2000). Community pharmacists in a Canadian province completed a questionnaire including stage of change, decisional balance, demographics, and agreement with current legislative status of pharmacists-only products. Most of the respondents were staff pharmacists in independent pharmacies. Demographic variables had no significant effect on readiness for change, and the majority were not ready to adopt the proposed new behaviors. As hypothesized, the pros and cons varied across the stages.

Summary

The majority of the studies in the area of health care provider behavior have examined the behavior of pharmacists. Decisional balance and stages of change have been examined with readiness for rendering pharmaceutical care, and readiness to adopt new assessment standards. Interventions based on the TTM have been developed and examined in a variety of populations including nurse practitioners and internal medicine residents. Further research in this area is required to further examine and validate measures of TTM constructs applied to changing health care provider behavior.

OTHER BEHAVIORS

The TTM has been applied to other behaviors. Some research has been applied to general stages of change in therapy (McConnaughy et al., 1983; Prochaska, Rossi, & Wilcox, 1991), as well as to understanding treatment for specific disorders such as phobias (Prochaska, 1991). Several studies have examined application of the TTM to pain management, and a questionnaire has been developed to assess individuals' readiness to adopt a self-management approach to chronic pain conditions (Kerns, Rosenberg, Jamison, Caudill, & Haythornthwaite, 1997; Jensen, Nielson, Romano, Hill, & Turner, 2000). A study using cluster analysis examined patients' adoption of a self-management approach to their arthritis found five stages of change (Keefe et al., 2000). Other behavioral areas that have been examined include readiness to perform cardiopulmonary resuscitation (Nolan et al., 1999), bulimia (Levy, 1997; Treasure et al., 1999), batterer treatment (Levesque, Gelles, & Velicer, 2000), and breast feeding (Humphreys, Thompson, & Miner, 1998; Kloeblen, Thompson, & Miner, 1999). The TTM is also beginning to be applied to areas outside the health arena. Initial studies in the area of organizational change (Prochaska, Prochaska, & Levesque, in press) have examined family service agencies' intentions to adopt time-limited therapy (Prochaska, 2000) and integrated service delivery (Levesque, Prochaska, & Prochaska, 1999). Another study examined the stages of changing financial behavior with individuals in New York (O'Neil, Brisotow, & Brennan, 1999).

OVERVIEW/SUMMARIZING REMARKS

This review provided a comprehensive, though not thoroughly exhaustive, review of the research of the TTM as applied to several problem behavior domains. Some summarizing remarks are in order.

1. *Scope.* The TTM has demonstrated broad scope. Several problem behaviors were considered in some detail (smoking cessation and acquisition, safer sex, alcohol/drug cessation and acquisition, diet (fat intake, fruit/vegetable/fiber consumption, and weight control), stress management, sun exposure, screening behaviors, medication compliance, and health care provider behavior) to which application of the TTM has shown promise. Additionally, the TTM is being or has been applied in other areas not specifically discussed here. Stage of change and processes of change have been successful in predicting client termination or completion of psychotherapy (Brogan, Prochaska, & Prochaska, 1999). It is being used in organizational change and for effecting change at the community level. Several researchers have shown that the stages of change (precontemplation, contemplation, preparation, action, and maintenance), the 10 processes of change (consciousness raising, dramatic relief, self-reevaluation, environmental reevaluation, social liberation, counterconditioning, helping relationships, reinforcement management, self-liberation, and stimulus control), decisional balance (the pros and cons of either adopting or ceasing a behavior), and self-efficacy (both confidence and temptation) are valid across a wide range of behaviors (Nigg et al., 1999; Prochaska et al., 1994; Rossi, 1992a, 1992b). "Strong and Weak principles of change" (the *strong principle* is that there is a one standard deviation increase in pros from precontemplation to action; the *weak principle* is that cons decrease by approximately one half of a standard deviation from precontemplation to action) have been found to be consistent across a number of different problem behaviors (Prochaska, Velicer, et al., 1994).

The evidence suggests that the TTM has broad scope and models that tailor interventions to stage of readiness to change can be applied to a vast number of problem health behaviors.

2. *Validation of TTM for problem behaviors other than smoking cessation.* Although research has demonstrated validity of the TTM constructs, the need for additional research remains a top priority. Smoking cessation remains the prototype for behavior change using the TTM, and the extensive statistical analyses involved in the validation of TTM constructs for smoking cessation should be the model for validation of the TTM with other problem behaviors. These analyses, including the validation of the model in diverse populations, the use of longitudinal analysis methods for verifying the movement of individuals through the stages of change, and the development of interventions including expert systems, have resulted in a behavior change model that has progressed rapidly in terms of theory development. Similar intensive research is needed to further validate the utility of the model with other health behavior domains

3. *The stage of change variable.* Although model constructs appear to be consistent across a number of health behaviors, there is no clear consensus that the stage of change variable "fits" all behaviors as originally posited in the TTM. It appears that, particularly for alcohol cessation, there might be other ways of staging individuals that would result in more effective tailoring of interventions. However, more research is needed to determine if this is true. One should not become confused by the various measures for alcohol use that may, on the surface, appear different (such as SOCRATES). The TTM was unique in its staging of individuals based on their readiness to change, and virtually all of the variants retain one common factor—each stages individuals with the goal of ultimately finding the best "fit" for movement closer to adoption or cessation of the problem behavior. There is really no reason to assume that the TTM should be applied to each problem behavior in exactly the same way.

The number of stages has its most importance in terms of intervention. Expert systems interventions based on tailoring behavior to one's readiness to change smoking behavior are based on five stages of change. However, there does not seem to be consensus in the other behaviors, such as drug and alcohol addiction, for a five-stage model. As noted earlier, research in smoking cessation has found that there is variability within stages, and that certain processes tend to be more important in certain stages but also at certain points with a particular stage. Hedeker, Mermelstein, and Weeks (1999) have found evidence for a thresholds of change model in which self-efficacy is an important discriminating variable in the transition state between precontemplation and contemplation (the contemplation threshold) and between contemplation and action (the action threshold). Research with adolescents has necessitated the inclusion of *acquisition* stages to account for trying substance use behaviors (Kelly et al., 1999; Pallonen, Prochaska, et al., 1998; Werch, 1997). These models, then, incorporate multiple stages that describe the acquisition of a problem behavior like alcohol consumption and cessation of that behavior.

Also, as noted in the discussion of alcohol cessation, some researchers are finding fewer stages of change than the traditional five-stage model. Pierce, Farkas, and Gilpin (1998) found eight levels in the smoking cessation continuum from precontemplation to advanced maintenance (precontemplation, contemplation, early preparation, intermediate preparation, advanced preparation, action, early maintenance, and advanced maintenance); an analysis of the stages indicates that the eight stages are mostly consistent with and represent a more "refined" five-stage model.

The bottom line here is an exciting one, and useful for two main reasons. First, more fine-tuned analysis of the stages will provide the opportunity to tailor interventions even more specifically to the unique needs of the individual trying to change his or her behavior. This would probably result in more people making progress in the behavior change process. Discovery of additional stages should be seen as a potentially beneficial result for the task of behavior change. Second, variance in number of stages provides additional evidence that researchers need to proceed with caution when adapting the model that has been successful with smoking cessation to other behavior domains. It may be, as research in staging of alcohol addiction is indicating, that there are fewer important stages that discriminate problem drinkers.

4. *Diverse populations.* Special attention needs to be paid to application of the TTM to different populations. For example, gay men and people of color are at disproportionate risk for HIV, yet the model has rarely been tested in these populations. In one study Lafferty et al. (1999), in their work with Asian American smokers,

found relationships between pros and cons different from that predicted by the TTM. Complications in older age can often be avoided through preventive behaviors such as proper exercise, diet, and moderation in substance use; little research has been done using the TTM with older adults (see Nigg et al., 1999 for an application of the TTM to 10 problem behaviors in older adults). There is much room for continued testing of the TTM in ethnic populations. Prochaska (1992) indicated that health behavior change among minority populations is targeted toward those in the action stage of change, and that these groups would be better served by tailoring the intervention specific to the individual readiness for change.

Using another example, sexuality has various constructions that are culture dependent. Several researchers have pointed to the impact of culture on sexual behavior, such as ideas of "machismo" in the Latino culture (Diaz, 1998). The TTM does not explicitly take these constructions into account. More research is needed to determine if these factors add unique variance beyond what can be explained by stage and processes of change, and decisional balance, alone.

5. *Are there other variables important to the model?* Further analysis will be required to determine if the current TTM measures—stage of change, processes of change, decisional balance, and self-efficacy (confidence and temptation) are the principle variables required to explain the variability in behavior change. Some have advocated other measures including perceived risk (Harlow, Quina, Morokoff, Rose, & Grimley, 1993). Burkholder (2000) found some support for perceived risk adding additional variance to models including decisional balance and stage of change measure. Some researchers, such as Redding and Rossi (1999), and Brown, Melchoir, Panter, Slaughter, and Huba (2000), have recognized differences with populations of women due to their unique circumstances of relationship power, assertiveness for using condoms, and domestic violence. The relationship between interpersonal factors and HIV/AIDS risk has been demonstrated for sexual assertiveness (for birth control use, for refusal and initiation of sex, and for communication of preferences to sex partners) as well as for interpersonal violence in the context of the relationship (Harlow et al., 1993; Morokoff et al., 1997; Quina, Harlow, Morokoff, & Saxon, 1997; Quina, Harlow, Morokoff, Burkholder, & Dieter, 1999; Zierler & Krieger, 1997).

Rosenthal, Hall, and Moore (1992) echoed these findings in their study of adolescents. Another variable of interest may be that of willingness. In studies of adolescents (Gibbons & Gerrard, 1995, 1997: prototype/willingness model), it was found that behavioral willingness added significant variance (that beyond models with behavioral intention alone) to models predicting risk behavior. This appeared to be important for adolescents whose behavior is, for the most part, unplanned (Gibbons, Gerrard, Blanton, & Russell, 1998). It may be that all, some, or none of these important variables will explain additional, unique variance in behavior change.

6. *Definition of "action."* For some behaviors the criteria for being in the action stage are relatively clear. In smoking cessation we define someone to be in action who has ceased smoking cigarettes for less than 6 months. In most other behaviors, determination of the criteria is more difficult. For example, a common criteria for action on dietary fat is "I have eaten a lower fat diet for 6 months or less"; most algorithms involve some combination of perceived fat intake, previous attempts to eat a lower fat diet, and intention to change diet (Kristal et al., 1999). Most staging models show a very high percentage of the population in either action or maintenance stages. There also could be controversy in the alcohol addiction domain, for there are those who believe that the learning of controlled drinking is better for some people than total abstinence. In the HIV risk domain, the use of condoms every time a person has sex may not always be appropriate, particularly if the person is in a monogamous, long-term relationship. In the context of a marriage or a steady, committed relationship, partners may choose not to use condoms. Are they in precontemplation, contemplation, preparation, action, or maintenance? These are some examples of the issues faced by public health leaders and researchers in trying to decide the criteria for action that usually escape clear definition (unlike smoking cessation). The important point here is that the action stage of change will be defined differently for different behaviors, and studies that include interventions will help researchers to refine the criteria for action.

CONCLUSION

The science of behavior change is an exciting and challenging endeavor. The TTM has established itself as a viable, cost-effective means of helping people to change problem behaviors. While there has been much research using this model, much remains to be investigated in its application to the broad spectrum of problem behaviors. In a short period of approximately 20 years, the TTM has progressed rapidly into a well-developed theory. Rapid advances strongly advocate the need for rapid dissemination of results of research, particularly interventions, using the TTM. It is further empirical research (as well as feedback from practitioners who may work with clients using basic TTM principles) that will be required to keep theory development alive.

The following chapters show some of the ways that researchers have adapted the TTM to exercise behavior, a relatively understudied domain, and to older adults, an understudied population. The description of the TTM provided in chapter 3, and the extensive overview provided here, should give the reader an understanding of what the model is and what it can potentially do in the important area of exercise behavior with older adults.

REFERENCES

Ahijevych, K., & Parsely, L. A. (1999). Smoke constituent exposure and stage of change in Black and White women cigarette smokers. *Addictive Behaviors, 24,* 115–120.

Anderson, J. E., Cheney, R., Faruque, S., & Long, A. (1996). Stages of change for HIV risk behavior: Injecting drug users in five cities. *Drugs & Society, 9,* 1–17.

Bane, C. M., Ruggiero, L., Dryfoos, J. M., & Rossi, J. S. (1999). Development of a pregnancy-tailored decisional balance measure for smoking cessation. *Addictive Behaviors, 24,* 795–799.

Barnum, B. J. S. (1990). *Nursing theory: Analysis, application, evaluation* (3rd ed.). Glenview, IL: Scott, Foresman, and Company.

Berger, B. A., & Grimley, D. (1997). Pharmacists' readiness for rendering pharmaceutical care. *Journal of the American Pharmaceutical Association, 5,* 535–542.

Bowen, D. J., Meischke, H., & Tomoyasu, N. (1994). Preliminary evaluation of the processes of changing to a low-fat diet. *Health Education Research, 9,* 85–94.

Bowen, A. M., & Trotter, R. (1995). HIV risk in intravenous drug users and crack cocaine smokers: Predicting stage of change for condom use. *Journal of Consulting and Clinical Psychology, 63,* 238–248.

Brogan, M. M., Prochaska, J. O., & Prochaska, J. M. (1999). Predicting termination and continuation status in psychotherapy using the transtheoretical model. *Psychotherapy, 36,* 105–113.

Brown, V., Mechior, L. A., Panter, A. T., Slaughter, R., & Huba, G. J. (2000). Women's steps of change and entry into drug abuse treatment: A multidimensional stages of change model. *Journal of Substance Abuse Treatment, 18,* 231–240.

Brug, J., Glanz, K., & Kok, G. (1997). The relationship between self-efficacy, attitudes, intake compared to others, consumption, and stages of change related to fruit and vegetable consumption. *American Journal of Health Promotion, 12,* 25–30.

Burbank, P. M., Padula, C. A. & Nigg, C. R. (2000). Changing health behaviors of older adults. *Journal of Gerontological Nursing, 26,* 26–33.

Burkholder, G. J. (2000). *Integrating theories and methods in assessing longitudinal change in heterosexual HIV risk among women.* Unpublished doctoral dissertation, University of Rhode Island.

Carney, M. M., & Kivlahan, D. R. (1995). Motivational subtypes among veterans seeking substance abuse treatment: Profiles based on stages of change. *Psychology of Addictive Behaviors, 9,* 135–142.

Cassidy, C. A. (1999). Using the transtheoretical model to facilitate behavior change in patients with chronic illness. *Journal of the American Academy of Nurse Practitioners, 11*(7), 281–287.

Catania, J. A., Kegeles, S. M., & Coates, T. J. (1990). Towards an understanding of risk behavior: An AIDS risk reduction model (ARRM). *Health Education Quarterly, 17,* 53–72.

CDC (Centers for Disease Control and Prevention). (1997, December). *HIV/AIDS Surveillance Report, 9*(2), 1–43.

CDC (Centers for Disease Control and Prevention). (1999, December). *HIV/AIDS Surveillance Report, 11,* 1–43.

Clark, M. M., Abrams, D. B., Niaura, R. S., Eaton, C. A., & Rossi, J. S. (1991). Self-efficacy in weight management. *Journal of Clinical and Consulting Psychology, 59,* 739–744.

Curry, S. J., Kristal, A. R., & Bowen, D. H. (1992). An application of the stage model of behavior change to dietary fat reduction. *Health Education Research, 7,* 319–325.

Diaz, R. (1998). *Latino gay men and HIV.* New York: Routledge.

DiClemente, C. C., & Hughes, S. O. (1990). Stages of change profiles in outpatient alcoholism treatment. *Journal of Substance Abuse, 2,* 217–235.

DiClemente, C. C., & Prochaska, J. O. (1982). Self-change and therapy change of smoking behavior: A comparison of processes of change in cessation and maintenance. *Addictive Behaviors, 7,* 133–142.

DiClemente, C. C., Prochaska, J. O., & Gilbertini, M. (1985). Self-efficacy and the stages of self-change of smoking. *Cognitive Therapy and Research, 9,* 181–200.

Dijkstra, A., DeVries, H., & Bakker, M. (1996). Pros and cons of quitting, self-efficacy, and the stages of change in smoking cessation. *Journal of Clinical and Consulting Psychology, 64,* 758–763.

Donovan, R. J., Jones, S., Holman, C. D. J., & Corti, B. (1998). Assessing the reliability of a stage of change scale. *Health Education Research, 13,* 285–291.

Driskell, M. M., Evers, K. E., Johnson, J. L., Johnson, S. S., & Prochaska, J. M., (2001, March). *Stages of change for cancer screening behaviors.* Presented at the 22nd Annual Scientific Sessions of the Society of Behavioral Medicine, Seattle, WA.

Earp, J. A., Altpeter, M., Mayne, L., Viadro, C. I., & O'Malley, M. S. (1995). The North Carolina Breast Cancer Screening Program: Foundations and design of a model for reaching older, minority, rural women. *Breast Cancer Research and Treatment, 35,* 7–22.

Edens, J. F., & Willoughby, F. W. (1999). Motivational profiles of polysubstance-dependent patients: Do they differ from alcohol-dependent patients? *Addictive Behaviors, 24,* 195–206.

Emmett, C., & Ferguson, E. (1999). Oral contraceptive pill use, decisional balance, risk perception and knowledge: An exploratory study. *Journal of Reproductive and Infant Psychology, 17,* 327–343.

Etter, J., & Perneger, T. (1999). A comparison for two measures of stage of change for smoking cessation. *Addiction, 94,* 1881–1889.

Evers, K. E., Evans, J. L., Fava, J. L., & Prochaska, J. O. (2000, April). *Development and validation of Transtheoretical Model variables applied to stress management.* Presented at the 21st Annual Scientific Sessions of the Society of Behavioral Medicine, Nashville, TN.

Evers, K. E., Harlow, L. L., Redding, C. A., & LaForge, R. G. (1998). Longitudinal changes in stages of change for condom use in women. *American Journal of Health Promotion, 13,* 19–25.

Evers, K. E., & Padula, J. (2001, March). *A population-based stress management program: From science to practice.* Presented as part of a symposium at the 22nd Annual Scientific Sessions of the Society of Behavioral Medicine, Seattle, WA.

Fava, J. L., Norman, G. J., Levesque, D. A., Redding, C. A., Johnson, S., Evers, K., & Reich, T. (1998, March). *Measuring decisional balance for stress management.* Paper presented at the Nineteenth Annual Scientific Sessions of The Society of Behavioral Medicine, New Orleans, LA.

Fava, J. L., Norman, G. J., Redding, C. A., Levesque, D. A., Evers, K., & Johnson, S. (1998, March). *A processes of change measure for stress manage-*

ment. Paper presented at the Nineteenth Annual Scientific Sessions of The Society of Behavioral Medicine, New Orleans, LA.

Fava, J. L., Rossi, J. S., Redding, C. A., Ding, L., & Prochaska, J. O. (1994). *Progress toward cessation for smokers in precontemplation*. Presented at the 15th Annual Meeting of the Society for Behavioral Medicine. Boston, MA.

Fawcett, J. (1999). *The relationship of theory and research*. Philadelphia: F. A. Davis Company.

Galavotti, C., Cabral, R. J., Lansky, A., Grimley, D. M., Riley, G. E., & Prochaska, J. O. (1995). Validation of measures of condom and other contraceptive use among women at high risk for HIV infection and unintended pregnancy. *Health Psychology, 14*, 570–578.

Gibbons, F. X., & Gerrard, M. (1995). Predicting young adults' health risk behavior. *Journal of Personality and Social Psychology, 69*, 505–517.

Gibbons, F. X., & Gerrard, M. (1997). Health images and their effects on health behavior. In B. P. Buunk & F. X. Gibbons (Eds.), *Health, coping, and well-being: Perspectives from social comparison theory* (pp. 63–94). Mahwah, NJ: Erlbaum.

Gibbons, F. X., Gerrard, M., Blanton, H., & Russell, D. W. (1998). Reasoned action and social reaction: Willingness and intention as independent predictors of health risk. *Journal of Personality and Social Psychology, 5*, 1164–1180.

Glanz, K., Kristal, A. R., Tilley, B. C., & Hirst, K. (1998). Psychosocial correlates of healthful diets among male auto workers. *Cancer Epidemiological Biomarkers Prevention, 7*, 119–126.

Glanz, K., Patterson, R. E., Kristal, A. R., DiClemente, C. C., Heimendinger, J., Linnan, L., & McLerran, D. F. (1994). Stages of change in adopting healthy diets: Fat, fiber, and correlates of nutrient intake. *Health Education Quarterly, 21*, 499–519.

Gottlieb, N. H., Galavotti, C., McCuan, R. A., & McAlister, A. L. (1990). Specification of a social-cognitive model predicting smoking cessation in a Mexican-American population: A prospective study. *Cognitive Therapy & Research, 14*, 529–542.

Greene, G. W., & Rossi, S. R. (1998). Stages of change for reducing dietary fat intake over 18 months. *Journal of the American Dietetic Association, 98*, 529–534.

Greene, G. W., Rossi, S. R., Reed, G. R., Willey, C., & Prochaska, J. O. (1994). Stages of change for reducing dietary fat to 30% of energy or less. *Journal of the American Dietetic Association, 94*, 1105–1110.

Grimley, D. M., Prochaska, G. E., & Prochaska, J. O. (1993). Condom use assertiveness and the stages of change with main and other partners. *Journal of Applied Biobehavioral Research, 1*, 152–173.

Grimley, D. M., Prochaska, G. E., & Prochaska, J. O. (1997). Condom use adoption and continuation: A transtheoretical approach. *Health Education Research: Theory and Practice, 12,* 61–75.

Grimley, D. M., Prochaska, G. E., Prochaska, J. O., Velicer, W. F., Galavotti, C., Cabral, R. J., & Lansky, A. (1996). Cross-validation of measures assessing decisional balance and self-efficacy for condom use. *American Journal of Health Behavior, 20,* 406–416.

Grimley, D. M., Prochaska, J. O., Velicer, W. F., & Prochaska, G. E. (1995). Contraceptive and condom use adoption and maintenance: A stage paradigm approach. *Health Education Quarterly, 22,* 20–35.

Hargreaves, M. K., Schlundt, D. G., Buchowski, M. S., Hardy, R. E., Rossi, S. R., & Rossi, J. S. (1999). Stages of change and the intake of dietary fat in African American women: Improving stage assignment using the eating styles questionnaire. *Journal of the American Dietetic Association, 99,* 1392–1399.

Harlow, L. L., Prochaska, J. O., Redding, C. A., Rossi, J. S., Velicer, W. F., Snow, M. G., Schnell, D., Galavotti, C., O'Reilley, K., & Rhodes, R. (1999). Stages of condom use in a high HIV-risk sample. *Psychology and Health, 14,* 143–157.

Harlow, L. L., Quina, K., Morokoff, P. J., Rose, J. G., & Grimley, D. M. (1993). HIV risk in women: A multifaceted model. *Journal of Applied Biobehavioral Research, 1,* 3–38.

Hedeker, D., Mermelstein, R. J., & Weeks, K. A. (1999). The thresholds of change model: An approach to analyzing stages of change data. *Annals of Behavioral Medicine, 21,* 61–70.

Humphreys, A. S., Thompson, J. J., & Miner, K. R. (1998). Assessment of breast-feeding intention using the Transtheoretical Model and the Theory of Reasoned Action. *Health Education Research, 13*(3), 331.

Isenhart, C. E. (1994). Motivational subtypes in an inpatient sample of substance abusers. *Addictive Behaviors, 19,* 463–475.

Jaekle, C., Keller, S., Baum, E., & Basler, H. (1999). Scales for the measurement of self-efficacy and decisional balance in the process of behavioral change in smokers. *Diagnostica, 45,* 138–146.

Janis, I. L., & Mann, L. (1977). *Decision-making: A psychological analysis of conflict, choice, and commitment.* New York: Free Press.

Jensen, M. P., Nielson, W. R., Romano, J. M., Hill, M. L., & Turner, J. A. (2000). Further evaluation of the pain stages of change questionnaire: Is the transtheoretical model of change useful for patients with chronic pain? *Pain, 86*(3), 255–264.

Johnson, S. S. (1998). *Oral Contraceptive Adherence: The Application of the Transtheoretical Model.* Unpublished doctoral dissertation. University of Rhode Island, Kinston: RI.

Johnson, S. S., Grimley, D. M., & Prochaska, J. O. (1998a). Prediction of adherence using the Transtheoretical Model: Implications for pharmacy care practice. *Journal of Social and Administrative Pharmacy, 15*(3), 135–148.

Johnson, S. S., Grimley, D. M., & Prochaska, J. O. (1998b, March). *The development and validation of a processes of change measure for medication compliance.* Paper presented at the 19th annual convention of Society of Behavioral Medicine, New Orleans, LA.

Johnson, S. S., Norman, G. J., & Fava, J. L. (1998, March). *Are subjects in maintenance for stress management at risk for relapse?* Paper presented at the Nineteenth Annual Scientific Sessions of The Society of Behavioral Medicine, New Orleans, LA.

Joseph, J., Breslin, C., & Skinner, H. (1999). Critical perspectives on the transtheoretical model and stages of change. In J. A. Tucker, D. M. Donovan, & G. A. Marlatt (Eds.), *Changing addictive behavior: Bridging clinical and public health strategies* (pp. 160–190). New York: Guilford Press.

Keefe, F. J., Lefebvre, J. C., Kerns, R. D., Rosenberg, R., Beaupre, P., Prochaska, J., Prochaska, J. O., & Caldwell, D. S. (2000). Understanding the adoption of arthritis self-management: Stages of change profiles among arthritis patients. *Pain, 87*(3), 303–313.

Kelaher, M., Gillespie, A. G., Allotey, P., Manderson, L., Potts, H., Sheldrake, M., & Young, M. (1999). The Transtheoretical Model and cervical screening: Its application among culturally diverse communities in Queensland, Australia. *Ethnicity and Health, 4,* 259–264.

Keller, S., Nigg, C. R., Jaekle, C., Baum, E., & Basler, H. (1999). Self-efficacy, decisional balance, and the stages of change for smoking cessation in a German sample. *Swiss Journal of Psychology, 58,* 101–110.

Kelly, R. M., Denny, G., & Young, M. (1999). Modified stages of acquisition of gateway drug use: A primary prevention application of the stages of change model. *Journal of Drug Education, 29,* 189–203.

Kerns, R. D., Rosenberg, R., Jamison, R. N., Caudill, M. A., & Haythornthwaite, J. (1997). Readiness to adopt a self-management approach to chronic pain: The Pain Stages of Change Questionnaire (PSOCQ). *Pain, 72*(1–2), 227–234.

Kloeblen, A. S., Thompson, N. J., & Miner, K. R. (1999). Predicting breastfeeding intention among low-income pregnant women: A comparison of two theoretical models. *Health Education and Behavior, 26,* 675–688.

Kristal, A. R., Glanz, K., Curry, S. J., & Patterson, R. E. (1999). How can stages of change be best used in dietary interventions? *Journal of the American Dietetic Association, 99,* 679–684.

Kristal, A. R., Shattuck, A. L., & Henry, P. J. (1990). Patterns of dietary behavior associated with selecting diets low in fat: Reliability and validity of a behavioral approach to dietary assessment. *Journal of the American Dietetic Association, 90,* 215–220.

Lafferty, C. K., Heaney, C. A., & Chen, M. S. (1999). Assessing decisional balance for smoking cessation among Southeast Asian males in the U.S. *Health Education Research, 14,* 139–146.

Lauby, J. L., Semaan, S., Cohen, A., Leviton, L., Gielen, A., Pulley, L. V., Walls, C., & O'Campo, P. (1998). Self-efficacy, decisional balance and stages of change for condom use among women at risk for HIV infection. *Health Education Research: Theory and Practice, 13,* 343–356.

Levesque, D. A., Gelles, R. J., & Velicer, W. F. (2000). Development and validation of a stages of change measure for men in batterer treatment. *Cognitive Therapy and Research, 24,* 175–199.

Levesque, D. A., Prochaska, J. M., & Prochaska, J. O. (1999). Stages of change and integrated service delivery. *Consulting Psychology Journal: Practice and Research, 51*(4), 226–241.

Levy, R. K. (1997). The Transtheoretical Model of Change: An application to bulimia. *Psychotherapy, 34*(3), 278.

Lipkus, I. M., Rimer, B. K., & Strigo, T. S. (1996). Relationships among objective and subjective risk for breast cancer and mammography stages of change. *Cancer Epidemiology, Biomarkers and Prevention, 5,* 1005–1011.

Maddock, J. E., Rossi, J. S., Redding, C. A., Meier, K. S., Velicer, W. F., & Prochaska, J. O. (1998, March). *Development of transtheoretical model constructs for sun protection behaviors among adolescents.* Paper presentation at the 19th annual meeting of the Society of Behavioral Medicine, New Orleans, LA.

Mah, Z., & Bryant, H. E. (1997). The role of past mammography and future intentions in screening mammography usage. *Cancer Detection and Prevention, 21,* 213–220.

Mann, J. M., Tarantola, D. J. M., & Netter, T. W. (1992). *AIDS in the world.* Cambridge, MA: Harvard University Press.

Martin, R. A., Velicer, W. F., & Fava, J. L. (1996). Latent transition analysis to the stages of change for smoking cessation. *Addictive Behaviors, 21,* 67–80.

McConnaughy, B. A., Prochaska, J. O., & Velicer, W. F. (1983). Stages of change in psychotherapy: Measurement and sample profiles. *Psychotherapy: Theory, Research, and Practice, 20,* 368–375.

Migneault, J. P., Pallonen, U. E., & Velicer, W. F. (1997). Decisional balance and stage of change for adolescent drinking. *Addictive Behavior, 22,* 339–351.

Migneault, J. P., Velicer, W. F., Prochaska, J. O., & Stevenson, J. F. (1999). Decisional balance for immoderate drinking in college students. *Substance Use & Misuse, 34,* 1325–1346.

Miller, D. L., & Weinstock, M. A. (1994). Nonmelanoma skin cancer in the United States: Incidence. *Journal of the American Academy of Dermatology, 30,* 774–777.

Miller, W. R., & Tonigan, J. S. (1996). Assessing drinkers' motivation for change: The stages of change readiness and treatment eagerness scale (SOCRATES). *Psychology of Addictive Behaviors, 10,* 81–89.

Milstein, B., Lockaby, T., Fogarty, L., Cohen, A., & Cotton, D. (1998). Processes of change in the adoption of consistent condom use. *Journal of Health Psychology, 3,* 349–368.

Montoya, I. D. (1997). Attitudes, norms, self-efficacy, and state of change among out-of-treatment female crack cocaine users: A pilot study. *AIDS Education and Prevention, 9,* 421–441.

Morera, O. F., Johnson, T. P., Feels, S., Parsons, J., Crittendon, K. S., Flay, B. R., & Warnecke, R. B. (1998). The measure of stage of readiness to change: Some psychometric considerations. *Psychological Assessment, 10,* 182–186.

Morokoff, P. J., Quina, K., Harlow, L. L., Whitmire, L. E., Grimley, D. M., Gibson, P., & Burkholder, G. J. (1997). Sexual assertiveness scale (SAS) for women: Development and validation. *Journal of Personality and Social Psychology, 73,* 790–804.

Nigg, C. R., Burbank, P. M., Padula, C., Dufresne, R., Rossi, J. S., Velicer, W. F., Laforge, R. G., & Prochaska, J. O. (1999). Stages of change across ten health risk behaviors for older adults. *Gerontologist, 39,* 473–482.

Nolan, R. P., Wilson, E., Shuster, M., Rowe, B. H., Stewart, D., & Zambon, S. (1999). Readiness to perform cardiopulmonary resuscitation: An emerging strategy against sudden cardiac death. *Psychosomatic Medicine, 61*(4), 546–551.

Norman, G. J., Fava, J. L., Levesque, D. A., Redding, C. A., Johnson, S., Evers, K., & Reich, T. (1997). An inventory for measuring confidence to manage stress. *Annals of Behavioral Medicine, 19*(Supplement), 78.

Norman, G. J., Velicer, W. F., Fava, J. L., & Prochaska, J. O. (1998). Dynamic typology clustering within the stages of change for smoking cessation. *Addictive Behaviors, 23,* 139–153.

Northwestern National Life Insurance Company. (1991). *Employee burnout: America's newest epidemic.* Minneapolis, MN: Northwestern National Life Insurance Company.

O'Connor, E. A., Carbonari, J. P., & DiClemente, C. C. (1996). Gender and smoking cessation: A factor structure comparison of processes of change. *Journal of Consulting and Clinical Psychology, 64,* 130–138.

O'Neil, B., Bristow, B., & Brennan, P. (1999). Changing financial behavior: Implications for family and consumer sciences professionals. *Journal of Family and Consumer Sciences, 4,* 43–48.

O'Reilly, K. R., & Higgins, D. L. (1991). AIDS community demonstration projects for HIV prevention among hard-to-reach groups. *Public Health Reports, 106,* 714–720.

Pallonen, U. E., Fava, J. L., Salonen, J. T., & Prochaska, J. O. (1992). Readiness for smoking change among middle-age Finnish men. *Addictive Behaviors, 17,* 415–423.

Pallonen, U. E., Leskinen, L., Prochaska, J. O., Willey, C. J., Kaariainen, R., & Salonen, J. T. (1994). A 2-year self-help smoking cessation manual intervention among middle-aged Finnish men: An application of the Transtheoretical Model. *Preventive Medicine, 23,* 507–514.

Pallonen, U. E., Murray, D. M., Schmid, L., Pirie, P., & Luepker, R. V. (1990). Patterns of self-initiated smoking cessation among young adults. *Health Psychology, 9,* 418–426.

Pallonen, U. E., Prochaska, J. O., Velicer, W. F., & Prokhorov, A. V. (1998). Stages of acquisition and cessation for adolescent smoking: An empirical investigation. *Addictive Behaviors, 23,* 303–324.

Pallonen, U. E., Velicer, W. F., Prochaska, J. O., Rossi, J. S., Bellis, J. M., Tsoh, J., Migneault, J. P., Smith, N. F., & Prokhorov, A. V. (1998). Computer-based smoking cessation interventions in adolescents: Description, feasibility, and six month follow-up findings. *Substance Use & Misuse, 33,* 935–965.

Pearlman, D. N., Rakowski, W., Clark, M. A., Ehrich, B., Rimer, B. K., Goldstein, M. G., Woolverton, H. 3rd, & Dube, C. E. (1997). Why do women's attitudes toward mammography change over time? Implications for physician-patient communication. *Cancer Epidemiology, Biomarkers and Prevention, 6,* 451–457.

Pearlman, D. N., Rakowski, W., Ehrich, B., & Clark, M. A. (1996). Breast cancer screening practices among black, Hispanic, and white women: Reassessing differences. *American Journal of Preventive Medicine, 12,* 327–337.

Perz, C. A., DiClemente, C. C., & Carbonari, J. P. (1996). Doing the right thing at the right time? The interaction of stages and processes of change in successful smoking cessation. *Health Psychology, 15,* 462–468.

Peteet, J. R., Brenner, S., Curtiss, D., Ferrigno, M., & Kaufmann, J. (1998). A stage of change approach to addiction in the medical setting. *General Hospital Psychiatry, 20,* 267–273.

Pierce, J. P., Farkas, A. J., & Gilpin, E. A. (1998). Beyond stages of change: The quitting continuum measures progress towards successful smoking cessation. *Addiction, 93,* 277–286.

Pololi, L. H., & Potter, S. (1996). Behavioral change in preventive medicine. An efficacy assessment of a physician education module. *Journal of General Internal Medicine, 11*(9), 545–547.

Prochaska, J. M. (2000). A Transtheoretical Model for assessing organizational change: A study of family service agencies' movement to time-limited therapy. *Families in Society, 81*(1), 76.

Prochaska, J. M., Prochaska, J. O., & Levesque, D. A. (in press). A transtheoretical approach to changing organizations. *Administration and Policy in Mental Health.*

Prochaska, J. O. (1979). *Systems of psychotherapy: A transtheoretical analysis.* Homewood, IL: Dorsey Press.

Prochaska, J. O. (1991). Prescribing to the stage and level of phobic patients. *Psychotherapy, 28,* 463–469.

Prochaska, J. O. (1992). A transtheoretical model of behavior change: Implications for diet interventions. *Proceedings for promoting dietary change in communities: Applying existing models of dietary change to population-based interventions.* Seattle, WA: Fred Hutchinson Cancer Research Institute.

Prochaska, J. O. (1994). Strong and weak principles for progressing from precontemplation to action on the basis of twelve problem behaviors. *Health Psychology, 13,* 47–51.

Prochaska, J. O., & DiClemente, C. C. (1982). Transtheoretical therapy: Toward a more integrative model of change. *Psychotherapy: Theory, Research, and Practice, 19,* 276–288.

Prochaska, J. O., & DiClemente, C. C. (1983). Stages and processes of self-change in smoking: Towards an integrative model of change. *Journal of Consulting and Clinical Psychology, 51,* 390–395.

Prochaska, J. O., & DiClemente, C. C. (1984). *The transtheoretical approach: Crossing traditional boundaries of change.* Homewood, IL: Dorsey Press.

Prochaska, J. O., DiClemente, C. C., & Norcross, J. C. (1992). In search of how people change: Applications to addictive behaviors. *American Psychologist, 9,* 1102–1114.

Prochaska, J. O., DiClemente, C. C., Velicer, W. F., Ginpil, S., & Norcross, J. C. (1985). Predicting change in smoking status for self-changers. *Addictive Behaviors, 10,* 395–406.

Prochaska, J. O., DiClemente, C. C., Velicer, W. F., & Rossi, J. S. (1993). Standardized, individualized, interactive, and personalized self-help programs for smoking cessation. *Health Psychology, 12,* 399–405.

Prochaska, J. O., Norcross, J. C., Fowler, J. L., Follick, M. J., & Abrams, D. B. (1992). Attendance and outcome in a work site weight control program: Processes and stages of change as process and predictor variables. *Addictive Behaviors, 17,* 35–45.

Prochaska, J. O., Redding, C. A., & Evers, K. E. (1997). The transtheoretical model and stages of change. In K. Glanz, F. M. Lewis, & B. K. Rimer (Eds.), *Health behavior and health education: Theory, research, and practice* (2nd ed., pp. 60–84). San Francisco, CA: Jossy-Boss.

Prochaska, J. O., Redding, C. A., Harlow, L. L., Rossi, J. S., & Velicer, W. F. (1993). The transtheoretical model of change and HIV prevention: A review. *Health Education Quarterly, 21,* 471–486.

Prochaska, J. O., Redding, C. A., Harlow, L. L., Rossi, J. S. & Velicer, W. F. (1994). The transtheoretical model of change and HIV prevention: A review. *Health Education Quarterly, 21,* 471–486.

Prochaska, J. O., Rossi, J. S., & Wilcox, N. S. (1991). Change processes and psychotherapy outcome in integrative case research. *Journal of Psychotherapy Integration, 1,* 103–119.

Prochaska, J. O., Velicer, W. F., DiClemente, C. C., & Fava, J. S. (1998). Measuring processes of change: Applications to the cessation of smoking. *Journal of Consulting and Clinical Psychology, 56,* 520–528.

Prochaska, J. O., Velicer, W. F., Guadagnoli, E., & Rossi, J. S. (1991). Patterns of change: Dynamic typology applied to smoking cessation. *Multivariate Behavioral Research, 26,* 83–107.

Prochaska, J. O., Velicer, W. F., Rossi, J. S., Goldstein, M. G., Marcus, B. H., Rakowski, W., Fiore, C., Harlow, L. L., Redding, C. A., Rosenbloom, D., & Rossi, S. R. (1994). Stages of change and decisional balance for 12 problem behaviors. *Health Psychology, 13,* 39–46.

Prokhorov, A. V., Pallonen, U. E., Prochaska, J. O., Alexandrov, A. A., Velicer, W. F., & Allard, G. A. (1995). Readiness to change smoking behavior in different social environments. In K. Slama (Ed.), *Tobacco and health* (pp. 639–642). New York: Plenum.

Public Health Service: The Surgeon General's Report on Nutrition and Health. (1988). DHHS (PHS) Publication No 88-50210.

Quina, K., Harlow, L. L., Morokoff, P. J., Burkholder, G. J., & Deiter, P. J. (2000). Sexual communication in relationships: When words speak louder than actions. *Sex Roles, 42,* 523–549.

Quina, K., Harlow, L. L., Morokoff, P. J., & Saxon, S. E. (1997). Interpersonal power and women's HIV risk. In N. Goldstein & J. L. Manlowe (Eds.), *The gender politics of HIV/AIDS in women* (pp. 188–206). New York: NYU Press.

Quinlan, K. B., & McCaul, K. D. (2000). Matched and mismatched interventions with young adult smokers: Testing a stage theory. *Health Psychology, 19,* 165–171.

Rakowski, W., Andersen, M. R., Stoddard, A. M., Urban, N., Rimer, B. K., Lane, D. S., Fox, S. A., & Costanza, M. E. (1997). Confirmatory analysis of opinions regarding the pros and cons of mammography. *Health Psychology, 16,* 433–441.

Rakowski, W., Clark, M. A., Pearlman, D. N., Ehrich, B., Rimer, B. K., Goldstein, M. G., Dube, C. E., & Woolverton, H. 3rd. (1997). Integrating pros and cons for mammography and pap testing: Extending the construct of decisional balance to two behaviors. *Preventative Medicine, 26,* 664–673.

Rakowski, W., Dube, C. E., Marcus, B. H., Prochaska, J. O., Velicer, W. F., & Abrams, D. A. (1992). Assessing elements of women's decisional about mammography. *Health Psychology, 11,* 111–118.

Rakowski, W., Ehrich, B., Dube, C. A., Pearlman, D. N., Goldstein, M. G., Rimer, B. K., Woolverton, H., & Peterson, K. K. (1996). Screening mammography and constructs from the transtheoretical model: Associations using two-definition of the stages of adoption. *Annals of Behavioral Medicine, 18,* 91–100.

Rakowski, W., Fulton, J. P., & Feldman, J. P. (1993). Women's decision making about mammography: A replication of the relationship between stages of adoption and decisional balance. *Health Psychology, 12,* 209–214.

Redding, C. A., Meier, K. S., Noar, S. M., White, S. L., Rossi, J. S., Doherty-Iddings, P., Gazabon, S. A., Morokoff, P. J., & Mayer, K (2001, March). *The transtheoretical model for condom use in a community sample of at-risk men and women.* Paper accepted for presentation at the Twenty-Second Annual Scientific Sessions of the Society of Behavioral Medicine, Seattle, WA.

Redding, C. A., Prochaska, J. O., Pallonen, U. E., Rossi, J. S., Velicer, W. F., Rossi, S. R., Greene, G. W., Meier, K. S., Evers, K. E., Plummer, B. A., & Maddock, J. E. (1999). Transtheoretical individualized multimedia expert systems targeting adolescents' health behaviors. *Cognitive and Behavioral Practice, 6,* 144–153.

Redding, C. A., & Rossi, J. S. (1993). The processes of safer sex adoption. *Annals of Behavioral Medicine, 15:S106* (Abstract).

Redding, C. A., & Rossi, J. S. (1999). Testing a model of situational self-efficacy for safer sex among college students: Stage of change and gender-based differences. *Psychology and Health, 14,* 467–486.

Redding, C. A., Rossi, J. S., Velicer, W. F., & Prochaska, J. O. (1989). *The pros and cons of safer sex: A measurement model.* Presented at the 97th Annual Convention of the American Psychological Association. New Orleans, LA.

Rhodes, F., & Malotte, C. K. (1996). Using stages of change to assess intervention readiness and outcome in modifying drug-related and sexual HIV risk behaviors of IDU's and crack users. *Drugs & Society,* *9,* 109–136.

Riley, T. A., Toth, J. M., & Fava, J. L. (2000). The transtheoretical model and stress management practices in women at risk for, or infected with, HIV. *Journal of the Association of Nurses in AIDS Care, 11*(1), 67–77.

Robbins, M. L., Fava, J. L., Norman, G. J., Velicer, W. F., Redding, C., & Levesque, D. B. (1998, March). *Stages of change for stress management in three samples.* Paper presented at the Nineteenth Annual Scientific Sessions of The Society of Behavioral Medicine, New Orleans, LA.

Rollnick, S., Heather, N., Gold, R., & Hall, W. (1992). Development of a short "readiness to change" questionnaire for use in brief, opportunistic interventions among excessive drinkers. *British Journal of Addiction, 87,* 743–754.

Rosenthal, D. A., Hall, C., & Moore, S. M. (1992). AIDS, adolescents, and sexual risk taking: A test of the health belief model. *Australian Psychologist, 27,* 177–171.

Rossi, J. S. (1992a). *Common processes of change across nine problem behaviors.* Presented at the 100th Annual Convention of the American Psychological Association, Washington, DC.

Rossi, J. S. (1992b). *Stages of change for 15 health risk behaviors in an HMO population.* Presented at the 13th meeting of the Society for Behavioral Medicine, New York, NY.

Rossi, J. S., Blais, L. M., Redding, C. A., & Weinstock, M. A. (1995). Preventing skin cancer through behavior change: Implications for interventions. *Dermatologic Clinics, 13*(3), 613–622.

Rossi, J. S., Blais, L. M., & Weinstock, M. A. (1994). The Rhode Island Sun Smart Project: Skin cancer prevention reaches the beaches. *American Journal of Public Health, 84,* 1–2.

Rossi, S. R., Greene, G. W., Reed, G., Prochaska, J. O., Velicer, W. F., & Rossi, J. S. (1993). *A comparison of four stage of change algorithms for dietary fat reduction.* Presented at the 13th annual convention of the Society for Behavioral Medicine, San Francisco, CA.

Rossi, J. S., Prochaska, J. O., & DiClemente, C. C. (1988). Processes of change in heavy and light smokers. *Journal of Substance Abuse, 1,* 1–9.

Rossi, J. S., Rosenbloom, D., Monti, P. M., Rohsenow, D. J., Prochaska, J. O., & Martin, R. A. (1993). *Transtheoretical model of behavior change for cocaine use.* Presented at the 101st Annual Convention of the American Psychological Association, Ontario, Canada.

Rossi, S. R., & Rossi, J. S. (1993). *Processes of change for dietary fat reduction.* Presented at the 13th Annual Convention of the Society for Behavioral Medicine, San Francisco, CA.

Ruggiero, L., Redding, C. A., Rossi, J. S., & Prochaska, J. O. (1997). A stage-matched smoking cessation program for pregnant smokers. *American Journal of Health Promotion, 12*, 31–33.

Schorling, J. B. (1995). The stages of change of rural African-American smokers. *American Journal of Preventive Medicine, 11*, 170–177.

Shilling, S., & Brackbill, R. M. (1987). Occupational health and safety risks and potential health consequences perceived by U.S. workers. *Public Health Rep., 102*, 36–46.

Snow, M. G., Prochaska, J. O., & Rossi, J. S. (1994). Processes of change in alcoholics anonymous maintenance factors in long-term sobriety. *Journal of Studies on Alcohol, 55*, 362–371.

Stark, M. J., Tesselaar, H. M., O'Connell, A. A., Person, B., Galavotti, C., Cohen, A., & Walls, C. (1998). Psychosocial factors associated with the stages of change for condom use among women at risk for HIV and STD's: Implications for intervention development. *Journal of Consulting and Clinical Psychology, 66*, 967–978.

Taylor, J., Berger, B., Anderson-Harper, H., & Grimley, D. (2000). Pharmacists' readiness to assess consumers' over the-counter product selections. *Journal of the American Pharmaceutical Association, 40*(4), 487–494.

Tejero, A., Trujols, J., Hernandez, E., de los Cobos, J. P., & Casas, M. (1997). Processes of change assessment in heroin addicts following the Prochaska and DiClemente Transtheoretical Model. *Drug & Alcohol Dependence, 47*, 31–37.

Treasure, J. L., Katzman, M., Schmidt, U., Troop, N., Todd, G., & de Silva, P. (1999). Engagement and outcome in the treatment of bulimia nervosa: First phase of a sequential design comparing motivation enhancement therapy and cognitive behavioural therapy. *Behaviour Research and Therapy, 37*(5), 405–418.

U.S. Department of Health and Human Services. (1991). *Healthy People 2000: National Health Promotion and Disease Prevention Objectives.* Washington, DC. (PHS 91-50212).

U.S. Department of Health and Human Services. (2000, January). *Healthy People 2010 (Conference Edition, in Two Volumes).* Washington, DC.

Velicer, W. F., DiClemente, C. C., Prochaska, J. O., & Brandenburg, N. (1985). A decisional balance measure for assessing and predicting smoking status. *Journal of Personality and Social Psychology, 48*, 1279–1289.

Velicer, W. F., Fava, J. L., Prochaska, J. O., Abrams, D. B., Emmons, K. M., & Peirce, J. P. (1995). Distribution of smokers by stage in three representative samples. *Preventive Medicine, 24*, 401–411.

Velicer, W. F., Hughes, S. L., Fava, J. L., Prochaska, J. O., & DiClemente, C. C. (1995). An empirical typology of subjects within stage of change. *Addictive Behavior, 20*, 299–320.

Velicer, W. F., Norman, G. J., Fava, J. L., & Prochaska, J. O. (1999). Testing 40 predictions from the transtheoretical model. *Addictive Behaviors, 24,* 455–469.

Velicer, W. F., Prochaska, J. O., Bellis, J. M., DiClemente, C. C., Rossi, J. S., Fava, J. L., & Steiger, J. H. (1993). An expert system integration for smoking cessation. *Addictive Behaviors, 18,* 269–290.

Velicer, W. F., Prochaska, J. O., Fava, J. L., Norman, G. J., & Redding, C. A. (1998). Smoking cessation and stress management: Applications of the Transtheoretical Model of behavior change. *Homeostasis, 38,* 216–233.

Weinstock, M. A., & Rossi, J. S. (1998). The Rhode Island Sun Smart Project: A scientific approach to skin cancer prevention. *Clinical Dermatology, 16,* 411–413.

Weinstock, M. A., Rossi, J. S., Redding, C. A., Maddock, J. E., & Cottrill, S. D. (2000). Sun protection behaviors and stages of change for the primary prevention of skin cancers among beachgoers in southeastern New England. *Annals of Behavioral Medicine, 22*(4), 1–8.

Werch, C. E. (1997). Expanding the stages of change: A program matched to the stages of alcohol acquisition. *American Journal of Health Promotion, 12,* 34–37.

Willey, C. (1999). Behavior-changing methods for improving adherence to medication. *Current Hypertensive Reports, 1,* 477–481.

World Cancer Research Fund/American Institute for Cancer Research. (1997). *Food, nutrition and the prevention of cancer: A global perspective.* Washington, DC: American Institute for Cancer Research.

Zierler, S., & Krieger, N. (1997). Reframing women's risk: Social inequalities and HIV infection. *Annual Review of Public Health, 18,* 401–436.

CHAPTER 5

The Transtheoretical Model: Research Review of Exercise Behavior and Older Adults

Claudio R. Nigg and Deborah Riebe

"An active mind cannot exist in an inactive body."

~General George Patton

The Transtheoretical Model of Behavior Change (TTM) is an effective way of changing behavior. The previous chapter reviewed how the TTM has been successful in helping individuals to quit smoking, lower dietary fat, and stay out of the sun. Exercise differs from other behaviors in that it is an acquisition behavior rather than a cessation behavior. Rather than quitting smoking, lowering dietary fat intake, or staying out of the sun, exercise involves adopting and maintaining an active lifestyle.

In the past, exercise research has attempted to look at whether individuals were exercising regularly or not (Courneya, 1995a), even though in the 1980s experts recommended that exercise should be considered in a more complex framework (Dishman, 1988; Sallis &

Hovell, 1990; Sonstroem, 1988). They argued that exercise is a dynamic behavior including individuals who are not exercising at all, individuals who are in the process of starting, individuals who are regularly exercising and have been doing so for a while, and individuals who are regressing or relapsing. Theories and models were supposed to encompass the dynamic nature of exercise. The theories and models should be about exercise behavior change, not exercise behavior *per se.*

Further, exercise can take several forms including lifestyle activities (e.g., gardening), scheduled classes (e.g., tai chi, group exercise classes), team sports and games, individual activities, and competitions. This points to many aspects of motivation, some more self-centered and some more socially focused, some more fun versus achievement oriented. To this end, a model used to explain exercise behavior and to motivate individuals to engage in exercise should include a range of mechanisms to get people to start thinking about, begin, and continue to exercise.

The TTM is one model that embraces the dynamic nature of behaviors (see chapter 3 for a description). During the past decade, many researchers have applied the TTM to exercise. This chapter will describe what has been learned from these investigations and will focus specifically on the body of TTM work targeting older adults.

THE FIRST GENERATION OF TTM AND EXERCISE RESEARCH

In the early 1990s, Marcus and her colleagues applied the TTM to exercise behavior in work site settings (e.g., Marcus, Selby, Niaura, & Rossi, 1992; Marcus & Simkin, 1993). This body of research focused on adapting the instruments from existing measures in other health behavior areas to assess the core TTM constructs for exercise behavior. In general, the instruments revealed results similar to the TTM instruments that existed for other health behavior areas. The research showed that:

- self-efficacy increased from precontemplation to maintenance,
- the pros increased from precontemplation to maintenance,
- the cons decreased from contemplation to maintenance,

- the experiential processes were more important in the earlier stages, and
- the behavioral processes were more important in the later stages.

The Marcus group also reported the first intervention study, which was community based including young, middle-aged, and older adults. They implemented a six-week, stage-targeted intervention consisting of self-help materials, a resource manual describing activity options, weekly fun walks, and activity nights. Briefly, a *targeted* approach involves defining a particular population group, usually based on one or more demographic characteristics shared by all its members. The targeted approach assumes that the members of the defined group are similar enough for one message to sufficiently communicate with all its members. For example, within the TTM five interventions are created—one for each stage of change. It has been noted that it is important to define appropriate groups for proactive communication for physical activity promotion, given that many individuals are not seeking to change their physical activity behavior (Marcus, Rossi, Selby, Niaura, & Abrams, 1992).

The results of this study showed that the percentage of people in the early stages (contemplation and preparation) decreased while the percentage of people in action increased. This demonstrated that individuals were significantly more active after the intervention (Marcus, Banspach, et al., 1992). This pilot study opened the door for using the TTM to motivate people to consider and to actually start exercising.

THE NEXT STEP—EXPANDING THE APPLICATION OF THE TTM

In the mid 1990s, several research studies were published using the TTM in exercise. The major focus was to apply the components of the TTM to other populations to see if it is generalizable to different groups. The stage construct was validated for adolescents, young, middle-aged, and older adults (Cardinal, 1995b, 1995c, 1997; Courneya, 1995a; Gorely & Gordon, 1995; Marcus & Simkin, 1993; Wyse, Mercer, Ashford, Buxton, & Gleeson, 1995). In general, the validation measures increased from precontemplation to maintenance.

Studies found that as individuals moved through the stages, they reported doing more exercise and were found to be more fit in those studies that used physiological measurements such as body mass index, frequency of sweating, and percent body fat.

One of the main limitations with this body of work is that the time descriptors used for the stages of exercise were adapted from the smoking work. The time frame used in the adapted stage instruments is 6 months. The definitions make intuitive sense: 6 months is about how far people can plan any life decision, which corresponds to the contemplation definition, and maintaining regular exercise for more than 6 months does roughly correspond to exercising beyond a season (e.g., summer activities, or sport seasons). This has actually never been tested, however, and the question remains whether the time frames used are the optimal ones for exercise staging.

Another weakness in early studies was that there was no consistent stage assessment among studies. Formats used to assess stages of exercise behavior change included: (1) an interview algorithm with yes/no response format (Courneya, Estabrooks, & Nigg, 1997; Courneya, Nigg, & Estabrooks, 1998); (2) one question with five responses—one for each stage, where the participant selects the most applicable response (Courneya, 1995a, 1995b; Gorely & Gordon, 1995; Nigg, Norman, Rossi, & Benisovich, 1999); (3) a 32-item scale designed to assess four stages of change (Barké & Nicholas, 1990), which resembles the original stages of change scale, the University of Rhode Island Change Assessment (McConnaughy, Prochaska, & Velicer, 1983); and (4) other algorithms where the individual stage definitions are not entirely consistent with the theory (e.g., Lee, 1993; Hellman, 1997). Given the possibility of non- or misclassification and in the interest of theoretical consistency, the first two methods are recommended. Reed, Velicer, Prochaska, Rossi, and Marcus (1997) also concluded this, adding that the more clearly defined the criteria behavior is, the more accurate the resulting stage distribution. The two stage measures are presented in Figure 5.1.

Processes of change have been the least investigated of the TTM constructs in exercise research. In general, it has been shown that as individuals progress through the stages of change, they use different processes to modify their behavior (Gorely & Gordon, 1995; Marcus, Rossi, et al., 1992; Nigg & Courneya, 1998). The use of experiential

Exercise Stage Assessment (recommended for interviews)
Regular Exercise: is any *planned* physical activity (e.g., brisk walking, jogging, bicycling, swimming, line-dancing, tennis, etc.) performed to increase physical fitness. Such activity should be performed *3 or more times* per week for *20 or more minutes* per session at a level that increases your breathing rate and causes you to break a sweat. According to the definition above:

1. Do you currently engage in regular exercise?   YES   NO
      Skip Pattern: If YES go to 4; If NO go to 2
2. Do you intend to engage in regular exercise in the next 6 months?   YES   NO
      Skip Pattern: If YES go to 3; If NO end
3. Do you intend to engage in regular exercise in the next 30 days?   YES   NO
      Skip Pattern: If YES or NO end
4. Have you been exercising regularly for the past 6 months?   YES   NO
      Skip Pattern: If YES or NO end

Scoring
If item 1 = NO and item 2 = NO   **Precontemplation**
If item 1 = NO and item 2 = YES and item 3 = NO   **Contemplation**
If item 1 = NO and item 2 = YES and item 3 = YES   **Preparation**
If item 1 = YES and item 4 = NO   **Action**
If item 1 = YES and item 4 = YES   **Maintenance**

Exercise Stage Assessment (recommended for questionnaires)
The following five statements will assess how much you currently exercise in your leisure time (exercise done outside of a job). **Regular Exercise** is any *planned* physical activity (e.g., brisk walking, jogging, bicycling, swimming, line-dancing, tennis, etc.) performed to increase physical fitness. Such activity should be performed *3 or more times* per week for *20 or more minutes* per session at a level that increases your breathing rate and causes you to break a sweat.
Do you exercise regularly according to the definition above? **Please mark only ONE of the five statements**.

1 ____No, and I do not intend to begin exercising regularly in the next 6 months.
2 ____No, but I intend to begin exercising regularly in the next 6 months.
3 ____No, but I intend to begin exercising regularly in the next 30 days.
4 ____Yes, I have been, but for less than 6 months.
5 ____Yes, I have been for more than 6 months.

Scoring: Item 1 = Precontemplation; Item 2 = Contemplation; Item 3 = Preparation; Item 4 = Action; Item 5 = Maintenance

FIGURE 5.1   Recommended methods for assessing stage.

processes have a tendency to increase in precontemplation to contemplation, stay the same in preparation, increase from preparation to action, and decrease in maintenance, whereas behavioral processes increase from precontemplation to action and level off (Marcus, Rossi, et al., 1992). Furthermore, the use of processes has been found to increase for adopters, decrease for relapsers, and remain the same for stable active or inactive groups (Marcus, Simkin, Rossi, & Pinto, 1996).

Several problems are evident in the body of work on processes. Researchers have yet to look at which process is important for the individual stage changes (e.g., from precontemplation to contemplation; from contemplation to preparation, etc.). Also, the stage definition used for preparation (irregular exercise) is not theoretically appropriate (Prochaska & Velicer, 1997) and allows for irregular exercisers who have absolutely no intention of becoming regular exercisers to be classified in the preparation stage. The appropriate definition for preparation should include *immediate intention* for regular exercise (see chapter 3). Finally, the process scale used (Marcus, Rossi, et al., 1992) was adapted from the smoking process scale and lacks face validity. Simply put, items do not make sense to individuals filling in the process scale. Therefore, a new process scale was developed based on a random sample representing the general population. A new item pool was generated by a small group of psychologists, exercise scientists, exercisers, and non-exercisers. A sample of New Englanders ($n = 346$; age range = 18 to 75; 62% female; 95% white) participating in random telephone interviews completed the 68-item inventory. The final scales were internally consistent (alpha range = .64 to .86), possess strong face and content validity, and fit the same process measurement model (Nigg, Norman, Rossi, & Benisovich, 1999). These results were replicated in college students (Nigg, Norman, et al., 1999) and older adults (Nigg et al., 2001). This demonstrates the robustness of the processes of change for exercise behavior. Further, the development of a sound, general processes of change measure may curtail the need for sample-specific measures (see Figure 5.2 for the process items).

Self-efficacy has been shown to increase from precontemplation to maintenance in older adults (Gorely & Gordon, 1995), middle-aged adults (Herrick, Stone, & Mettler, 1997; Marcus & Owen, 1992), young adults (Wyse et al., 1995) and adolescent populations (Nigg &

Processes of Change

The following experiences can affect the exercise habits of some people. Think of similar experiences you may be currently having or have had **during the past month**. Then rate how frequently the event occurs by circling the appropriate number. Please answer using the following 5-point scale:

1	2	3	4	5
Never	**Seldom**	**Occasionally**	**Often**	**Repeatedly**

1. I read articles to learn more about exercise. 1 2 3 4 5

2. I get upset when I see people who would benefit from exercise but choose not to exercise. 1 2 3 4 5

3. I realize that if I don't exercise regularly, I may get ill and be a burden to others. 1 2 3 4 5

4. I feel more confident when I exercise regularly. 1 2 3 4 5

5. I have noticed that many people know that exercise is good for them. 1 2 3 4 5

6. When I feel tired, I make myself exercise anyway because I know I will feel better afterwards. 1 2 3 4 5

7. I have a friend who encourages me to exercise when I don't feel up to it. ..1 2 3 4 5

8. One of the rewards of regular exercise is that it improves my mood. 1 2 3 4 5

9. I tell myself that I can keep exercising if I try hard enough. 1 2 3 4 5

10. I keep a set of exercise clothes with me so I can exercise whenever I get the time. 1 2 3 4 5

11. I look for information related to exercise. 1 2 3 4 5

12. I am afraid of the results to my health if I do not exercise. 1 2 3 4 5

13. I think that by exercising regularly I will not be a burden to the health care system. 1 2 3 4 5

14. I believe that regular exercise will make me a healthier, happier person. ...1 2 3 4 5

15. I am aware of more and more people who are making exercise a part of their lives.. 1 2 3 4 5

16. Instead of taking a nap after work, I exercise. 1 2 3 4 5

17. I have someone who encourages me to exercise. 1 2 3 4 5

FIGURE 5.2 Processes of change, decisional balance, and self-efficacy stems and items.

18. I try to think of exercise as a time to clear my mind as well as a workout
    for my body. 1   2   3   4   5

19. I make commitments to exercise. 1   2   3   4   5

20. I use my calendar to schedule my exercise time 1   2   3   4   5

21. I find out about new methods of exercising. 1   2   3   4   5

22. I get upset when I realize that people I love would have better health
    if they exercised. 1   2   3   4   5

23. I think that regular exercise plays a role in reducing health care costs. 1   2   3   4   5

24. I feel better about myself when I exercise 1   2   3   4   5

25. I notice that famous people often say that they exercise regularly. 1   2   3   4   5

26. Instead of relaxing by watching TV or eating, I take a walk or exercise. 1   2   3   4   5

27. My friends encourage me to exercise. 1   2   3   4   5

28. If I engage in regular exercise, I find that I get the benefit of
    having more energy. 1   2   3   4   5

29. I believe that I can exercise regularly. 1   2   3   4   5

30. I make sure I always have a clean set of exercise clothes. 1   2   3   4   5

Scoring

Consciousness Raising – 1, 11, 21   Counterconditioning – 6, 16, 26
Dramatic Relief – 2, 12, 22   Helping Relationships – 7, 17, 27
Environmental Reevaluation – 3, 13, 23   Reinforcement Management – 8, 18, 28
Self-Reevaluation – 4, 14, 24   Social Liberation – 9, 19, 29
Self-Liberation – 5, 15, 25   Stimulus Control – 10, 20, 30

FIGURE 5.2   *(continued)*

Confidence

This part looks at how confident you are to exercise when other things get in the way. Read the following items and fill in the circle that best expresses how each item relates to you in your leisure time. Please answer using the following 5-point scale:

1	2	3	4	5
Not at all Confident	**Somewhat Confident**	**Moderately Confident**	**Very Confident**	**Completely Confident**

I am confident I can participate in regular exercise when:

1. It is raining or snowing or icy 1 2 3 4 5

2. I am under a lot of stress 1 2 3 4 5

3. I feel I don't have the time... 1 2 3 4 5

4. I have to exercise alone.. 1 2 3 4 5

5. I don't have access to a place for exercise 1 2 3 4 5

6. I am spending time with friends 1 2 3 4 5

Scoring

All 6 items are a general Self-Efficacy scale representing the six factors. The long form (3 items per factor) may be obtained from the primary author.

FIGURE 5.2   *(continued)*

Decisional Balance

This section looks at positive and negative aspects of exercise. Read the following items and indicate how important each statement is with respect to your decision to exercise or not to exercise in your leisure time by filling in the appropriate circle. Please answer using the following 5-point scale:

1	2	3	4	5
Not At All Important	**Somewhat Important**	**Moderately Important**	**Very Important**	**Extremely Important**

1. I would have more energy for my family and friends if I
    exercised regularly. 1   2   3   4   5

2. I would feel embarrassed if people saw me exercising. 1   2   3   4   5

3. I would feel less stressed if I exercised regularly. 1   2   3   4   5

4. Exercise prevents me from spending time with my friends........................... 1   2   3   4   5

5. Exercising puts me in a better mood for the rest of the day. 1   2   3   4   5

6. I feel uncomfortable or embarrassed in exercise clothes 1   2   3   4   5

7. I would feel more comfortable with my body if I exercised regularly. 1   2   3   4   5

8. There is too much I would have to learn to exercise...................................... 1   2   3   4   5

9. Regular exercise would help me have a more positive outlook on life. 1   2   3   4   5

10. Exercise puts an extra burden on my significant other 1   2   3   4   5

Scoring
PROS – 1, 3, 5, 7, 9   CONS – 2, 4, 6, 8, 10

FIGURE 5.2   *(continued)*

Courneya, 1998). The increase of self-efficacy across stages does not seem to depend upon the scale used or the population studied, supporting the universality of the self-efficacy construct. The main issue with the self-efficacy research portion of the TTM is that only a unidimensional self-efficacy scale was used (Marcus, Selby, et al., 1992). Self-efficacy has been described as a multidimensional construct (McAuley & Mihalko, 1998) that would allow for different types of self-efficacy to be important at different stages. For example, self-efficacy to start an exercise program is hypothesized to be more important in the contemplation/preparation stages, and self-efficacy to exercise regularly when certain barriers (bad weather or social events) may interfere is thought to be more important in the action stage. Benisovich, Rossi, Norman, and Nigg (1998) developed and validated a multidimensional measure of exercise self-efficacy and showed that six different components of self-efficacy were able to predict exercise behavior. The components were labeled Negative Affect, Excuse Making, Exercising Alone, Access to Equipment, Resistance from Others, and Weather. Results suggest that a multidimensional approach to self-efficacy is better able to address the dynamic nature of exercise behavior. Results with this scale in older adults are encouraging (Nigg et al., 2001; see Figure 5.2 for the self-efficacy items).

For decisional balance, in general, pros increase and cons decrease across the stages of change, regardless of populations studied and measures used (Gorely & Gordon, 1995; Herrick, et al., 1997; Marcus, Rossi, et al., 1992; Marcus & Owen, 1992; Nigg & Courneya, 1998). It is important to consider that the majority of these populations have consisted of work-site samples. In addition, the crossover of pros and cons, the decisional balance point, appeared to occur between the contemplation and action stages (Gorely & Gordon, 1995; Herrick et al., 1997; Marcus, Rossi, et al., 1992; Marcus & Owen, 1992). From this body of work one can conclude that the decisional balance construct is very robust and important early in the change process (items of a decisional balance scale are presented in Figure 5.2).

CURRENT GENERATION OF TTM WORK IN EXERCISE—INTERVENTION RESEARCH

More rigorous intervention work started in 1995 (Cardinal & Sachs, 1995). They describe an intervention study designed to increase the amount of physical activity in a population of healthy young urban female employees (n = 81; mean age = 36.9, SD = 7.2; 63% African American, 27% white, 9% Latino, 1% Native American). Three different types of exercise packets were developed: group (a) stage-based lifestyle exercise packet; group (b) stage-based structured exercise packet; and group (c) control packet (fitness feedback), which were randomly distributed. Cardinal and Sachs found the interventions to be advantageous, particularly for those in the early stages, regardless of the exercise packet (lifestyle or structured) received. Independent of group, most of the people increased their stage of change (43.2%) or maintained their stage (42%), whereas only 14.8% regressed in stage. This study demonstrated that an inexpensive method of stage-based material delivery can be effective, especially with less motivated individuals. Similar results were noted when evaluating the relatively short-term effects of a 50-day work-site intervention with a three-level incentive program for 1,192 employees working in a federal agency (Cole, Leonard, Hammond, & Fridinger, 1998). They reported that only a small percentage (6.5%) of participants regressed one or more stages, 30.3% maintained their stage, and 21.1% progressed one or more (14.3%) stages.

Several sources have agreed and recommended tailoring interventions to the individuals' needs. A tailored intervention approach custom fits message content to each individual within a targeted group based on individualized assessment along variables believed to be important in the behavior change process. These data are then used to produce messages that respond to individual variations along the important variables (Nigg, Riebe, Rossi, Velicer, & Prochaska, 1999). One of the main advantages of individually tailoring print communications is that it increases the probability that the material is read and considered (Brinberg & Axelson, 1990; Skinner, Strecher, & Hospers, 1994). In addition to increasing attention to the material, individual tailoring appears to be more effective than generic print materials for producing actual behavior change across health behavior domains, including smoking, diet and exercise (e.g., Brug, Steenhuis, van Assema, & de Vries, 1996; Marcus, Bock, et al., 1998; Prochaska, DiClemente, Velicer, & Rossi, 1993; Rakowski et al., 1997; Strecher et al., 1994).

Marcus, Emmons, et al. (1998) compared stage-tailored interventions (motivationally tailored, printed self-help exercise promotion materials) to standard printed materials (supplied by the American Heart Association) to increase exercise in 1,559 employees. The motivationally tailored intervention resulted in more stage progressors (37 vs. 27%), less stage maintainers (52 vs. 58%), and less stage regressors (11 vs. 15%) than the standard intervention. Marcus, Bock, and colleagues (1998) reported on an intervention with 150 primarily white, middle-class female high school graduates who received either an individually tailored or a standard intervention. Results of this study suggest that individualized, motivationally tailored intervention increases physical activity participation significantly more than standard self-help manuals. Participants in the tailored intervention were more likely to reach the action stage. Among those who were in precontemplation and contemplation at baseline, the individualized approach was more effective.

It is evident that the TTM is a very promising framework for motivating individuals to consider and to engage in exercise behaviors. What follows is an examination of the TTM research that has been conducted with older adults.

THE TTM FOR EXERCISE IN OLDER ADULTS

The studies addressing the TTM in exercise for older adults are summarized in Table 5.1.

The exercise stages of change have been validated with older adults. Active groups placed themselves further along the stages of exercise compared to inactive groups (Barké & Nicholas, 1990). Exercise behaviors increased from precontemplation to maintenance in a sample of older U.S. adults with cardiac diagnoses after discharge from a cardiac rehabilitation inpatient program (Hellman, 1997), and in older Australians (Gorely & Gordon, 1995). The stages of exercise behavior change have been found to be reliable in a sample of older Canadians (2-week test–retest = .79; Courneya, 1995a). Although the validity and reliability data to date is encouraging, more rigorous investigations are called for incorporating objective measures such as pedometers or measurement of VO_2max. The validity and reliability research to date has focused on measures defining the preparation stage as irregular behavior. Defining preparation as immediate intention maximizes treatment appropriateness,

TABLE 5.1 Summary of Studies Examining the Transtheoretical Model in the Exercise Domain

Study	Sample	Design	Measures	Results
Barké & Nicholas (1990)	59 participants aged 59–80 years: an elderhostel group ($n = 21$), an exercise program participants group ($n = 18$) and matched retiree group ($n = 20$)	Cross-sectional	Stages of change	Higher stages (A and M) were associated with the more active groups and lower stages (PC) were associated with the retiree group
Lee (1993)	286 older Australian women aged 50–64	Cross-sectional	Demographics; exercise knowledge; attitudes and opinions; exercise preferences and availability; exercise recall; and stages of change	The telephone survey revealed moderate to low levels of activity among the study group. Exercise knowledge, perceived family support, and perceived psychological benefits of exercise distinguished the A group from PC, whereas perceived barriers were the major difference between C and A groups.

TABLE 5.1 *(continued)*

Study	Sample	Design	Measures	Results
Courneya (1995a)	288 older participants; mean age = 71, SD = 6.3; 63% female; 46% married; 68% completed high school; 85% with family income less than $40,000	Cross-sectional	Subjective norm; attitude; perceived behavioral control; intention; stages of change	Moderate to high correlations were found between the theory of planned behavior constructs and the stages of change. Intention, attitude, perceived behavioral control, and subjective norm shared variances of 54%, 31%, 29%, and 21%, respectively, with stage. The overall explained variance in stage of change was 63%. All stages could be differentiated using the theory of planned behavior constructs, except for A from M. Furthermore, path analysis identified direct paths for intention, attitude, and perceived behavioral control on stage of exercise.

(continued)

TABLE 5.1 *(continued)*

Study	Sample	Design	Measures	Results
Gorely & Gordon (1995)	583 older Australian adults aged 50–65 years; 49.8% male; 55.1% (employed full time)	Cross-sectional	Stages of change and the processes of change, self-efficacy, and decisional balance	Self-reevaluation, consciousness raising, counterconditioning, self-liberation, stimulus control, self-efficacy, pros and cons significantly and independently contributed to the discrimination among stages. Tukey's post hoc analysis revealed that the use of the processes of change fluctuated across the stages, that self-efficacy increased from PC to M, and that the balance between the pros and cons changed from PC to M.
Courneya (1995b)	$n = 270$; 64% female; 45% married; 72% completed high school; 87% had an income of less than $40,000; mean age of 71.3, SD = 6.2	Cross-sectional	Visibility; rate of onset and time of onset of a disease; perceived severity of physical inactivity; stages of change	M was over-represented with 58% of the sample. Perceived severity discriminated PC from all other stages and discriminated P from A and M. Visibility had similar results, except that it failed to discriminate PC from C. Path analysis indicated that the effects of the perceived severity dimensions on the stages of change were mediated by perceived severity and that visibility made the strongest contribution to perceived severity.

TABLE 5.1 (*continued*)

Study	Sample	Design	Measures	Results
Cardinal (1995a)	8 women and 6 men; mean age = 63.1, SD = 8.8; all completed high school or more	Cross-sectional	*Educational Materials Review Form* examined production quality, content, credibility, attractiveness, ability to convey information, ability to change attitudes, ability to elicit appropriate action, and overall rating	The lifestyle material consistently outperformed the structured exercise packets, however, the results were not statistically significant. The reason given for the nonsignificant results was low statistical power owing to the low number of participants and a mean effect size of .46.
Courneya, Estabrooks, & Nigg (1997)	*n* = 147; 55% female; mean age = 71.7, SD = 6.0; 46% married; 67% completed high school	3-year naturalistic longitudinal	Baseline: Attitude, perceived behavioral control, subjective norm, intention, and stage; Follow-up: stage via telephone	Participants were classified as: resisters (inactive at both time points; *n* = 17); maintainers (active at both time points; *n* = 91); adopters (inactive then active; *n* = 17); and relapsers (active then inactive; *n* = 22). Adopters had higher perceptions of control at baseline compared to resisters, and maintainers had more positive attitudes, higher perceptions of control, and stronger intentions at baseline than relapsers.

(continued)

TABLE 5.1 (*continued*)

Study	Sample	Design	Measures	Results
Hellman (1997)	349 older adults aged 65+ with a cardiac diagnosis after discharge from a cardiac rehabilitation inpatient program	Cross-sectional	Stages of change; physical activity in the past week; perceived health status; barriers and benefits of exercise; perceived self-efficacy; interpersonal support for exercise; processes of change	Perceived self-efficacy, benefits of exercise, interpersonal support for exercise, and barriers to exercise were significant predictors and accounting for 50% of the variance in stage of exercise adherence. Further, the theoretical ordering of the stages was supported by the significant increase in exercise time from PC to M. Interpersonal support was a significant predictor whereas the processes of change from the TTM were not.
Courneya, Nigg, & Estabrooks (1998)	131 elderly Canadians; mean age = 71.5, SD = 6.0; 56% female; 45% married; 71% completed at least high school	3-year naturalistic longitudinal	Baseline: attitude, perceived control, subjective norm, intention and stage; 3-year follow-up: stage and exercise behavior	Path analyses revealed that (a) the theory of planned behavior constructs were significant predictors of the stages of change; (b) intention mediated the effects of theory of planned behavior constructs on stage; and (c) exercise behavior was best predicted by intention rather than stage.

TABLE 5.1 (continued)

Study	Sample	Design	Measures	Results
Nigg, Burbank, Padula, Dufresne, Rossi, Velicer, Laforge, & Prochaska (1999)	19,266 adults from RI and MA; 14,972 < 55 years (54.7% female); 1,924 55–64 years (53.1% female); 1,194 65–74 years (53% female); 421 75+ years (58.9% female).	Cross-sectional	Stages of change for 10 health behaviors: seat belt use, avoidance of high fat food, eating a high fiber diet, losing weight, exercising regularly, avoiding sun exposure, sunscreen use, reducing stress, stopping smoking, and conducting cancer self-exams.	The stage paradigm was found to apply to older adults for all 10 behaviors. Precontemplators had the highest or second highest percentage across all 5 stages. The prevalence of maintaining a low fat/high fiber diet appears to increase with age. A pattern was displayed where distributions increased toward extreme stages as age increased. The behaviors of losing weight, sunscreen use, and exercise consist of most individuals in precontemplation and fewest in maintenance.

however, whether this can be made operational has yet to be validated. Further, with the recent emphasis on physical activity (United States Department of Health and Human Services [USDHHS], 1996), the distinction between exercise and physical activity needs to be more thoroughly investigated. Minimally, the differences in the definitions of exercise and physical activity need to be explicitly described when staging individuals.

Processes of Change

Studies addressing the processes of change in older adults (Gorely & Gordon, 1995; Hellman, 1997) have used the scale developed on a work-site sample (Marcus, Rossi, et al., 1992). The studies, however, report differing results. Gorely and Gordon (1995) found that five of the 10 processes, self-reevaluation, consciousness raising, counterconditioning, self-liberation, and stimulus control significantly and independently contributed to the discrimination among stages. Conversely, Hellman (1997) reported that the processes of change from the TTM were not significant predictors of the stages of change. Both of these studies used prediction analyses on cross-sectional data sets. This technique was quite different than that used by Marcus, Rossi, et al. (1992) and may not have been appropriate. Considering that the studies are cross-sectional, the validity of their results are questioned. Further, predictive analyses assume linear relationships between independent variables and dependent variables. As stated earlier, the processes are curvilinear across the stages (Marcus, Rossi, et al., 1992; Nigg & Courneya, 1998; Prochaska & Velicer, 1997). Therefore, the most appropriate predictive and longitudinal change analyses should be conducted with adjacent stage transitions (e.g., precontemplation-contemplation, contemplation-preparation, etc.), not across all the stages.

Self-Efficacy

Self-efficacy for exercise within the TTM has shown consistent results. Self-efficacy significantly and independently contributed to the discrimination among stages and increased from precontemplation to maintenance (Gorely & Gordon, 1995; Hellman, 1997). This increase does not seem to depend on the scale used or the population studied, exemplifying the universality of exercise self-efficacy (Nigg & Courneya, 1998).

Decisional Balance

The balance between the pros and cons changed from precontemplation to maintenance in older Australians, consistent with theory (Gorely & Gordon, 1995). Pros increased and cons decreased across the stages and the decisional balance point (the crossover) was between contemplation and action. The barriers and benefits of exercise (along with perceived self-efficacy and interpersonal support for exercise) were significant predictors of stage of exercise adherence for older U.S. adults (Hellman, 1997). These variables accounted for 50% of the variance in stage of exercise adherence.

The findings from the reviewed studies illustrate the generalizability of the processes of change, self-efficacy, and decisional balance as conceptualized by the TTM across different populations. However, the questionnaires employed in the majority of the studies were developed on adult work-site samples (e.g., Marcus, Rakowski, & Rossi, 1992; Marcus, Rossi, et al., 1992; Marcus, Selby, et al., 1992). The possibility that the number of important decision-making constructs vary for different populations was highlighted by the findings of Gorely and Gordon (1995) and Hellman (1997). In future studies, questionnaires should be developed, not only stemming from the definitions established for other health behaviors, but also with the TTM constructs as envisioned by exercise focus groups. Questionnaires should be developed in the same rigorous manner as the Marcus, Rossi, et al. (1992) study, ensuring that the most appropriate variables are identified for each population. Potential implications are that interventions may need to address unique items, content, or variables for unique populations to maximize intervention efficacy.

OTHER CONSTRUCTS INVESTIGATED IN THE TTM FRAMEWORK

Studies investigating other variables in relation to the TTM have all employed the stages-of-change framework. The theory that has received the most attention is the Theory of Planned Behavior

(TOPB) (Ajzen, 1988; Fishbein & Ajzen, 1975). The TOPB proposes that intention is the best predictor of behavior. Intention is directly influenced by attitude, subjective norm, and perceived behavioral control. Attitude focuses on an individual's positive or negative evaluation of a specific behavior, while subjective norm reflects the perceived social pressure felt by the individual to perform (or not) a particular behavior. Perceived behavioral control assesses the presumed ease or difficulty of performing a behavior and is thought to be an approximation of one's actual situational control (Ajzen, 1991).

Courneya (1995a) found moderate to high correlations between the TOPB constructs and the stages of change in older, relatively active participants. All stage transitions could be differentiated using the TOPB constructs except those from action to maintenance. Path analysis identified direct paths for intention, attitude, and perceived behavioral control to stage of exercise, explaining 63% of the stage variance.

Courneya and colleagues also applied the TOPB to understand exercise stage change over 3 years in older Canadian adults (Courneya, Estabrooks, & Nigg, 1997; Courneya, Nigg, & Estabrooks, 1998). Exercise adopters had higher perceptions of control at baseline compared to resisters, and maintainers had more positive attitudes, higher perceptions of control, and stronger intentions at baseline than relapsers. Further, (a) the TOPB constructs were significant predictors of the stages of change; (b) intention mediated the effects of TOPB constructs on stage; and (c) exercise behavior was best predicted by intention rather than stage. These studies show that it may be beneficial to integrate the TOPB with the stages of change model in providing an understanding of the beliefs across the stages of behavior change as there is evidence for the long-term predictive validity of the TOPB in the exercise domain.

Lee (1993) determined, in a sample of older Australian women who reported low to moderate levels of activity, that exercise knowledge, perceived family support, and perceived psychological benefits of exercise distinguished the action group from precontemplators, whereas perceived barriers were the major difference between contemplation and action groups.

Courneya (1995b) found that perceived severity for an illness or disease due to a lack of exercise (from the Health Belief model and Protection Motivation Theory) discriminated precontemplation from all other stages and discriminated preparation from action and maintenance. This shows that perceived severity should be addressed when getting people to think about starting to exercise. The effect of perceived severity dimensions (visibility of the illness or disease and rate of onset) on the stages of change were mediated by perceived severity, and visibility made the strongest contribution to perceived severity.

Hellman (1997) revealed that interpersonal support for exercise and other TTM variables (self-efficacy, pros, and cons) were significant predictors of and accounted for 50% of the variance in stage of exercise adherence. This study showed that interpersonal support (similar to social support or helping relationships) along with one's confidence level and the decisional balance may be important components of exercise interventions targeting older adults. It is noteworthy that a variable not presently included in the TTM, interpersonal support, was a significant predictor whereas the processes of change from the TTM were not.

Preliminary evidence has been found when incorporating constructs from other theories with the stages of change framework (e.g., Courneya et al., 1997, 1998). Along with variables from the TOPB, which help us identify underlying beliefs about why one changes behavior, other theories and models (e.g., Health Belief Model, Self-Determination Theory, Relapse Prevention Model) may provide useful variables for understanding, explaining, and predicting stage change. Although the TTM has been developed based on numerous different theories of therapy (Prochaska & DiClemente, 1982), it is recommended that rigorous comparisons of the TTM constructs with other leading variables in the exercise area be conducted. Furthermore, personality variables are not addressed under the TTM. It is possible that certain personalities may respond more successfully to different processes of change. Suggestions for possible personality variables to be investigated within the TTM framework are self-concept, locus of control, extroversion-introversion, and self-motivation among others.

TTM, EXERCISE, AND OLDER ADULTS—INTERVENTION RESEARCH

Although Cardinal (1995a) documented the successful development and evaluation of written stage-based intervention materials by 14 elderly individuals, few TTM intervention studies have been conducted specifically targeting older adults. To understand the process of exercise adoption and maintenance, and to clarify causal relationships among the TTM variables, more longitudinal, naturalistic, and experimental designs are needed. The entire TTM should be employed to maximize the interpretability of the results and to identify constructs that have the most important impact on stage change over time. When intervention studies are proposed, appropriate control groups and legitimate follow-up procedures need to be incorporated. Benchmarking is also endorsed, comparing TTM interventions to other leading exercise interventions, as a strict test for identifying the best interventions possible. It is important that these interventions be systematic and based on past findings to be most effective.

An integral aspect of the TTM is that it allows interventions to be stage targeted (one intervention for each stage) and, more importantly, stage tailored. Stage tailoring consists of feedback supplied from questionnaires assessing all constructs of the TTM. Within each stage the individual receives feedback based on her/his process, self-efficacy, and decisional balance levels compared to norms. Follow-up reports supply normative (compared to population norms) and ipsative (compared to the individual's past answers) feedback, based on current and previous responses from the individual. The delivery of this type of feedback is through an *expert system* (Marcus, Nigg, Riebe, & Forsyth, 2000; Nigg, Riebe, et al., 1999; Velicer et al., 1993).

Expert system interventions mimic the reasoning of human experts by basing their feedback on decision rules predetermined either by qualified professionals or statistically. An expert system contains a series of feedback sections based on the constructs deemed important for behavior change—for maximum understanding and explanation of behavior change the constructs should stem from a theory or model. Assessment of the variables provides the necessary data for the computer expert system to produce individualized feedback reports both for the normative components and the ipsative components. This type of system allows for a large number of individual feedback possibilities (paragraph combinations). Expert systems allow for about 300 different feedback variations at baseline and this increases exponentially to about 19,000 potential combinations by the third feedback. Preliminary work is being done in the exercise area using expert system technology (Marcus, Bock, et al., 1998; Marcus, Emmons, et al., 1998; Nigg, Norman, Prochaska, Riebe, & Stillwell, 1997). The first intervention studies have demonstrated that tailored interventions seem to be effective at changing physical activity behaviors (Marcus, Bock, et al., 1998; Marcus, Emmons, et al., 1998). The following section will describe the author's current program of research applying the TTM to older adult exercise motivation.

A TTM-BASED RESEARCH PROGRAM MOTIVATING OLDER ADULTS TO EXERCISE

The University of Rhode Island's Aging and Health Promotion Partnership began preliminary research on a community sample of 70 residents at a senior housing site in Rhode Island (Nigg et al., submitted). The assessment instrument included items on participant demography, nutrition (DETERMINE screen), and physical, emotional, and social functional assessment (Short Form Health Survey). The quantity and duration of exercise along with exercise stage were incorporated to test the applicability of the TTM of health behavior change in this older population. The Tinetti Balance and Gait test, which measures physical functioning (Tinetti, 1986), was administered to a subsample of 38 individuals. The project was a single group feasibility trial. The exercise program consisted of approximately 45 minutes of group exercise conducted twice a week at the site and included range of motion, aerobic, lower extremity strengthening, and coordination and balance exercises. To help those in the precontemplation or contemplation stage move forward in their behavior, stage-targeted educational material was developed and distributed to residents who were not in the exercise program.

Of participants in the maintenance stage, 72% continued to be in maintenance after 7 months in the exercise program. Thirty-two percent of the participants improved their stage of change and 19% declined in their stage of change level over this period. The data were further grouped according to movement through stage level from baseline to the 7-month interview: progressors were individuals who improved in their exercise stage level, maintainers were individuals who maintained their stage level, and relapsors were those participants who moved backward in stage. Persons who either maintained or progressed in their stage reported a significantly better overall physical function, and those persons who attended the exercise program at least partially improved significantly in their overall Tinetti score in contrast to persons not attending the exercise program. The results from this pilot research showed: (1) 90% improved their stage of change suggesting that we are able to improve adoption, and (2) of those participants who were in action or maintenance of exercise, only 11% relapsed to an inactive stage.

These results are impressive for any population of exercise participants, but even more so given the characteristics of the group (mean age of 78) who were impaired in their physical function (22% were at high risk on the Tinetti). These results also suggest that functional improvements as assessed by the Short Form Health Survey occurred: (1) people who maintained or progressed in exercise stage had more improved overall health ratings than people who relapsed in stage, (2) physical functioning ratings improved in people who either maintained or progressed in exercise stage level; this was supported by the overall Tinetti scores which increased in individuals who attended the exercise program, and (3) people who maintained or progressed in their exercise stage level reported less bodily pain and rated themselves higher in overall health after the 7-month exercise program than did individuals who relapsed in stage level. Although a pilot study with an over-representation of active participants, this promising result led to development of a TTM-based intervention for a larger population.

The Senior*cise* Study (Jones et al., Submitted)

The URI Aging and Health Promotion Partnership were interested to see if the pilot study's results could be replicated on a population basis. This meant that a public health approach needed to be taken, incorporating the TTM-based intervention. To achieve this the efficacy of an inexpensive educational print exercise intervention based on the TTM for older adults was examined. Secondary objectives of this study were to examine the quality of the print intervention and possible ways to improve it through a survey technique to identify positive and negative aspects of the booklet and intervention process.

One hundred thirty-three posters and over 5,280 pamphlets with postcards (for the Senior*cise* booklet) were delivered to senior housing communities and recreation centers in Rhode Island over a period of 9 months in 1999. With each poster, 40 pamphlets were included, of which 20 were placed in the poster pocket, and 20 were given to the contact person for restocking. In each pamphlet, a postcard was inserted to complete if individuals were interested in the Senior*cise* booklet. When the postcard was completed and mailed in, the interested individual received the ten-page, stage-based Senior*cise* exercise booklet. The goal was to provide 100 booklets to older Rhode Islanders and to interview no less than 34 persons in order to have an acceptable review of the quality and efficacy of the booklet, based on a standard expectation of a one third population return (Fowler, 1988). Ninety-eight booklets were sent out to individuals requesting it and 54 individuals competed the survey. Self-reported exercise revealed that the study group was currently completing approximately 4.5 hours of exercise per week (planned activity to impact health or fitness).

The booklet provided information about exercise for participants in the earlier stages of change and helped them think about the pros and cons of remaining active. For participants in the later stages of change, the booklet contained a series of illustrations, suggestions for becoming active and remaining active, instructions on particular exercises and stretches, different suggestions on how to reward themselves on their efforts, and finally, additional information on the various other exercise programs provided in the community.

A series of 15 questions was developed to evaluate the booklet based on many of the factors cited by the Educational Materials Review Form produced by the National Cancer Institute to efficiently evaluate educational materials (National Cancer Institute, Office of Cancer Communication). The factors examined were: (a) overall rating, (b) appearance, (c) organization, (d) interactive rating, (e) clarity, (f) ability to change attitudes, and (g) ability to elicit the desired behavior change. Phone calls were made to all that had requested the exercise booklet within 2 weeks of mailing.

Seniorcise Results

The mean age of the participants was 73 (SD = 3.5) years and included 47 females and 7 males. The majority of the participants rated the booklet good or very good (93%) overall. The majority of participants also rated the booklet's general appearance good or very good (84%), and its organization as good or very good (95%). The interactive/write-in sections of the booklet were also graded good or very good (77%), as was the quality of the directions (95%). The majority of participants felt that the number of write-in areas should stay the same (57%) and overwhelmingly desired more illustrations (90%). Of the participants, 98% stated that the booklet helped them to think about exercise and 72% were inspired to actually participate in exercise.

Qualitative analysis of the booklet revealed more positive than negative aspects, although many participants chose not to complete these questions. The most common positive comments about the booklet included the presentation and quality of the exercise instructions. The motivational quality and the understandability of the booklet were also common positive comments expressed by the participants. The most common negative aspects of the booklet were the small number of illustrations, the lack of a Spanish version, and the unexpected difficulty in writing on the back cover action planner of the booklet due to the type of paper used.

This work shows that an intervention like the Senior*cise* program can be accomplished with a minimum amount of staffing (two research assistants) to cover a large geographical area with educational materials. The interest and response the booklet created exemplified that a minimally artistic, two-color reading intervention can make a difference. Although the Senior*cise* program was not an exceptionally large study, some learning issues did arise that may improve other such print intervention studies. The main suggestion for improvement is to know the culture of study areas. Many subjects in the Senior*cise* program desired a Spanish version of the booklet, which was unavailable. Understanding the culture of the people that are included in a future study will help include as many potential participants as possible. Education of the study population is also a factor that should be considered. In order for a print intervention to have a successful outcome, participants must first be able to read and understand the print materials. Also pictures can explain exercises and concepts more clearly than words depending on the reading ability of the participants. These pictures do not have to be bright and flashy, but just need to convey the ideas represented in the print material.

The SENIOR Project

These preliminary studies have led directly to the funding (from the National Institute on Aging) of a large community-based intervention. The Study of Exercise and Nutrition in Older Rhode Islanders (the SENIOR project) represents a multidisciplinary (psychology, exercise science, food science and nutrition, gerontology, nursing, pharmacy, and public health) collaboration to address multiple health behavior changes in older adults.

The SENIOR project is designed to focus on one primary and two secondary questions: Primary (1) Is a two-behavior intervention based on the TTM more effective than either one alone in improving nutrition and exercise behaviors in community-dwelling older persons?; Secondary (2) What are the effects on functional ability and general health outcomes of stage-based physical activity and nutrition interventions singly and in combination?; Secondary (3) How do older adults change their health-related behaviors?

The SENIOR project is a 2X2 experimental design with the following groups: (1) physical activity intervention only, (2) nutrition intervention only, (3) combined physical activity and nutrition, and (4) control group (receiving fall prevention materials). Educational materials based on the TTM expert system—including a manual, newsletters, expert system reports, and coaching phone calls—make up the 1-year intervention of groups 1 through 3. Outcome measures include objective and subjective physical activity and nutrition assessments; and stage and processes of change, decisional balance, and self-efficacy assessments; and the Medical Outcomes Study Short Form SF-36.

The target population is comprised of community-dwelling older persons 65 years of age and older from the city of East Providence, Rhode Island, and others who meet the inclusion criteria. East Providence has the highest percentage of older persons in the state (20%) and a high percentage of minorities represented. The interventions will be delivered by mail and telephone. At the time of this writing, the study is in recruitment and beginning data-collection stages. Results will be determined in 2002.

SUMMARY

The TTM has been successfully adapted to the exercise area even though exercise is an acquisition behavior. Overall, the research on the TTM shows that the stages of decisional balance and self-efficacy apply to older adults. Processes of change, however, need more investigation. Intervention studies have been effective in stage progression and assisting individuals to adopt a more active lifestyle. TTM interventions with older adults, although preliminary, show promise. There are some limitations and unanswered questions in the current body of TTM and exercise literature, which call for more research.

REFERENCES

Ajzen, I. (1988). *Attitudes, personality, and behavior.* Chicago, IL: Dorsey Press.

Ajzen, I. (1991). The theory of planned behavior. *Organizational Behavior and Human Processes, 50,* 179–211.

Barké, C. R., & Nicholas, P. R. (1990). Physical activity in older adults: The stages of change. *The Journal of Applied Gerontology, 9,* 216–223.

Benisovich, S. V., Rossi, J. S., Norman, G. J., & Nigg, C. R. (1998). Development of a multidimensional measure of exercise self-efficacy. *Annals of Behavioral Medicine, 20,* S190.

Brinberg, D., & Axelson, M. L. (1990). Increasing the consumption of dietary fiber: A decision theory analysis. *Health Education Research, 5,* 409–420.

Brug, J., Steenhuis, I., van Assema, P., & de Vries, H. (1996). The impact of a computer-tailored nutrition intervention. *Preventive Medicine, 25,* 236–242.

Cardinal, B. J. (1995a). Development and evaluation of stage-matched written materials about lifestyle and structured physical activity. *Perceptual and Motor Skills, 80,* 543–546.

Cardinal, B. J. (1995b). The stages of exercise scale and stages of exercise behavior in female adults. *Journal of Sport Medicine and Physical Fitness, 35,* 87–92.

Cardinal, B. J. (1995c). Behavioral and biometric comparisons of the preparation, action, and maintenance stages of exercise. *Wellness Perspectives: Research, Theory, and Practice, 11*(3), 36–43.

Cardinal, B. J. (1997). Construct validity of stages of change for exercise behavior. *American Journal of Health Promotion, 12*(1), 68–74.

Cardinal, B. J., & Sachs, M. L. (1995). Prospective analysis of stage-of-exercise movement following mail-delivered, self-instructional exercise packets. *American Journal of Health Promotion, 9*(6), 430–432.

Courneya, K. S. (1995a). Understanding readiness for regular physical activity in older individuals: An application of the theory of planned behaviour. *Health Psychology, 14,* 80–87.

Courneya, K. S. (1995b). Perceived severity of the consequence of physical inactivity across the stages of change in older adults. *Journal of Sport and Exercise Psychology, 17,* 447–457.

Courneya, K. S., Estabrooks, P. A., & Nigg, C. R. (1997). Predicting change in exercise over a three-year period: An application of the theory of planned behavior. *Avante, 3*(1), 1–13.

Courneya, K. S., Nigg, C. R., & Estabrooks, P. A. (1998). Relationships among the theory of planned behavior, stages of change, and exercise behavior in older persons over a three-year period. *Psychology & Health, 13,* 355–367.

Cole, G., Leonard, B., Hammond, S., & Fridinger, F. (1998). Using the "stages of behavioral change" constructs to measure the short-term effects of a worksite-based intervention to increase moderate physical activity. *Psychological Reports, 82,* 615–618.

Dishman, R. K. (1988). Exercise adherence research: Future directions. *American Journal of Health Promotion, 3,* 52–56.

Fowler, F. J. (1988). *Survey research methods.* Sage Publications: Newbury Park.

Fishbein, M., & Ajzen, I. (1975). *Belief, attitude, intention and behavior: An introduction to theory and research.* Reading, MA: Addison-Wesley.

Gorely, T., & Gordon, S. (1995). An examination of the transtheoretical model and exercise behavior in older adults. *Journal of Sport and Exercise Psychology, 17,* 312–324.

Hellman, E. A. (1997). Use of the stages of change in exercise adherence model among older adults with a cardiac diagnosis. *Journal of Cardiopulmonary Rehabilitation, 17,* 145–155.

Herrick, A. B., Stone, W. J., & Mettler, M. M. (1997). Stages of change, decisional balance, and self-efficacy across four health behaviors in a worksite environment. *American Journal of Health Promotion, 12,* 49–56.

Jones, N. D., DellaCorte, M. R., Nigg, C. R., Clark, P. G., Burbank, P. M., Garber, C. E., & Padula, C. (submitted). Senior*cise*: A Print Exercise Intervention in Older Adults.

Lee, C. (1993). Attitudes, knowledge and stages of change: A survey of exercise patterns in older Australian women. *Health Psychology, 12,* 476–480.

Marcus, B. H., Banspach, S. W., Lefebvre, R. C., Rossi, J. S., Carleton, R. A., & Abrams, D. B. (1992). Using the stage of change model to increase the adoption of physical activity among community participants. *American Journal of Health Promotion, 6,* 424–429.

Marcus, B. H., Bock, B. C., Pinto, B. M., Forsyth, L. H., Roberts, M. B., & Traficante, R. M. (1998). Efficacy of an individualized, motivationally-tailored physical activity intervention. *Annals of Behavioral Medicine, 20,* 174–180.

Marcus, B. H., Emmons, K. M., Simkin-Silverman, L. R., Linnan, L. A., Taylor, E. R., Bock, B. C., Roberts, M. B., Rossi, J. S., & Abrams, D. B. (1998). Evaluation of motivationally tailored vs. standard self-help physical activity interventions at the workplace. *American Journal of Health Promotion, 12,* 246–253.

Marcus, B. H., Nigg, C. R., Riebe, D., & Forsyth, L. H. (2000). Interactive communication strategies: Implications for population-based physical activity promotion. *American Journal of Preventive Medicine, 19,* 121–126.

Marcus, B. H., & Owen, N. (1992). Motivational readiness, self-efficacy and decision-making for exercise. *Journal of Applied Social Psychology, 22,* 3–16.

Marcus, B. H., Rakowski, W., & Rossi, J. S. (1992). Assessing motivational readiness and decision-making for exercise. *Health Psychology, 11,* 257–261.

Marcus, B. H., Rossi, J. S., Selby, V. C., Niaura, R. S., & Abrams, D. B. (1992). The stages and processes of exercise adoption and maintenance in a worksite sample. *Health Psychology, 11*(6), 386–395.

Marcus, B. H., Selby, V. C., Niaura, R. S., & Rossi, J. S. (1992). Self-efficacy and the stages of exercise behavior change. *Research Quarterly for Exercise and Sport, 63,* 60–66.

Marcus, B. H., & Simkin, L. R. (1993). The stages of exercise behaviour. *Journal of Sports Medicine and Physical Fitness, 33,* 83–88.

Marcus, B. H., Simkin, L. R., Rossi, J. S., & Pinto, B. M. (1996). Longitudinal shifts in employees' stages and processes of exercise behavior change. *American Journal of Health Promotion, 10*(3), 195–200.

McAuley, E., & Mihalko, S. L. (1998). Measuring exercise-related self-efficacy. In J. L. Duda (Ed.), *Advances in sport and exercise psychology measurement* (pp. 371–390). Morgantown, WV: Fitness Information Technology, Inc.

McConnaughy, E. N., Prochaska, J. O., & Velicer, W. F. (1983). Stages of change in psychotherapy: Measurement and sample profiles. *Psychotherapy: Theory, Research, and Practice, 20,* 368–375.

National Cancer Institute, Office of Cancer Communication (1989). *Making health communication programs work: A planner's guide.* Bethesda, MD: National Institutes of Health.

Nigg, C. R., Burbank, P., Padula, C., Dufresne, R., Rossi, J. S., Velicer, W. F., Laforge, R. G., & Prochaska, J. O. (1999). Stages of change across ten health risk behaviors for older adults. *The Gerontologist, 39,* 473–482.

Nigg, C. R., & Courneya, K. S. (1998). Transtheoretical Model: Examining adolescent exercise behavior. *Journal of Adolescent Health, 22,* 214–224.

Nigg, C., English, C., Owens, N., Burbank, P., Dufresne, R., Fey-Yensan, N., Luisi, A., Padula, C., Saunders, S., & Clark, P. (submitted). Health correlates of exercise behavior and stage change in a community-based exercise intervention for the elderly: A pilot study.

Nigg, C. R., Norman, G. J., Prochaska, J. O., Riebe, D., & Stillwell, K. M. (October, 1997). *Adopting and maintaining physical activity in a clinic based weight management program.* Paper presented at Physical Activity Interventions, The Cooper Institute Conference Series, American College of Sports Medicine Specialty Conference, Dallas, TX.

Nigg, C. R., Norman, G. J., Rossi, J. S., & Benisovich, S. V. (1999). Processes of exercise behavior change: Redeveloping the scale. *Annals of Behavioral Medicine, 21,* S79.

Nigg, C. R., Riebe, D., Rossi, J. S., Stillwell, K. M., Garber, C. E., Burbank, P. M., & Clark. P. G. (2001). Do the transtheoretical model instruments for exercise behavior apply to older adults? *Medicine and Science in Sports and Exercise, 33*(5), S149.

Nigg, C. R., Riebe, D., Rossi, J. S., Velicer, W. F., & Prochaska, J. O. (1999). Individualized expert system interventions for adopting and maintaining physical activity. Presentation at ACSM Special Event: Demonstrations of New Information Technology to Promote Physical Activity. *Medicine and Science in Sports and Exercise, 31*(5), S157.

Nigg, C. R., Rossi, J. S., Norman, G. J., & Benisovich, S. V. (1998). Structure of decisional balance for exercise adoption. *Annals of Behavioral Medicine, 20,* S211.

Prochaska, J. O., & DiClemente, C. C. (1982). Transtheoretical therapy: Toward a more integrative model of change. *Psychotherapy: Theory, Research and Practice, 19*(3), 276–288.

Prochaska, J. O., DiClemente, C. C., Velicer, W. F., & Rossi, J. S. (1993). Standardized, individualized, interactive, and personalized self-help programs for smoking cessation. *Health Psychology, 12*(5), 399–405.

Prochaska, J. O., & Velicer, W. F. (1997). The Transtheoretical Model of behavior change. *American Journal of Health Promotion, 12,* 38–48.

Rakowski, B., Ehrich, L., Dube, C., Goldstein, M., Paterson, J., Pearlman, L., Clark, M., Reimer, B., Prochaska, J., & Velicer, W. (April, 1997).

Individualized messages for increasing mammography screening. San Francisco, CA: Society for Behavioral Medicine.

Reed, G. R., Velicer, W. F., Prochaska, J. O., Rossi, J. S., & Marcus, B. H. (1997). What makes a good staging algorithm: Examples from regular exercise. *American Journal of Health Promotion, 12*(1), 57–66.

Sallis, J. F., & Hovell, M. F. (1990). Determinants of exercise behaviour. In K. B. Pandolph & J. O. Holloszy (Eds.), *Exercise and Sport Sciences Reviews, Vol. 18* (pp. 307–330). Baltimore, MD: Williams & Wilkins.

Skinner, C. S., Strecher, V. J., & Hospers, H. (1994). Physicians' recommendations for mammography: Do tailored messages make a difference? *American Journal of Public Health, 84,* 43–49.

Sonstroem, R. J. (1988). Psychological models. In R. Dishman (Ed.), *Exercise adherence* (pp. 125–154). Champagne, IL: Human Kinetics Publishing.

Strecher, V. J., Kreuter, M., Denboer, D. J., Kobrin, S., Hospers, H. J., & Skinner, C. S. (1994). The effects of computer-tailored smoking cessation messages in family practice settings. *Journal of Family Practice, 39*(3), 262–270.

Tinetti, M. (1986). Performance-oriented assessment of mobility problems in elderly patients. *Journal of the American Geriatrics Society, 34,* 119–126.

U.S. Department of Health and Human Services Centers for Disease Control and Prevention, National Center for Chronic Disease Prevention and Health Promotion. (1996). *Physical activity and health: A report of the Surgeon General.* Atlanta, GA: Author.

Velicer, W. F., Prochaska, J. O., Bellis, J. M., DiClemente, C. C., Rossi, J. S., Fava, J. L., & Steiger, J. H. (1993). An expert system intervention for smoking cessation. *Addictive Behaviors, 18,* 269–290.

Wyse, J., Mercer, T., Ashford, B., Buxton, K., & Gleeson, N. (1995). Evidence for the validity and utility of the stages of exercise behavior change scale in young adults. *Health Education Research, 10*(3), 365–377.

CHAPTER 6

Applying the Transtheoretical Model: Tailoring Interventions to Stages of Change

Patricia J. Jordan and Claudio R. Nigg

"Things do not change, we change."

~Henry David Thoreau

Each day more than 12 billion display advertisements appear in daily newspapers across the United States; another 6 billion are printed in magazines; 2.6 billion radio spots are broadcast; and 330 million commercials are shown on television (Plous & Neptune, 1997). Each one of them is designed to get people to change behavior. Change the brand of paper towels they use. Change the amount of milk they drink. Change the channel. Switch the dial. Join the club. "Just Do It!" And most people will not change.

Why do some messages motivate people to take action while others fail? Why do some patients begin a regular exercise program when asked by their doctors and others sink deeper into the couch? The answer is *readiness*. Everyone has different levels of readiness for changing certain behaviors. Everyone is different. That's just the way it is. But there are ways to motivate people to change certain behaviors by respecting their level of readiness and gradually moving them through the various stages of change.

The major success of the Transtheoretical Model (TTM) in behavior change is based on tailoring interventions to the individual's stage of change. Applications of the TTM to both healthy adults and caregivers of older adults have been described by other researchers (Burbank, Padula, & Nigg, 2000; Riebe & Nigg, 1998). This chapter describes in detail the application of the TTM to exercise in healthy older adults with an emphasis on tailoring to stage of change.

Traditional approaches to health behavior change have focused mainly on education—the assumption being that given enough information people will spontaneously change their behavior. Not surprisingly, these types of approaches have produced low participation rates and high rates of relapse (Prochaska, DiClemente, & Norcross, 1992).

The stages of change have their roots in psychotherapy (Prochaska, 1979) and were further established through research with individuals who were trying to quit smoking (DiClemente & Prochaska, 1982; Prochaska & DiClemente, 1983). Over time, the stages of change evolved into the existing five-stage model and include: precontemplation, contemplation, preparation, action, and maintenance (DiClemente, Prochaska, Fairhurst, Velicer, Velasquez, & Rossi, 1991). Individuals are generally thought to progress in a spiral manner from precontemplation to contemplation, contemplation to preparation, and so on. This means that most older adults attempting a health behavior change will relapse and recycle through previous stages, gradually learning how to successfully progress to maintenance (Prochaska et al., 1992). Although there are those who will progress straight from precontemplation through maintenance, it is a relatively rare phenomenon.

Assessing a person's stage of change and then tailoring behavior change interventions has received support in several research studies. For example, Marcus et al. (1992) found that a 6-week intervention program using written materials tailored to the stages of change increased the stage of exercise adoption for most participants. Furthermore, matching interventions to include all variables of the

TTM, not only stage, has been found to be effective for a vast array of health behaviors (see chapter 4).

THE TRANSTHEORETICAL MODEL

The relationships between the stages of change and the other TTM variables (i.e., pros and cons, self-efficacy, and processes of change) are described in detail in chapter 3, so they will be examined only briefly here.

Pros and Cons

Based on Janis and Mann's (1977) model of decision making, the TTM incorporates the decisional balance concept by evaluating an individual's relative assessment of the benefits (pros) and costs (cons) of changing a specific behavior (Velicer, DiClemente, Prochaska, & Brandenburg, 1985). A cross-sectional examination of 12 health behaviors (Prochaska et al., 1994) confirmed the importance of the relationship between the pros and cons and an individual's progress through the stages of change. For all 12 behaviors, the cons of behavior change outweighed the pros for individuals at the precontemplation stage, whereas the reverse was found to be true for those at action and maintenance. The decisional balance point, or crossover between the two, is most often found between the contemplation and preparation stages of change (Prochaska et al., 1994).

Self-Efficacy

Adapted from the work of Bandura (1977), self-efficacy has been integrated into the stages of change model as one of the most important constructs for assessing intermediate outcome and predicting future success (DiClemente, Prochaska, & Gilbertini, 1985; Velicer, DiClemente, Rossi, & Prochaska, 1990). Within the TTM, self-efficacy is assessed in two parts: confidence and temptations. Confidence in this case is situation specific, whereby an individual judges her/his ability to deal with high-risk situations without engaging in a specific behavior (Velicer et al., 1990). Temptations are described as an individual's rating of the strength of his/her desire to engage in a specific behavior when faced with various high-risk situations (Prochaska, Redding, & Evers, 1997; Velicer et al., 1990).

Across the stages, confidence scores have been shown to increase almost linearly from precontemplation to maintenance for a number of health behaviors (Prochaska, Velicer, Guadagnoli, Rossi, & DiClemente, 1991). This means that precontemplators have very low self-efficacy to change a particular behavior. Confidence increases to reach its maximum at the maintenance stage (Prochaska & Marcus, 1994). Temptations generally decrease across the stages of change, with the most obvious decline occurring between the preparation to maintenance stages (Hausenblas et al., in press; Prochaska & DiClemente, 1984; Velicer et al., 1990).

Processes of Change

Processes of change are the various strategies that people use to transform their experiences and environments in order to change behavior (Prochaska, Velicer, DiClemente, & Fava, 1988; Prochaska et al., 1992). The processes used by individuals in the early stages of change are often described as cognitive or *experiential*, and include consciousness raising, dramatic relief, environmental reevaluation, self-reevaluation, and social liberation (Prochaska & Velicer, 1997). Those further along in the change process rely more heavily on *behavioral* processes, such as counterconditioning, helping relationships, reinforcement management, self-liberation, and stimulus control (Prochaska & Velicer, 1997). (A summary of the processes of change and their definitions can be found in Table 3.1 in chapter 3.)

One aspect of this TTM that often goes unrecognized is that it is the processes of change that drive movement through the stages of change (Prochaska & DiClemente, 1984; Redding et al., 1999). In fact, investigations of the integration of the stages of change with the processes of change have demonstrated a consistent pattern in process use by individuals at different stages (DiClemente & Prochaska, 1982; Prochaska & DiClemente, 1983). For example, individuals at the preparation stage, who are starting to engage in the new behavior, use behavioral processes more than those at the contemplation stage. People at the action stage will tend to show a slight decrease in the overall use of experiential processes but increase their use of behavioral processes compared with those at preparation. A decrease in the use of certain experiential and behavioral processes has been found to set apart individuals at maintenance stage from those at the action stage.

HOW IS STAGE OF CHANGE ASSESSED?

It is extremely important to accurately assess stage of change prior to introducing a behavior change program. Prochaska et al. (1992) found that the amount of progress people made in a behavior change program was directly related to their stage of change before they began participating in the program. More importantly, however, research has shown that while stage-matched programs are effective for inciting change, stage-mismatched programs can actually have negative effects on an individual's motivation to change (Prochaska & Velicer, 1997; Blissmer, 1999).

Using the series of questions shown in the previous chapter in Figure 5.1 can help more accurately determine an older individual's stage of change for exercise. This type of question format is called a staging algorithm. One group of researchers (Reed, Velicer, Prochaska, Rossi, & Marcus, 1997) examined several criteria in order to determine the best components of a good staging algorithm for exercise and concluded that it should include:

1. a complete definition of exercise, including frequency, duration, and intensity;
2. measurement criteria that is understandable so that individuals can accurately stage themselves; and
3. a true/false or five-choice response format for the algorithm.

The most important part of the staging algorithm is the behavioral definition. It is critical to the success of any TTM-based program that the determination of stage of change for a given population be both accurate and consistent. Only when stage of change has been determined can stage-appropriate messages be delivered. The remainder of this chapter provides stage-by-stage guidelines for health care professionals, caregivers, or family members who are helping seniors establish or continue a regular exercise program.

THE PRECONTEMPLATION STAGE

Precontemplation is the stage at which an individual has *no intention of changing behavior* in the near future, usually measured as the next 6 months. It is important to define what is meant by having no intent to change behavior. Refer back to the exercise staging algorithm provided in Figure 5.1. Before any staging questions are presented, there is a precise behavioral definition that identifies the specific criteria for exercise. Precontemplators will have no intention of meeting *those* behavioral criteria in the next 6 months. That is not to say that a precontemplator will not change behavior in the next 6 months, but he or she will have no *intention* of meeting the specified behavioral criteria.

For example, assume a researcher is creating a TTM intervention to help seniors brush their teeth at least 3 times per day, every day of the week. A 65-year-old male who brushes his teeth once before bed each evening and has absolutely *no intention* of changing that behavior would be classified at the precontemplation stage. If this person is revisited 4 months later and he occasionally brushes his teeth in the morning before going to work, how is his stage of change classified? If he still has *no intention* of brushing his teeth 3 times per day in the next 6 months, he is still a precontemplator. He may have a slightly different view of the pros and cons of dental hygiene, and he may even be using more of certain processes of change; but he is still a precontemplator.

Older adults at the precontemplation stage for exercise may be underinformed or completely uninformed about the consequences of their behavior (Prochaska, Redding, & Evers, 1997). It is also possible that they have become demoralized about their ability to change, perhaps based on certain physical limitations or prior failed attempts to engage in an exercise program (Prochaska et al., 1992). Precontemplators are often characterized as resistant or unmotivated and tend to avoid information, discussion, or thought with regard to the targeted health behavior (Prochaska et al., 1992)—in this case, exercise.

People at the precontemplation stage rate the cons (or drawbacks) of exercise as being more important than the pros (or benefits). Precontemplators do not think of themselves as exercisers, they do not look for information about exercise, and rarely pay attention to the consequences of not exercising. As a result, older adults at the precontemplation stage can be extremely difficult to motivate. It is unlikely that their lifestyle is structured in such a way that exercise could be conveniently added to their weekly routine. They may even be defensive about their sedentary habits.

For older individuals at the stage of precontemplation who do not intend to change their behavior, the goal is to increase awareness of the need to change. The following strategies have been found to prompt precontemplators to consider exercise, and help them move to the contemplation stage.

Ponder the Pros

Most sedentary individuals do not place a great deal of importance on the pros of exercise. In addition to that, they often place far too much emphasis on the cons of exercise. The goal for older adults at the precontemplation stage is to become more aware of the pros. One way to do this is to mentally list 10 pros of exercise. (It is better to write them down, of course, but not necessary.) Older adults may not realize that regular exercise can help them sleep better, which in turn leads to other major benefits such as increased energy and improved concentration. Caregivers and other health care professionals can start the behavior change process by simply inviting discussion about the pros of exercise as a means of introducing those that are specific to older adults. There are hundreds of benefits from exercise; at least 25 of them are listed in Table 6.1. Coming up with 10 may be difficult at first, but once the process has started it becomes much easier to recognize and appreciate them.

Knowledge Is Power

The most important process of change at this stage is *consciousness raising*—increasing awareness and understanding about exercise. For older adults, this may mean reading magazine articles that promote

TABLE 6.1   25 Pros of Exercise for Older Adults

1. Exercise is good for my heart.
2. Exercise gives me energy.
3. Exercise helps me sleep.
4. Exercise curbs my appetite.
5. Exercise is good for my bones.
6. Exercise helps control my blood pressure.
7. Exercise gives me something to do.
8. Exercise keeps me fit.
9. Exercise makes me feel good about myself.
10. Exercise makes me a good role model for others.
11. Exercise impresses other people.
12. Exercise keeps me from getting sick.
13. Exercise helps me think more clearly.
14. Exercise lets me spend time with friends.
15. Exercise helps me manage my weight.
16. Exercise helps me relax.
17. Exercise keeps me strong.
18. Exercise helps me recover faster from colds and flu.
19. Exercise is good for my lungs.
20. Exercise is good for my joints.
21. Exercise puts me in a good mood.
22. Exercise improves my balance.
23. Exercise helps me remain self-sufficient.
24. Exercise gives me self-confidence.
25. Exercise helps me feel young.

exercise in people aged 65 and above, visiting Web sites about health and exercise for the elderly, watching television shows that include physically fit seniors, and listening to others who have successfully made exercise a part of their lives. In addition to learning about exercise in general, precontemplators should pay attention to the various kinds of activities that are classified as exercise. Along with more strenuous sports like tennis and running, some older adults may prefer some less common forms of exercise, such as swimming, walking outdoors, or ballroom dancing.

It is important not to suggest behaviorally oriented activities to people at the precontemplation stage (e.g., go to the library and get a book about exercise). Precontemplators should not feel pressured to take action too soon. For most, it is tougher to change one's mind than change one's behavior. More cognitive or mental activities are required at this stage to facilitate change.

Face Those Fears

A second process of change that is valuable in moving precontemplators to the next stage of change is *dramatic relief.* Most older adults will have a strong emotional response when they are made aware of the negative consequences of not exercising. For example, there are a greater number of health risks for sedentary people, such as myocardial infarction and exacerbation of chronic health problems such as arthritis or high blood pressure. Even simple things like shortness of breath or lack of energy can be alleviated by regular exercise.

Media messages, personal experience, and talking to others can prompt an emotional reaction in a precontemplator. What is crucial is that precontemplators are aware that exercise can help to abate their concerns. They need to feel the worry about their sedentary lifestyle and experience the emotional relief that thinking about exercise can bring.

Think About Others

A third process of change that has been shown to influence change in precontemplators is *environmental reevaluation.* Environmental re-evaluation combines both affective and cognitive considerations of how one's sedentary behavior may affect one's social environment. Some examples for older adults could include: Does the lack of activity make it difficult to play with grandchildren? Has it made you a burden on your spouse? Are you setting a poor example for your children? This process can often be combined with dramatic relief to maximize impact. Imagining that a change in one's behavior can have a positive effect on others can be a powerful motivational tool.

Summary

Precontemplators *can* and *do* change. One of the most important things to remember is that the goal of a precontemplator is to become a contemplator, not move immediately to action. Strategies for older individuals at the precontemplation stage should include the following:

- *Increasing the pros*—establish the importance of the many benefits of exercise.
- *Consciousness raising*—increase awareness and understanding about exercise.
- *Dramatic relief*—elicit strong affective responses when considering the negative consequences of a sedentary lifestyle.
- *Environmental reevaluation*—consider how a sedentary lifestyle affects the people around them.

THE CONTEMPLATION STAGE

Individuals at the contemplation stage openly state their intent to change behavior *within the next 6 months*. They are more aware of the pros of changing, but remain highly aware of the cons (Prochaska et al., 1997). Contemplators are often described as ambivalent to change or procrastinators (Prochaska & DiClemente, 1984). Returning to the previous dental hygiene example can help to illustrate another point. Consider the same individual, who is brushing his teeth only once per day. When faced with an action criterion of brushing at least 3 times per day, he recognizes that he does not meet our criteria but *intends to do so* in the next 6 months. This person is at the contemplation stage. When he is visited 3 months later, he is still brushing only once per day, but he still *intends* to increase to 3 times per day within the next 6 months. He therefore remains a contemplator.

Any older individual at the contemplation stage is aware that a sedentary lifestyle is problematic and is thinking about adopting exercise. The individual has not yet made a commitment to take action in the near future and needs to make an informed decision to start an exercise program. The goal for seniors in this group is to increase their motivation and their self-confidence in their ability to change. It is important to provide contemplators with as much relevant information as possible to assist them in making a healthy decision.

In addition to continuing the strategies that were effective at the precontemplation stage, consider adding the following strategies when dealing with older adults at the contemplation stage.

Make the Pros Outweigh the Cons

Where it was most important at the precontemplation stage to increase the pros, the concentration at the contemplation stage is on decreasing the importance of the cons. In fact, by the time an individual moves to the preparation stage, there is an emergence of parity between the pros and cons of exercise. Older adults can start by jotting down a listing of all the pros and cons of exercise that are relevant to them. These lists should include potential benefits and costs to themselves and others, as well as possible feelings of approval and disapproval from themselves and others. It is now timely to introduce the idea that many of the cons can be countered by alternative thinking. For example, some older adults may be concerned that they are too frail to exercise. These people can benefit from the information that even mild exercise on a regular basis can actually help strengthen muscles and joints and lessen their risk for falls and injuries. Sometimes the best way to contradict a con on the list is to point to a pro. For example, another common con reads: "I don't have enough time for exercise." One of the pros that could be highlighted is the fact that regular exercise can be easily incorporated into any lifestyle. For example: park the car a little farther away from the shopping center; get off the bus at least one stop early; or walk around the house a little during the TV commercials. Once the individual is able to cognitively reduce the importance of each of the cons on his or her list, it will be easier to focus on the importance of each of the pros.

One Step at a Time

In the same way the Berlin Wall was torn down—one brick at a time—so must an individual's *self-efficacy* to exercise be built. Self-efficacy increases linearly from the precontemplation to maintenance stages. Most older adults at the early stages of change are not only resistant to change, they do not believe they can do it. A wall of confidence needs to be built one brick at a time, so that these individuals can gradually imagine exercise becoming a part of their lives. The difficulty of increasing confidence at this stage is the reluctance of the individual to take action. In this way, it is important to help build self-efficacy through the use of more cognitive activities, not behavioral ones. Seniors may find it useful to identify times in the past where they have been able to accomplish a set goal (e.g., eating better, reading a thick book, finishing a crafts project, raising a child). What were the barriers that needed to be overcome? How worthwhile was the feeling of accomplishment? These experiences can be compared to that of starting an exercise program.

Think Differently

An important process of change at this stage is *self-reevaluation*. Older individuals at the contemplation stage do not think of themselves as exercisers, which makes introducing exercise into their lifestyle counterintuitive to their own self-image. There are a variety of ways to help a contemplator change his or her self-image. Both visualization and role-playing can be used to begin this process. Ask the individual to think about how his or her life might be different if he or she were a regular exerciser. (This is an ideal time to examine the pros and cons again.) Help the individual identify other older adults whom he or she admires for their commitment to exercise (e.g., friends, family, celebrities, etc.). Find out what is stopping the person from viewing him or herself as an exerciser. (This may also be time to approach the problem of low self-efficacy.)

Pay Attention

Another process of change that is useful at the contemplation stage is *social liberation*—the awareness of opportunities that exist to encourage regular exercise in older adults. This could mean looking into exercise classes that are held only for older adults. Check out walking or bike trails in the neighborhood. When are the senior swim times at the pool? Remember, at the contemplation stage it is not necessary to *do* anything, just get the information. There is no need to join the gym—just find out where it is.

Summary

Contemplators are often described as procrastinators who are ambivalent to change. The goal for older adults in this group is to increase their motivation and self-confidence in their own ability to begin an exercise program. It is important to provide contemplators with as much relevant information as possible to assist them in making a healthy decision. Refer to Figure 6.1 for an example of a stage-matched newsletter. In addition to the recommendations made for those at the precontemplation stage, strategies for individuals at the contemplation stage should include the following:

- *Pros outweigh the cons*—continue to increase the importance of the pros and focus on decreasing the importance of the cons.
- *Increase self-efficacy*—begin building self-efficacy through the use of more cognitive activities.
- *Self-reevaluation*—help them change their self-image.
- *Social liberation*—increase awareness of opportunities that exist to encourage regular exercise in older adults.

THE PREPARATION STAGE

Preparation is the stage at which individuals *intend to change* their behavior, usually *within the next month* (DiClemente et al., 1991). These individuals are starting to take small steps toward becoming a regular exerciser and may have already made minor adjustments in their thought patterns and behaviors, but typically do not reach the criteria for action (Prochaska et al., 1992). Due to its short 30-day duration, preparation is viewed as a transitional rather than a stable stage (Grimley, Prochaska, Velicer, Blais, & DiClemente, 1994). An important change at this stage is the decrease in use of experiential or cognitive processes of change and the gradual increase in reliance on behavioral processes of change. Of course, individuals may remain at the preparation stage for longer than 30

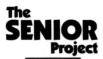 **The Exercise Connection...**

| **Thinking About Exercise** |

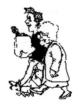

You are **thinking about starting to exercise.** You may not be sure about how to get started.

One Step at a Time

Start with small steps. Add some physical activity into your everyday routine.

- Park your car farther from the store and walk a little further

- When you are watching TV, get up and walk around your home during the commercials

- Each time you sit down on a chair, slowly raise and lower your arms and legs 10 times

- Take the stairs instead of the elevator

What Can You Do To Become More Active?

Are there some easy things that you could do to become more active? Write them down here.

_____

_____

_____

_____

Learn More About Exercise

The more you know about exercise, the more likely you are to participate. Learn as much as you can about exercise.

FIGURE 6.1   Sample stage-matched exercise newsletter for the contemplation stage.

*Adapted from: The Senior Project. A collaboration of: The City of East Providence, The University of Rhode Island, and the National Institute on Aging.
NIA Grant No. 1 RO1 AG16588, USDHHS

Where can you get information about exercise?

* Exercise: A Guide From the National Institute on Aging

  Provides information on exercise, nutrition, safety, and motivation, specific for seniors. This FREE guide is available by calling 1-800-222-2225

* Get in on the Action (and other materials)

  FREE and available by request from the American Heart Association

  The toll-free telephone number of the American Heart Association is:
  1-800-242-8721

  Can you think of any other places where you can get information about exercise? Write them here.

  _____.

  _____.

Think Differently: Think of Yourself as an Exerciser

It may be hard to imagine yourself exercising for 30 minutes. Instead, think about yourself doing smaller amounts of exercise.

Can you imagine yourself doing the following:

* Walking for 5 minutes without stopping

* Walking up the stairs without getting winded

* Lifting 1 or 2 pound weights up and down 10 times

* Walking to the store or post office instead of using your car

* Stretching your muscles for 5 minutes

  Remember – every little bit of exercise helps!

FIGURE 6.1   *(continued)*

days; what is most important here are the small steps toward change and the clear commitment to change in the foreseeable future.

Many of the strategies used at the precontemplation and contemplation stages should still be utilized at the preparation stage, but less reliance on cognition and more on behavior is needed. To help an individual progress to the action stage, several strategies are recommended.

Gaining Self-Efficacy

Confidence levels of those at the preparation stage have reached a midpoint. Emphasizing the gains in self-efficacy that have already been made and focusing on the individual's ability to continue taking small steps toward a regular exercise program will ensure increased confidence. One way of accomplishing this for older adults is to have them make a list of physical activities at three different levels: easy, moderate, and difficult. For example: buy running shoes (easy); walk around the block (moderate); walk a mile (difficult). Another example might include: talk to a friend about exercise (easy); make a plan to exercise with a friend (moderate); make a plan to exercise regularly with a friend (difficult). Let the individual decide how many of the easy items he or she can accomplish in the next week. Accomplishing these activities can be confidence building, and can help the individual accomplish more of the easy activities and attempt some of the moderate ones. Each time the stakes are raised, the individual increases her or his self-efficacy and moves toward action.

Let Others Lend Support

The process of change called *helping relationships* requires individuals to both seek and accept support for the change they are attempting to make. Older individuals should be encouraged to ask for support and encouragement from family and friends. This can be difficult for some; in fact, many people need to learn how to accept advice or suggestions from others. It can be especially difficult for those seniors who are ready to start exercising but lack a supportive community, or whose entire social network is a sedentary one. These individuals need to clearly state their needs and let others help. For example, one individual may find it helpful to inform his spouse not to serve dinner until he has walked for at least 15 minutes that day. Another individual may ask her daughter to walk with her to church each Sunday, so she will not be tempted to drive the short distance.

Make a Public Statement

Self-liberation is both the belief that one can change and the enduring commitment to do just that. Older adults at the preparation stage are ready to commit to exercise but they lack the resolve. Making a public commitment is one way to further that resolve and motivate these individuals to take action. New Year's resolutions are the most common sort of public commitment, but they may not be taken as seriously as some other forms of commitment. For example, have the person create and sign an "exercise contract," stating type of exercise, duration, and frequency of the activity. Suggest that a close friend or family member witness the signing, and post the contract in a prominent place. Alternatively, the individual can phone or e-mail five friends and announce that he or she is starting to exercise. Public declarations can be intensely motivating, particularly when an individual is at the preparation stage and is getting ready to act.

Drop Some Hints

Stimulus control becomes increasingly important at the preparation stage, as individuals begin to take small steps toward exercising on a regular basis. Older individuals should be encouraged to redesign their physical environment so they are increasingly reminded of their commitment to exercise. Some examples that are appropriate for older adults include:

1. purchasing a keychain of miniature running shoes. Adding this small reminder to a key ring can prompt some people to think more about exercise.
2. soliciting the help of family members and friends to rearrange furniture in the living room, so there is plenty of room to exercise.

3. posting inspirational messages or quotes on the refrigerator to help increase motivation.
4. placing exercise and health magazines, such as *Prevention*, in plain view. This strategy forms the impression that an exerciser lives in the home.

Substitute Alternatives

Another powerful process of change is called *counterconditioning*—substituting healthier alternatives for problem behaviors. In the case of exercise, look to provide older individuals with healthy activities when they are inactive. For example, instead of just sitting and watching television, the individual might do leg lifts or raise free weights while the show is on. Some older adults automatically take a nap when they are tired. Taking a brisk walk in the fresh air is an alternate way to get energized.

Summary

Individuals at the preparation stage are starting to take small steps towards becoming a regular exerciser and may have already made minor adjustments in their thought patterns and behaviors. One important change at this stage is the decrease in use of experiential or cognitive processes of change and the gradual increase in reliance on more behavioral processes of change. In addition to the recommendations made for those at the contemplation stage, strategies for seniors at the preparation stage should include the following:

- *Gains in self-efficacy*—emphasize the gains in self-efficacy that have already been made.
- *Helping relationships*—urge the individual to ask for support and encouragement from family and friends.
- *Self-liberation*—make a public commitment to begin exercising on a regular basis.
- *Stimulus control*—change the physical environment to include reminders of one's commitment to exercise.

- *Counterconditioning*—substituting healthier alternatives for sedentary behavior.

THE ACTION STAGE

The action stage is one at which the individual has made overt, perceptible lifestyle modifications for *fewer than 6 months* (Prochaska et al., 1997). Based on the staging algorithm in Figure 5.1, these individuals are exercising at least 3 times per week at a minimum of 20 minutes per session. Older adults at the action stage have high levels of self-efficacy and make good use of the behavioral processes of change to resist relapse and cement the new, healthier behavior into their lives. The first 6 months of regular exercise are the most difficult, and it will often be a struggle to remain active. Although all of the processes of change are being utilized to some degree, the behavioral processes of change and the pros are at peak levels, and self-efficacy is continuing to rise. The following strategies are recommended to help the individual maintain his or her status as a regular exerciser.

Rely on Increased Self-Confidence

Self-efficacy levels for people at the action stage are substantially higher than the previous three stages. This is the time to remind the individual how far he or she has come. At one point in time, these individuals were not thinking about regular exercise and did not believe they were capable of achieving such a goal. Older adults in the action stage are now well on their way to becoming a regular exerciser. Help these people to consider other healthy behaviors that have been a part of their lives for more than 6 months. This may include things such as not smoking cigarettes, not drinking alcohol, phoning grandchildren every Sunday, bathing or showering daily, and so on.

Develop a Reward System

Continuing to exercise regularly should be rewarded in some way—a process called *reinforcement management*. Older individuals should be encouraged to develop a reward system that provides smaller incentives for daily or weekly targets and larger ones for monthly goals. Because what constitutes a meaningful reward is often uniquely personal, individuals should develop their own standard. Small rewards, such as sleeping in on the weekend, renting a video, or buying a new book can serve as incentives for a week of regular exercise. Motivators such as a night at the movies, an evening at the theater, or a shopping trip may be used as rewards after a month of regular exercising.

Clean out the Attic

Individuals at the action stage are at risk for relapse because not only are they struggling to maintain a positive change in their exercise routine, they are battling the old voices in their heads telling them to give up. These unhealthy thoughts in the attic need to be cleaned out—another type of *counterconditioning.* Help the individual to establish a series of healthy "comebacks" to many of the pessimistic thoughts or worries that continue to crop up. This will give the new exercise habit a chance to grow stronger than the negative self-talk. For example, some older adults in the action stage revert to thoughts like: "I am too tired to exercise." Have them consider the idea that regular exercise is actually an energy booster. When the weather outside becomes a source of discouragement, help them think of several indoor activities.

Change Your Space

Stimulus control is of vital importance at this stage, when the individual should continue to remind her- or himself to exercise. In order to become a regular exerciser, their living space—both physical and mental—must become that of a regular exerciser. Older adults may find it helpful to prominently display calendars with exercise schedules on them; buy more than one pair of walking shoes, so they do not get bored wearing the same thing each day; or subscribe to an exercise magazine and leave it on prominent display.

Summary

The first 6 months of regular exercise are the most difficult, and it will be a struggle to remain active. Although all of the processes of change are being utilized to some degree, the behavioral processes of change and the pros are at peak levels and self-efficacy is continuing to rise. In addition to the recommendations made for those at the preparation stage, strategies for seniors at the action stage should include the following:

- *Reliance on self-efficacy*—Confidence levels are at an all-time high; remind the individual how far he or she has come.
- *Reinforcement management*—develop a reward system that provides incentives when goals are achieved.
- *Counterconditioning*—establish a list of positive responses to any pessimistic thoughts or worries that crop up.
- *Stimulus control*—create the physical and mental space of a regular exerciser by displaying reminders to exercise.

THE MAINTENANCE STAGE

The ultimate goal for everyone is to reach the maintenance stage. At maintenance, the individual is exercising regularly and has done so for *more than 6 months*, therefore the risk of relapse is substantially less than at any of the earlier stages of change. Those at maintenance are now working to prevent relapse and consolidate gains secured while at the action stage (Prochaska et al., 1992). Maintainers are distinguishable from those at the action stage in that they report the highest levels of confidence and report very little temptation to relapse (Prochaska & DiClemente, 1984; Hausenblas et al., in press). Seniors who are regular exercisers enjoy the positive results from exercising on a regular basis. Following are some techniques that can help maintain regular exercise behavior in older adults.

Enjoy This New-found Confidence

Individuals at the maintenance stage have established high levels of confidence because they have been regularly exercising for quite some time. This is an excellent time to review with them the types of things that have helped them continue to exercise in the face of many temptations to quit. When faced with temptations in the future, have them recall those strategies that have worked for them in the past.

Keep On Keeping On

Everyone has occasional doubts about their ability to continue with a new lifestyle change, but it is important to remember that exercise can help to clear those doubts. When people are feeling stressed or "down in the dumps," it's much easier to revert to unhealthy behaviors. Going for a walk or riding a bike instead of dwelling on those negative feelings are great ways to continue using *counterconditioning* techniques to one's advantage.

Show Self-Appreciation

Reinforcement management has been a strong motivator up to this point and should not be abandoned. Continuing to reinforce good exercise habits will continue to ensure good exercise habits. Incorporating *helping relationships* into the mix, by having family or friends provide additional rewards for ongoing maintenance of a regular exercise program, is a great way to strive for greater goals.

Keep Reminders Everywhere

Now that exercise has become a part of the maintainer's routine, many cues to exercise will already exist in and around the home. These reminders—based on the process of *stimulus control*—need to remain prominent. Older adults can make a list of the benefits of exercise and hang it on the fridge. Each day they can challenge themselves to add one new pro to the list until no more can fit. Setting out exercise clothes each night for the following morning can establish exercise as the first thing to do each day. Clipping motivational quotes about exercise and keeping them in one's wallet or stuck to the bathroom mirror can also provide reminders to exercise.

Think and Act Like an Exerciser

Older adults at the maintenance stage have a different view of themselves. They think of themselves as "exercisers"—not as people who "work out occasionally," or folks who are "trying to get fit"—an important change in their *self-reevaluation.* This means that they have earned the right to think and behave like an exerciser. It is essential that these individuals view being an exerciser as a positive thing. They can now serve as a role model for others in their immediate social circle and in their community. Older adults need more physically active role models, and now that he or she has reached the maintenance stage, it is important to uphold the commitment.

Summary

At the maintenance stage, the risk of relapse is substantially less than at any of the earlier stages of change. Those at maintenance are now working to prevent relapse and consolidate gains secured while at the action stage. Maintainers are discernible from those at the action stage in that they report the highest levels of confidence and report very little temptation to relapse. Strategies for seniors at the maintenance stage should include the following:

- *Keep confidence high*—review the things that have helped the individual resist temptation in the past.
- *Counterconditioning*—curb occasional doubts by thinking or doing something else.
- *Reinforcement management*—continue to reinforce good exercise habits with personal rewards.
- *Stimulus control*—keep prominent reminders and cues to exercise.
- *Self-reevaluation*—enjoy one's new self-image of an "exerciser."

RELAPSE

Relapse, slipup, setback—whatever it is called, it is not the end of the world. Although it is normal to recycle through the stages of change before reaching the maintenance stage, people need to learn from their setbacks in order to continue making progress. Research has shown that when individuals use the appropriate strategies outlined for each stage, they are less likely to slip back.

For older adults who slip back to precontemplation or contemplation, it is likely that they did not place enough importance on the pros of exercise before moving to the next stage. These individuals need to gather more information about how exercise can uniquely benefit them. For older adults who slip back to preparation, it is likely that they lacked confidence to resist several tempting situations, such as a run of bad weather or the demands of the holiday season. These barrier situations must first be identified and a plan of action to resist their temptation discussed. If individuals can recall what worked and did not work for them at each successive stage of change, they will be less likely to become discouraged from ever again attempting to engage in regular exercise.

THE TERMINATION STAGE

Is there anything after maintenance? Research on smoking cessation and alcohol abuse has identified a stage of change beyond maintenance—the *termination* stage. Termination is the stage at which individuals report 100% confidence and zero temptation (Prochaska & Velicer, 1997). Based on the fact that termination may not be a practical reality for a majority of individuals, it has not been the focus of much research. One study of former smokers and alcoholics found that fewer than 20% of individuals in each of these groups reported that they had reached the termination stage criteria (Snow, Prochaska, & Rossi, 1994). It is generally assumed that termination is common to addictions and other *cessation* behaviors, and does not appear to be evident in any of the *acquisition* behaviors, such as exercise. This may be because these behaviors require daily motivation to continue their implementation, whereas once a bad habit is removed, it no longer requires attention. Few studies have examined the existence of a termination stage for exercise (Cardinal, 1999, 2000). These studies found evidence that a sixth stage for exercise—the transformed stage—could exist. Similar to the findings of Snow and colleagues (1994), Cardinal found that approximately 16% of individuals had been in the maintenance stage for more than 5 years and remained 100% confident that they could maintain a regular exercise pattern for life. These people had a unique self-image in comparison to those at the maintenance stage. Certainly more research is needed regarding these conclusions, however, it is exciting to imagine that behavior change professionals can help individuals to not only change their exercise behavior but transform their self-image.

SUMMARY

Change is a process, not an event. Stages of change have predictable relationships with the pros and cons of behavior change, confidence in behavior change, temptation to relapse, and the processes of change (Redding et al., 1999). Success in behavior change should be measured in smaller increments because stage progression is the goal, rather than merely a dichotomous distinction of whether or not healthy behavior is practiced (Burbank, Padula, & Nigg, 2000). This allows for a more realistic, practical evaluation of progress toward health.

REFERENCES

Bandura, A. (1977). *Social learning theory.* Englewood Cliffs, NJ: Prentice-Hall.

Blissmer, B. J. (1999). *Integrating the theory of planned behavior and the transtheoretical model: A prospective study of lifestyle activity.* Unpublished dissertation, University of Illinois at Urbana-Champaign, Urbana-Champaign, IL.

Burbank, P. M., Padula, C. A., & Nigg, C. R. (March, 2000). Changing health behaviors of older adults. *Journal of Gerontological Nursing,* 26–33.

Cardinal, B. J. (1999). Extended stage model of physical activity behavior. *Journal of Human Movement Sciences, 37,* 37–54.

Cardinal, B. J. (2000). Are sedentary behaviors terminable? *Journal of Human Movement Sciences, 38,* 137–150.

DiClemente, C. C., & Prochaska, J. O. (1982). Self-change and therapy change of smoking behavior: A comparison of processes of change in cessation and maintenance. *Addictive Behaviors, 7,* 133–142.

DiClemente, C. C., Prochaska, J. O., Fairhurst, S. K., Velicer, W. F., Velasquez, M. M., & Rossi, J. S. (1991). The process of smoking cessation: An analysis of precontemplation, contemplation, and preparation stages of change. *Journal of Consulting and Clinical Psychology, 59,* 295–304.

DiClemente, C. C., Prochaska, J. O., & Gibertini, M. (1985). Self-efficacy and the stages of self-change in smoking. *Cognitive Therapy and Research, 9,* 181–200.

Grimley, D., Prochaska, J. O., Velicer, W. F., Blais, L. M., & DiClemente, C. C. (1994). The transtheoretical model of change. In T. M. Brinthaupt & R. P. Lipka (Eds.), *Changing the self: Philosophies, techniques and experiences* (pp. 201–227). Albany, NY: State University of New York Press.

Hausenblas, H. A., Nigg, C. R., Dannecker, E. A., Symons, D. A., Ellis, S. R., Fallon, E. A., Focht, B. C., & Loving, M. C. (2001). A missing piece of the transtheoretical model applied to exercise: Development and validation of the temptation to not exercise scale. *Research Quarterly of Exercise and Sports, 16*(4), 381–390.

Janis, I. L., & Mann, L. (1977). *Decision making: A psychological analysis of conflict, choice and commitment.* New York: Free Press.

Marcus, B. H., Banspach, S. W., Lefebvre, R. C., Rossi, J. S., Carleton, R. A., & Abrams, D. B. (1992). Using the stages of change model to increase the adoption of physical activity among community participants. *American Journal of Health Promotion, 6,* 424–429.

Plous, S., & Neptune, D. (1997). Racial and gender biases in magazine advertising. *Psychology of Women Quarterly, 21,* 627–644.

Prochaska, J. O. (1979). *Systems of psychotherapy: A transtheoretical analysis* (2nd ed.). Pacific Grove, CA: Brooks-Cole.

Prochaska, J. O., & DiClemente, C. C. (1983). Stages and processes of change of smoking: Toward an integrative model of change. *Journal of Consulting and Clinical Psychology, 51,* 390–395.

Prochaska, J. O., & DiClemente, C. C. (1984). *The transtheoretical approach: Crossing traditional boundaries of therapy.* Homewood, IL: Dow-Jones-Irwin.

Prochaska, J. O., DiClemente, C. C., & Norcross, J. C. (1992). In search of how people change: Applications to addictive behavior. *American Psychologist, 47,* 1102–1114.

Prochaska, J. O., & Marcus, B. H. (1994). The transtheoretical model: Applications to exercise. In R. Dishman, *Advances in exercise adherence* (pp. 161–180). Champaign, IL: Human Kinetics Press.

Prochaska, J. O., Redding, C. A., & Evers, K. E. (1997). The transtheoretical model and the stages of change. In K. Glanz, F. Marcus Lewis, & B. K. Rimer, *Health behavior and health education: Theory research and practice* (2nd ed.) (pp. 60–84). San Francisco, CA: Jossey-Bass.

Prochaska, J. O., & Velicer, W. F. (1997). The transtheoretical model of health behavior change. *American Journal of Health Promotion, 12*, 38–48.

Prochaska, J. O., Velicer, W. F., DiClemente, C. C., & Fava, J. (1988). Measuring processes of change: Applications to the cessation of smoking. *Journal of Consulting and Clinical Psychology, 56*, 520–528.

Prochaska, J. O., Velicer, W. F., Guadagnoli, E., Rossi, J. S., & DiClemente, C. C. (1991). Patterns of change: Dynamic typology applied to smoking cessation. *Multivariate Behavioral Research, 26*, 83–107.

Prochaska, J. O., Velicer, W. F., Rossi, J. S., Goldstein, M. G., Marcus, B. H., Rakowski, W., Fiore, C., Harlow, L. L., Redding, C. A., Rosenbloom, D., & Rossi, S. R. (1994). Stages of change and decisional balance for we problem behaviors. *Health Psychology, 13*, 39–46.

Redding, C. A., Prochaska, J. O., Pallonen, U. E., Rossi, J. S., Velicer, W. F., Rossi, S. R., Greene, G. W., Meier, K. S., Evers, K. E., Plummer, B. A., & Maddock, J., E. (1999). Transtheoretical individualized multimedia expert systems targeting adolescents' health behaviors. *Cognitive and Behavioral Practice, 6*, 144–153.

Reed, G., Velicer, W. F., Prochaska, J. O., Rossi, J. S., & Marcus, B. H. (1997). What makes a good staging algorithm: Examples from regular exercise. *American Journal of Health Promotion, 12*, 57–66.

Riebe, D., & Nigg, C. R. (1998). Setting the stage for healthy living: You really can help people adopt and maintain a healthy lifestyle. *ACSM's Health & Fitness Journal, 2*(3), 11–15.

Snow, M. G., Prochaska, J. O., & Rossi, J. S. (1994). Processes of change in AA: Maintenance factors in long-term sobriety. *Journal of Studies on Alcohol, 55*, 362–371.

Velicer, W. F., DiClemente, C. C., Prochaska, J. O., & Brandenburg, N. (1985). Decisional balance measure for assessing and predicting smoking status. *Journal of Personality and Social Psychology, 48*, 1279–1289.

Velicer, W. F., DiClemente, C. C., Rossi, J. S., & Prochaska, J. O. (1990). Relapse situations and self-efficacy: An integrative model. *Addictive Behaviors, 15*, 271–283.

Velicer, W. F., & Prochaska, J. O. (1999). An expert system for smoking cessation. *Patient Education and Counseling, 36*, 119–129.

CHAPTER 7

Applying the Transtheoretical Model: Challenges With Older Adults Across the Health/ Illness Continuum

Patricia M. Burbank, Cynthia A. Padula, and Mark A. Hirsch

> "Do what you can, with what you have, where you are."
>
> ~Theodore Roosevelt

Chronic illnesses are a significant health and financial burden not only for older adults but also for their families and the health care system. They frequently cause pain and suffering, are associated with increased use of medications, and most importantly, greatly affect quality of life by reducing functional abilities (Centers for Disease Control and Prevention, 1997). They increase dependency among older persons and necessitate the need for care and support services. The chronic illnesses of old age can be categorized into two types: those causing physical functional limitations and those affecting cognitive abilities, causing dementia. For some, a combination of both types of illnesses causes even more disability. This chapter addresses chronic illnesses and frailty among older adults with both cognitive and physical functional challenges. Exercise is discussed as the single most important general strategy for maintaining function and slowing decline for as long as possible. Application of the Transtheoretical Model (TTM) of behavior change is reviewed to assist the health care professional in promoting exercise behavior among older adults with these types of problems and their caregivers.

CHRONIC ILLNESSES AND DISABILITY

The majority of adults over age 65 have an average of four chronic illnesses, but are still able to carry out their everyday functional activities. Slightly over half are functionally limited in some way by the chronic disease (United States Department of Health & Human Services [USDHHS], 1999). The number of chronic illnesses and the degree of functional limitation increases with age, with the oldest (over 85 years of age) having the most limitations. Demographics indicate that this is also the fastest growing age group with estimates that it will reach nearly 9 million by 2030 (Bellenir, 1999). If chronic illness rates continue as they have, even more of our population may be functionally limited in the future and require caregivers and support services in order to complete simple activities of daily living.

The five leading causes of death among those aged 65 and older, in order of frequency, are heart disease, cancer, stroke, chronic obstructive pulmonary disease, and pneumonia. If only these diseases are considered, however, there is an inaccurate picture of the causes of disability and reduced quality of life among our elders. In contrast to the major causes of death, the most common chronic illnesses are arthritis, hypertension, heart disease, diabetes, respiratory disease, stroke, and cancer (see Figure 7.1). In 1995, 79% of noninstitutionalized people over age 70 had at least one of these seven chronic conditions (USDHHS, 1999).

The prevalence of most chronic conditions is increasing. Between 1984 and 1995 the prevalence of arthritis increased by 3%, heart

Percent

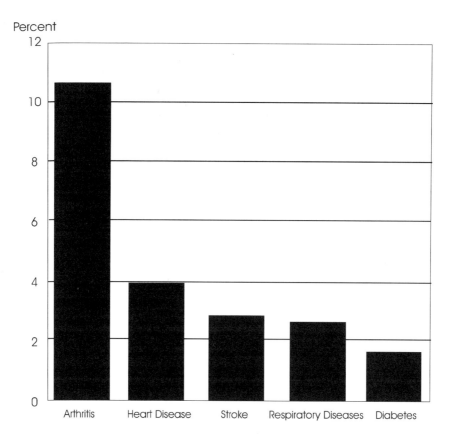

FIGURE 7.1

Notes: Based on interviews conducted between October 1994 and March 1996 with noninstitutionalized persons. Conditions are reported by persons who had any difficulty performing one or more activities of daily living (ADL). Multiple conditions may be reported. See Technical Notes for definitions of respiratory diseases and ADL.

Source: Centers for Disease Control and Prevention, National Center for Health Statistics, 1994 National Health Interview Survey, Second Supplement on Aging. See related figure 11 on chronic conditions and figure 15 for physical functioning and disability.

impaired. Speech often becomes more rambling and vacuous in meaning. The need for supervision increases as safety issues become important. Depression accompanies AD in the early stages for approximately one third of patients, with delusions and hallucinations occurring for a third of patients as the disease progresses (Kawa, 2000). In the later stages of the disease, the patient becomes bedridden and unable to speak. The course of the disease typically lasts between 10 and 15 years.

The term *frailty* is often used in the literature to refer to characteristics associated with extreme old age, disability, and presence of multiple chronic diseases or syndromes. An earlier review defined frailty as a state of reduced physiological reserves associated with increased susceptibility to disability (Buchner & Wagner, 1992). Fried and Walston (1999, p. 1389) expanded these definitions and defined frailty as a "state of age-related physiological vulnerability resulting from impaired homeostatic reserve and a reduced capacity of the organism to withstand stress." Frailty refers to a constellation of symptoms often manifested as chronic illnesses progress. These signs and symptoms include decreased muscle mass, balance and gait abnormalities, deconditioning, decreased bone mass, weight loss, fatigue, inactivity, and decreased food intake. It has been suggested that this decline in reserve occurs across multiple physiologic systems. Those symptoms believed to be central to the syndrome of frailty are neuromuscular changes resulting in sarcopenia (reduced muscle mass), problems with neuroendocrine regulation, and immunologic dysfunction (Fried & Walston, 1999).

Frailty seems to occur in a cycle or spiral with a spiraling cause-and-effect relationship between frailty and disability. Frailty likely causes a particular aspect of disability that results when a threshold severity of weakness and a level of decreased exercise tolerance is crossed. Declines in balance and slowed walking speed are associated with the frailty cycle. Falls are known to result from declines in strength and postural stability and thus increased risk of falls accompanies the cycle of frailty. Speechly and Tinetti (1991) supported this in their study where they defined frail individuals as having four or more of the following characteristics: over age 80, balance and gait abnormalities, infrequent walking for exercise, decreased strength in shoulder and/or knees, lower extremity disability, depression, sedative use, and near vision loss. Their findings showed that the frail group fell 3 times more frequently that the vigorous group. It should be noted, however, that frailty can also result exclusively from changes of aging and be unrelated to disease.

The widely accepted opinion about frail older adults and those with irreversible dementing diseases is that the course of their illness is a progressive downhill spiral with dramatic functional limitations, poor quality of life, and finally a death that ends the suffering. Caregiver issues become paramount and there is often a difficult burden for family members who care for these older adults. There is significant literature, however, that refutes the hopelessness and irreversibility of functional decline and documents that the cascade of decline can be slowed or sometimes even stopped by interventions such as a program of exercise and nutritional support.

EFFECTS OF EXERCISE

Exercise holds great potential for improving and maintaining function in older adults with chronic conditions. The widely held belief, however, is that it is too late for exercise to do any good at this stage, especially for people who have had lifelong habits of inactivity. Detailed information about the effects of exercise on older adults in general that refutes this belief can be found in chapter 1.

Research has documented dramatic positive effects related to increasing exercise among individuals who were sedentary (USDHHS, 1996). Loss of muscle mass, called sarcopenia, has been documented as an age-related change, along with an accompanying reduction in muscle strength. This carries significant consequences for functional capacity. Significant relationships have been found between muscle strength and walking speed (Bassey, Bendall, & Pearson, 1988; Bassey, Fiatarone, O'Neill, Kelly, Evans, & Lipsitz, 1992; Bennett, Carmack, & Gardner, 1982) suggesting that with advancing age and low activity levels, as often seen in frail and institutionalized older adults, muscle strength is a critical component of walking ability (American College of Sports Medicine [ACSM], 1998). Strength training, that is, training in which the resistance against which a muscle generates force is progressively increased over time, has been shown to increase muscle strength. This has been documented for older men and women as well with a two- to threefold increase in muscle strength accomplished within 3 to 4 months (Bevier et al., 1989; Frontera, Meredith, O'Reilly, & Evans, 1988). Fiatarone et al. (1990) found significant gains in muscle strength, size, and functional mobility among frail residents of a nursing home over age 90 following high-resistance weight training. Another study by McCool and Schneider (1999) found that frail older adults who participated in a 12-week program of leg strength training and physical therapy significantly improved their walking time and sit-to-stand time, and concluded that this type of program is practical and well tolerated by this group.

Declines in postural stability occur in this group of older adults with multiple chronic illnesses, cognitive impairment, and who are frail. Evidence that postural stability declines with age is well-documented (Woollacott & Shumway-Cook, 1990). The incidence of falls increases with advancing age and comorbidities with postural instability and balance problems contributing to this increased risk. A meta-analysis of the Fraility and injuries: Cooperative studies of intervention techniques (FICSIT) trials (Province et al., 1995), which studied the effects of exercise in frail older adults, found that those who were assigned to an exercise group experienced a decreased risk of falling, indicating an overall beneficial effect of exercise. Improvement in balance-related tests after participation in a variety of exercise programs (including Tai Chi) has been reported (Jarnlo, 1991; Judge, Lindsey, Underwood, & Winsemus, 1993; Wolf, Barnhart, Kutner, McNeely, Coogler, & Xu, 1996). Refer to chapter 1 for more information on exercise and falls.

Flexibility is also an important component of mobility. One of the most common chronic conditions, arthritis, often places significant limitations on flexibility. Although there is anecdotal information indicating that exercise improves flexibility, there is a paucity of research documenting the effects of exercise programs designed to improve flexibility, especially with older adults who are limited in physical or cognitive function. Further investigation is needed with this population group, but research is often more challenging with physically and cognitively impaired older adults due to frequent exacerbations of illnesses, changes in health status and deaths of participants, and difficulty studying those with cognitive impairments.

In one study by Brown et al. (2000), the effect of a 3-month, low-intensity exercise program on physical frailty in older adults was studied. They concluded that physical frailty is modifiable with a program of modest activities that can be performed by almost all older adults. They cautioned that although their findings suggest that frailty is modifiable, it is not likely to be completely eliminated with exercise, and recommended that intervention efforts be focused on prevention. Exercise, of course, is an essential component of prevention. Koroknay et al. (1995) initiated a program of daily walks for frail nursing home residents. After four months of walking, findings showed that ambulation improved significantly, with ambulation of cognitively impaired residents improving more than ambulation of cognitively intact residents. The proportion of residents who fell decreased from 25% before the walking program to 5% after the program.

Although there is also limited research documenting the effects of exercise on functional and cognitive abilities of Alzheimer's patients, exercise has been identified as a treatment focus. Exercise can help the person maintain mobility, strength, balance, and bone mass, thus reducing the risk of falling and potential injuries that may result. Sleep and bowel problems may also be alleviated by exercise, and it may be useful for reducing stress and aimless wandering (Hamdy, Turnbull, Edwards, & Lancaster, 1998). Findings from Russo-Neustadt, Beard, and Cotman's (1999) study of brain function in rats suggested that physical activity alone may have a positive effect on symptoms associated with AD and a potentiating effect when combined with antidepressants. A study by Teri et al. (1998) documented that persons with AD were impaired in the areas of physical performance and function compared to non-demented older adults. During a 12-week treatment program, caregivers were successfully taught to guide their family members with dementia in an individualized program of walking, strength training, balance, and flexibility exercises. Results showed that integration of exercise training into the care of persons with AD is both necessary and feasible. Exercise as a caregiver intervention has also been supported by Ham (1999).

To understand how exercise may positively affect cognitive functioning, a review of knowledge about the function of neurons and the brain is helpful. It has been widely believed that brain plasticity occurs more readily during the early developmental years and that neurons lack the ability to proliferate in adulthood; it was believed that they die and are not replaced resulting in a net loss of functional

nature of this relationship. Exercise has been found to have positive effects on depression, cognitive function, perception of control, and self-efficacy (ACSM, 1998). Rolland et al. (2000) studied the effects of a physical exercise program on autonomy, cognitive function, nutritional status, behavior problems, and risk of falls in patients with AD. Findings included improvement in cognitive function and nutritional status with decreased risk of falls and fewer behavioral problems. Dvorak and Poehlman (1998) studied patients with AD and concluded that higher levels of physical activity and energy intake are associated with increased skeletal muscle mass, indicating that nutritional and physical activity interventions may represent practical and inexpensive strategies in AD management. In studies that have examined the relationship between exercise and cognitive function among subjects without AD, however, the results have generally shown that aerobic training is not significantly associated with improved neuropsychological function (ACSM, 1998). A review of 34 studies (Anstey & Christensen, 2000) on the effect of physical activity on cognitive change found inconclusive results. More research is needed in this important area.

The effect of exercise on depression is much more well documented than the effects of exercise on cognitive function, with clear findings showing that exercise has a positive effect on depression (see chapter 1). Since rates of depression are even higher among older adults with functional as well as cognitive impairments, exercise can be very beneficial for this group.

GOALS OF EXERCISE

For younger people or people without physical limitations, the optimal goals of an exercise program are to achieve maximum cardiovascular and respiratory fitness through aerobic exercise and to maximize strength, flexibility, and balance through resistive exercises, stretching, and activities to improve balance. For people with specific problems, a rehabilitation program with individualized exercises designed to improve function in the areas of limitation is most appropriate. For the very old, people who are functionally impaired, people who are frail, and people who are cognitively impaired, the goals are different. As discussed here, exercise is still very beneficial. The goals are focused on maintaining the functional capacity that remains for as long as possible, improving it if possible, and slowing the process of further mental or physical decline. "Goals of exercise appropriate to younger adults, such as prevention of cardiovascular disease, cancer, and diabetes, and increases in life expectance, are replaced in the oldest adults with a new set of goals, which include minimizing biological changes of aging, reversing disuse syndromes, the control of chronic diseases, maximizing psychological health, increasing mobility and function, and assisting with rehabilitation from acute and chronic illness for many of the geriatric syndromes common to this vulnerable population" (ACSM, 1998, pp. 1000–1001).

The hazards of exercise in this population are not different from those contraindications with younger populations. Acute illnesses and unstable conditions, especially cardiac problems, need to be evaluated and stabilized if possible before an exercise program is begun. This is often difficult to accomplish as exercise is also a key factor that helps to resolve these problems. There are no reports to date of serious cardiovascular incidents, sudden death, myocardial infarction, exacerbation of metabolic control or hypertension among the frail older adults in nursing homes who have participated in studies on exercise. The major physiologic deficits that can be reversed with exercise include muscle weakness, low muscle mass, low bone density, cardiovascular deconditioning, poor balance, and gait (ACSM, 1998). The reader is referred to the ACSM (1998) position paper, which has specific recommendations for types of exercise for this population, as it is beyond the scope of this book include these recommendations here.

Whereas the first set of goals of improving cardiovascular fitness, strength, flexibility, and balance are more measurable, the latter goals for impaired older adults of slowing decline and maintaining function for as long as possible are much more difficult to evaluate. Because it is impossible to predict on an individual level what the illness trajectory will bring, it is impossible to measure outcomes related to the goals in this sense. It is necessary to be able to evaluate outcomes and more short-term goals need to be set. For instance, realistic goals such as the following may be set on a daily basis:

1. Mood will improve after an exercise session.
2. Evening agitation will decrease on days when the person exercises.

3. More food will be eaten in the meal following the exercise activity.
4. Sleep patterns on the nights following exercise sessions will be less disrupted.

Goals should be written using action verbs and specifying a time frame so that the method of evaluation is clearly a part of the goal. For example, with goal number two above, the length of time the person is normally agitated each day would be noted and evaluated in relation to days they exercise versus days they do not exercise.

Once health care personnel and family caregivers are given the necessary information to carry out and evaluate appropriate exercises, the next step is for the caregivers to include exercise in their care for every older person. To do this, behavior change is necessary both for the caregiver and the older person.

APPLICATION OF THE TRANSTHEORETICAL MODEL

The previous chapter discussed the application of the TTM to change exercise behaviors of healthy, functional older adults. This section will focus on the differences between application of the model with healthy older adults and with those with physical and cognitive limitations. Many people in this group receive assistance of some sort, either from family members, friends, or health care services if living at home, or from nursing care staff if living in institutions. For this group, the TTM needs to be utilized with both the older person and their primary caregiver or helper. For people with more advanced dementia, principles of TTM need to be utilized by their caregivers as this is a cognitively-based model and requires relatively intact cognitive function for application.

Over-burdened caregivers typically lack the motivation and knowledge to structure and supervise systematic exercise sessions. When bathing, feeding, and dressing are the major time-consuming activities, adding in time for exercise may become a luxury that the family caregiver cannot afford. In long-term care institutions, the staffing may be so minimal that no one has any time for extras such as exercise. Unless there is a commitment to exercise by administration in long-term care and support for it built into the system, it will not be accomplished. Creative ways of including exercise in daily care can help solve this problem. Use of volunteers may be an effective strategy. An elder rehabilitation program at the University of Arizona educates students to serve as rehabilitation partners and fitness supervisors for noninstitutionalized persons with dementia. They provide regular aerobics and weight training workouts, as well as memory and language-stimulation activities (Arkin, 1999). Such a volunteer program could be initiated in nursing homes as well. Another study provided a challenging exercise program to institutionalized older adults including those residents who were physically frail, incontinent, and/or had mild dementia. Their exercise program was designed to not only improve range of motion, as in typical nursing home exercise programs, but also to improve strength, balance, flexibility, mobility, and function. In addition to finding positive responses including significant improvements in mobility, balance, flexibility, and knee and hip strength, they concluded that this program demonstrated clear benefits over typical seated range of motion (ROM) exercises. Also, with minimal training, they found that such a program can be safely delivered at low cost by staff and volunteers (Lazowski et al., 1999). Neither of these studies, however, based their interventions on the TTM. Perhaps outcomes could have been improved further had interventions been tailored to stage of change and other concepts of the TTM. More intervention studies are needed to examine the effects of applying principles of the model to changing behavior with this population.

Assessment of stage of change is always the first step in application of the TTM in any situation. The stages of change, along with other components of the model, are described in detail in chapter 3. One needs to determine whether the person is exercising regularly or not. If they are not, their intentions need to be assessed. If they are not exercising and have no intentions of beginning to exercise any time in the future, they are in the precontemplation stage. The majority of older adults who are not exercising are in this stage. If they intend to exercise sometime in the future, sometime in the next 6 months, they are in the stage of contemplation. Those who are in the stage of preparation plan to begin to exercise sometime in the next 30 days. For those who are exercising, those who have been exercising for 6 months or less are in the action stage, while those who have been exercising for longer than 6 months are in the stage of maintenance. The goal with the TTM is progression through the stages rather than solely the behavior change of beginning an exercise program (changing from preparation to action). Progress can be made by stage progression even though the individual may still not be exercising.

The same assessment needs to be carried out with the family or staff caregivers. For this group of older adults who are physically or cognitively challenged, it is useful to think of the older adult and their caregiver as a dyad or team. Both members of the team need to be assessed for stage of change. Each person may be in a different stage of readiness to change. Until at least the client (with cognitively intact clients) is in the preparation stage, introduction of an exercise program or suggestions for exercises will be unsuccessful in changing behavior. With cognitively intact older persons and their caregivers, barriers or cons to change and processes used by each person to progress from one stage to the next may be different.

With cognitively impaired individuals, application of the TTM with the caregiver is even more imperative. For the person who is in the early stages of AD and minimally impaired, the caregiver/ older adult team approach with application of the model is most useful. However, as the disease advances, most of the emphasis needs to be shifted to the caregiver. Stage of change and barriers or cons should be assessed frequently as they may change as the disease progresses. For example, when she was experiencing only mild dementia, Mrs. S. exercised daily watching an exercise video geared for older adults while her daughter was preparing dinner. Often, she was not able to follow all the exercises, but she did move around to the music for about 20 minutes each day. As Mrs. S. became more confused and had trouble with complex tasks, she became frustrated with the video and refused to do her exercises. Her daughter was unable to convince her to try. Mrs. S. may have been able to change her activity and go for a walk with her daughter, but her daughter had no time to do this even though she believed it would help her mother. The barriers or "cons" became so overwhelming that Mrs. S. and her daughter relapsed into precontemplation, believing that nothing could improve the situation so that Mrs. S. could ever exercise again.

Self-Efficacy

To help understand the idea of self-efficacy, try visualizing the image of a person who is an "exerciser." When asked to do this, most people see an image of a young active person, either jogging or working out in a gym. Adjectives that might be used to describe this person are "young, strong, full of life, active, healthy, and vibrant." This is the opposite image from that of an older person who is frail, has chronic conditions, is functionally limited, and/or institutionalized. Such a discrepancy plays an important role in limiting exercise behavior for older adults. This negative image of older, functionally impaired people as exercisers greatly limits their own self-efficacy as well as the beliefs their caregivers have about their abilities to exercise. If an older person does not believe they can ever change their behavior to be a successful exerciser, then they have low self-efficacy for exercise. They will be in the precontemplation stage, even if their caregivers believe they may be able to exercise. If the caregiver does not believe that the older person is able to change their behavior and begin to exercise, the support needed for the older person to begin to exercise will be missing, even though the older person may believe that he or she could be a successful exerciser. Both the older adult and the caregiver must change their images of exercisers to include themselves! They must be able to believe that the older person can be a successful exerciser. Strong support for the importance of self-efficacy was found in a study by Resnick (2000) where outcome expectations and self-efficacy were found to be the only significant predictors of exercise behavior in a sample of residents in a long-term care setting.

Pros and Cons

In the precontemplation stage, the person has no intention of changing the behavior in the future. As people progress through the stages of change, they consider the pros and cons of behavior change. Stage progression comes when the pros become stronger than the cons and the balance tips in favor of the pros. Although there is a paucity of research in this area, experience leads one to conclude that the most difficult barrier or con, and one that keeps people in the precontemplation stage the longest, is probably the pervasive belief that it is not possible to benefit from exercise for those who are too old, too sick, or demented. Another extremely important con is the amount of time it takes to incorporate exercise into one's daily patterns for either older adults or their caregivers. The time and effort involved in even thinking about exercising is too much for many older adults and their caregivers. The thought of actually doing the exercises is beyond comprehension. It is a common experience for everyone, young and old alike, to avoid exercise when not feeling well. If exercise causes an initial increase in discomfort, as is often the case with arthritis, it is avoided. The amount of motivation required to exercise in the face of these difficulties is significant. A much stronger push is required to move through these barriers or cons into the action stage.

Based on the TTM, introduction of an exercise program to people who are in precontemplation or contemplation is of no use. Tailoring interventions to the stage of change is imperative. For precontemplators, the cons or reasons not to exercise outweigh the pros. Many older adults who are functionally limited and their caregivers who are in this stage cannot list any pros of exercise. Their list of cons, or reasons not to exercise, may be very long and seem insurmountable. Education about the pros of exercise specifically for this group, even individualized for each person with particular illnesses is very important. Without this information, there may be no pros! Older adults and their caregivers need evidence that exercise really works to help people in their situation.

Processes of Change

The processes used by people to change from one stage to the next are described in detail in chapters 3 and 6; the reader is referred to these chapters for more detailed discussions of these processes. In the first stage of preparation, the process of *consciousness raising* involves increasing awareness and understanding about exercise, gaining knowledge about the benefits of exercise for those older adults with chronic illness. Consciousness raising helps people identify more pros. In a second process called *dramatic relief,* the older person and their caregiver are helped to identify their fears about the negative consequences of not exercising. Once they experience an emotional reaction to the possible effects of being sedentary, they can think about the relief that they may feel when they begin to exercise and move toward changing their behavior. *Environmental reevaluation,* a third process of change, is where the older person thinks about the effect of his or her sedentary behavior on their social environment. For instance, an older woman who is being cared for by her daughter might ask, "What effect does my not exercising have on my daughter and her family? Does it make more work for her? Does it affect my ability to enjoy time with my grandchildren?" Most older adults value their independence a great deal and do not want to feel as thought they are a burden to their families. Imagining the positive effect that beginning to exercise may have on others can be a powerful motivator to exercise.

For those in contemplation, many of these very difficult blocks have been overcome. Contemplators are those people who are going to begin to exercise, but sometime in the next 6 months. Most older adults know that the diseases they have are progressive, so once some of the prohibitive cons of the precontemplation stage are eliminated, they may be more likely to plan to begin within the next 30 days than within the next 6 months. If they believe that exercise may be beneficial in slowing the chronic illness trajectory, putting off beginning to exercise would be seen as detrimental. Some common examples of cons for contemplators are the season (winter or rain), not feeling well, no transportation to their chosen place to exercise, and loss or unavailability of an exercise partner or program. An illustration of someone in this group would be Mr. B. whose mobility is severely limited by arthritis and emphysema. He knows he would benefit from exercise and has incorporated walking short distances into his daily life in the past. He recently became ill and was hospitalized with an upper respiratory infection that turned into pneumonia. Since returning home from the hospital, Mr. B. is extremely tired and finds it even more painful now to move around. His doctor told him to be patient, that it would probably take him several weeks before he could expect to feel less tired again. Although exercising may help relieve his fatigue, Mr. B. plans to start walking again, probably in a few months, when his arthritis pain subsides somewhat and he feels more energetic.

In the stage of contemplation, the pros of exercise have gotten stronger and the cons have decreased in importance. Health care professionals can help by looking at the older persons's list of cons, along with the family caregiver. Suggestions or information to respond positively to each con can be given. It is easier to focus on the pros once the power of the cons is reduced. Building confidence in the older person's ability to exercise is imperative. The older person and their caregiver must believe they can do it! The process of change called *self-reevaluation* helps them to think of themselves as exercisers. Visualization and role playing are two ways to facilitate this process. Examples and stories of other older adults with life circumstances and illnesses similar to theirs may help with this process. *Social liberation* is another process of change that is useful at the contemplation stage. It is important to know what options are available for exercise, should the older person decide to do that. For the health care professional, providing information about what kinds of exercises might be appropriate for the person and how they can get help to learn them is very useful. Identifying programs in the community such as day care programs where exercise is available and geared to the person's functional abilities is very useful. Specifics about transportation are also necessary because unless the suggestion is practical and actually able to be accomplished, it will not help the person to progress to the stage of preparation.

The next stage is preparation where the person is ready to make a change and to begin to exercise sometime in the next 30 days. In this stage, confidence levels have increased and the focus should be on strengthening the individual's ability to take small steps toward a regular exercise program. Just as with older adults who are not functionally impaired, persons in this group should be helped to make a list of activities that they could do to move toward beginning a regular exercise program. Then they can identify which things on this list are easy, moderately difficult, and difficult. The person can decide which of the easy items on the list they can accomplish within the next week. By doing this, self-efficacy will increase and both the older person and their caregiver will have even more confidence in the person's ability to succeed as an exerciser.

Processes important for change in the preparation stage include *helping relationships, self-liberation, stimulus control,* and *counterconditioning.* Although maintaining autonomy is important for most older adults, many people in this group have already accepted help from family members or others in order to manage successfully in their lives. Working as a partner with a caregiver is something that must be negotiated to be successful, however acceptance of helping relationships with regard to exercise can be an outgrowth of acceptance of help in other areas. *Self-liberation* is the belief that one *can* change and the actual commitment to making the change. A public commitment such as announcing to one's entire family that they will begin an exercise program next week is very motivating and helps the person move into action. *Stimulus control* refers to designing one's physical environment to include reminders of their commitment to exercise. Examples of reminders that can help the older person and caregiver are inspirational pictures of other functionally impaired athletes or older people who exercise, inspirational messages, or even a "prescription" from the health care provider for exercise. In *counterconditioning*, healthier alternatives are substituted for problem behaviors. With exercise, the problem behavior is being sedentary. An example of this process might be for the older person to do leg lifts and arm exercises during commercials instead of just sitting and watching TV.

In the action stage, the older person has begun to exercise but has not continued the exercise for longer than 6 months. Older adults who have exercised longer than 6 months are in the maintenance stage. For both of these stages, the pros always outweigh the cons, and the person must have increased confidence in their ability to exercise or they would not have been able to begin at all. The processes useful for the action and maintenance stages are *reinforcement management, counterconditioning, stimulus control, helping relationships, and self reevaluation.* Application of these processes for healthy older adults is discussed in detail in earlier chapters and is not different for older adults with functional impairments. What is different, however, is the consideration of the caregiver and the older adult as a team. These processes are more successful if both people are working together toward the same goal.

For people with progressive chronic illnesses, the course of the illness is uncertain with many exacerbations and remissions of symptoms. During times of exacerbation, or when another acute or chronic illness causes additional problems, relapse often occurs. The exacerbation or additional illness may leave the person at an even lower functional level than they had been previously. This can make recycling back to preparation and action even more difficult. Often depression or discouragement can make the cons loom large again and minimize any pros of exercise. Because these older adults have experienced a setback in their physical health, they may believe that exercise has not helped them and will not help if they begin it again. Energy levels may be depleted leaving them with little physical ability to exercise. In times like this, it is important to go back to basics. Identify what worked well to motivate the person to move from precontemplation to preparation and action before. If the person seems depressed, encouraging them to talk with their health care provider about antidepressant medications and other strategies may be useful. Use the same techniques that were successful in the past. The older person will need to rebuild their self-efficacy and reestablish the pros of exercise as more important than the cons. One of the keys to this is in taking small steps to begin to increase movement in any way. The older person, with the help of their caregiver, should be encouraged to begin to move their arms and legs as much as possible, even in bed, or in a chair or wheelchair. These small steps can evolve into an exercise program that is individualized for each person's functional abilities and goals, tailored for the person's new functional level, and practical in light of limitations presented.

SUMMARY

Exercise is a very beneficial intervention with broad-ranging benefits for older adults at all levels of functional ability. Most of these older adults and their caregivers, however, are not aware of these positive effects. In order to change behavior, health care professionals must be committed to educating older adults and families about the benefits of exercise and help them move through the stages of change. They also need the tools to learn safe, practical, and effective ways of exercising that are tailored to individual older adult's needs. The potential is great for positive outcomes when the TTM is applied to this group of chronically ill, frail, and demented older adults. Further research is needed to test the application of the TTM with this population group and answer questions about staging, self-efficacy, pros and cons, and processes of change. Such results are necessary to develop and then test specific interventions to assist older adults with functional limitations and their caregivers to maximize their potential through exercise.

REFERENCES

American College of Sports Medicine. (1998). Position stand on exercise and physical activity of older adults. *Medicine and Science in Sports and Exercise, 30,* 992–1008.

Anstey, K., & Christensen, H. (2000). Education, activity, health, blood pressure, and apolipoprotein E as predictors of cognitive change in old age: A review. *Gerontology, 46*(3), 163–177.

Arkin, S. M. (1999). Elder rehab: A student-supervised exercise program for Alzheimer's patients. *The Gerontologist, 39*(6), 729–735.

Bassey, E. J., Bendall, M. J., & Pearson, M. (1988). Muscle strength in the triceps surae and objectively measured customary walking activity in men and women over 65 years of age. *Clinical Science, 74,* 85–89.

Bassey, E. J., Fiatarone, M. A., O'Neill, E. F., Kelly, M., Evans, W. J., & Lipsitz, L. A. (1992). Leg extensor power and functional performance in very old men and women. *Clinical Science, 82,* 321–327.

Bellenir, K. (1999). *Alzheimer's disease sourcebook.* Detroit: Omnigraphics, Inc.

Bennett, J., Carmack, M. A., & Gardner, V. J. (1982). The effect of a physical exercise program on depression in older adults. *Physiology Education, 39,* 21–24.

Bevier, W. C., Wiswell, R. A., Pyka, K. C., Kozak, K. M., Newhall, K. M., & Marcus, R. (1989). Relationship of body composition, muscle strength, and aerobic capacity to bone mineral density on older men and women. *Journal of Bone Mineral Research, 4,* 421–432.

Brown, M., Sinacore, D. R., Ehsani, A. A., Binder, E. F., Holloszy, J. O., & Kohrt, W. M. (2000). Low-intensity exercise as a modifier of physical fraility in older adults. *Archives of Physical Medicine and Rehabilitation, 81*(7), 960–965.

Buchner, D. M., & Wagner, E. H. (1992). Preventing frail health. *Clinics in Geriatric Medicine, 7,* pp. 1–17.

Centers for Disease Control and Prevention, National Center for Chronic Disease Prevention and Health Promotion. (1997). *Unrealized preventions opportunities: Reducing the health and economic burden of chronic disease.* Atlanta, GA: Author.

Cummings, J. L., & Josie, D. V. (1999). Alzheimer's disease and its management in the year 2010. *Psychiatric Services, 50*(9), 1173–1177.

Dvorak, R.V., & Poehlman, E. T. (1998). Appendicular skeletal muscle mass, physical activity, and cognitive status in patients with Alzheimer's disease. *Neurology, 5*(15), 1386–1390.

Federal Interagency Forum on Aging-related Statistics. (2000). *Older Americans 2000: Key indicators of well-being.* Hyattsville, MD: Federal Interagency Forum on Aging-related Statistics.

Fiatarone, M. A., Marks, E. C., Ryan, N. D., Meredith, C. N., Lipsitz, L. A., & Evans, W. J. (1990). High-intensity strength training in nonagenarians. *Journal of the American Medical Association, 263*(22), 3029–3034.

Fried, L.P., & Walston, J. (1999). Frailty and failure to thrive. In W. R. Hazzard, J. P. Blass, W. H. Ettinger, J. B. Halter, & J. G. Ouslander, *Principles of geriatric medicine and gerontology* (4th ed.) (pp. 1387–1402). New York: McGraw Hill.

Frontera, W. R., Meredith, C. N., O'Reilly, K. P., & Evans, W. J. (1988). Strength training and determinants of VO_2max in older men. *Journal of Applied Physiology, 64,* 1038–1044.

Ham, R. J. (1999). Evolving standards in patient and caregiver support. *Alzheimers Disease Association, 13*(Suppl 2), S27–S35.

Hamdy, R. C., Turnbull, J. M., Edwards, J., & Lancaster, M. M. (1998) *Alzheimer's disease: A handbook for caregivers* (3rd ed.). St Louis: C. V. Mosby.

Hirsch, M. A., & Hirsch, H. V. (1998). Novel activities enhance performance of the aging brain. *Journal of Physical Education, Recreation and Dance, 69*(8), 15–19.

Hirsch, M. A., Ratliffe, T., & Vincent, J. (1997). Instructional strategies to help exercisers with Parkinson's disease, *Palaestra, 13,* 29–31, 46–49.

Jarnlo, G. B. (1991). Hip fracture patients: Background and function. *Scandinavian Journal of Rehabilitative Medicine, 24*(Suppl), 1–31.

Judge, J. O., Lindsey, C., Underwood, M., & Winsemus, D. (1993). Balance improvements in older women: Effects of exercise training. *Physical Therapist, 73,* 254–265.

Kastenbaum, R. J. (Ed.). (1995). The Georgia Centenarian Study (Special Issue). *International Journal of Aging and Human Development, 41*(2).

Kawas, C. H. (2000). Alzheimer's disease. In W. R. Hazzard, J. P. Blass, W. H. Ettinger, J. B. Halter, & J. G. Ouslander (Eds.), *Principles of geriatric medicine and gerontology* (4th ed., pp. 1257–1281). New York: McGraw-Hill.

Kempermann, G., & Gage, H. (1999). New nerve cells for the adult brain. *Scientfic American, 280*(5), 48–53.

Kempermann, G., Kuhn, H. G., & Gage, F. (1997). Experience-induced neurogenesis in the senescent dentate gyrus. *Journal of Neuroscience, 18,* 3206–3212.

Koroknay, V. J., et al. (1995). Maintain ambulation in the frail nursing home resident: A nursing administered walking program. *Journal of Gerontological Nursing, 21*(11), 18–24.

Knowles, M. (1884). *The adult learner: A neglected species.* Houston, TX: Gulf Publishing Company.

Lazowski, D. A., Ecclestone, N. A., Myers, A. M., Paterson, D. H., Tudor-Locke, C., Fitzgerald, C., Jones, G., Shima, N., & Cunnigham, D. A. (1999). *Journal of Gerontology-Biological Sciences and Medical Sciences, 54*(12), M621–M628.

Liepert, J., Bauder, H., Miltner, W. H. R., Taub, E., & Weiller, C. (2000). Treatment-induced cortical reorganization after stroke in humans. *Stroke, 31*, 1210–1216.

McCool, J. F., & Schneider, J. K. (1999). Home-based leg strengthening for older adults initiated through private practice. *Preventive Medicine, 28*(2), 105–110.

Murrell, W., Bushnell, G. R., Livesey, J., MacDonald, K. P. A., Bates, P. R., & Mackay, S. (1996). Neurogenesis in the adult human. *Neurology Report, 7*, 1189–1194.

Poon, L. W., Martin, P., Clayton, G. M., Messner, S., Noble, C. A., & Johnson, M. A. (1992). The influences of cognitive resources on adaptation and old age. *International Journal of Aging and Adult Development, 34*, 31–46.

Province, M. H., Hadley, E. C., Hornbrook, M. C., Lipsitz, L. A., Miller, J. P., Mulrow, C. D., Ory, M. G., Sattin, R. W., Tinetti, M. E., & Wolf, S. L. (1995). The effects of exercise on falls in elderly patients. *Journal of the American Medical Association, 273*(17), 1341–1347.

Resnick, B. (2000). Functional performance and exercise of older adults in long-term care settings. *Journal of Gerontological Nursing, 26*(3), 7–16.

Rolland, Y., Rival, L., Pillard, F., Lafont, C., Rivere, D., Albarede, J., & Vellas, B. (2000). *Journal of Nutrition and Health in Aging, 4*(2), 109–113.

Russo-Neustadt, A., Beard, R. C., & Cotman, C. W. (1999). Exercise, antidepressant medications, and enhanced brain derived neurotrophic factor expressions. *Neuropsychopharmacology, 21*(5), 679–682.

Scheibel, A. B. (1992). Structural changes in the aging brain. In E. Birren, R. B. Sloan, & G. D. Cohen, (Eds.), *Handbook of mental health and aging* (pp. 147–183). San Diego: Academic Press.

Speechly, M. N., & Tinetti, M. (1991). Falls and injuries in frail and vigorous community elderly persons. *Journal of the American Geriatrics Society, 39*, 46–51.

Taub, E., Crago, J. E., Burgio, L. D., Groomes, T. E., Cook, E. W., DeLuca, S. C., & Miller, N. E. (1994). An operant approach to rehabilitation medicine: Overcoming learned non-use by shaping. *Journal of Experimental Analysis of Behavior, 61*, 281–293.

Taub, E., Uswatte, G., & Pidikiti, R. (1999). Constraint-induced movement therapy: A new family of techniques with broad application to physical rehabilitation—A clinical review. *Journal of Rehabilitation Research and Development, 36*(3), 237–251.

Teri, L., McCurry, S. M., Buchner, D. M., Logsdon, R. G., LaCroix, A. Z., Kukull, W. A., Barlow, W. E., & Larsen, E. B. (1998). Exercise and activity level in Alzheimer's disease: A potential treatment focus. *Journal of Rehabilitation Research and Development, 35*(4), 411–419.

Toole, T., Hirsch, M, A., Forkink, A., Lehman, D. A., & Maitland, G. (2000). The effects of a balance and strength training program on equilibrium in Parkinsonism: A preliminary study. *NeuroRehabilitation, 14*(3), 1–10.

U.S. Department of Health & Human Services. (1999). *Health, United States, 1999: Health and Aging Chartbook.* DHHS Publication no. (PHS) 99-1232-1. Hyattsville, MD: Author.

U.S. Department of Health and Human Services, Centers for Disease Control and Prevention, National Center for Chronic Disease Prevention and Health Promotion, Surgeon General's Report. (1996). *Physical activity and health: A report of the Surgeon General.* Hyattsville, MD: Author.

Wolf, S. L., Barnhart, H. X., Kutner, N. G., McNeely, E., Coogler, C., & Xu, T. (1996). Reducing frailty and falls in older persons: An investigation of Tai Chi and computerized balance training—Atlanta FICSIT Group: Frailty and Injuries—Cooperative Studies of Intervention Techniques. *Journal of the American Geriatrics Society, 44*, 489–497.

Woolacott, M. H., & Shumway-Cook, A. (1990). Changes in posture control across the life span: A systems approach. *Physical Therapy, 20*, 799–807.

CHAPTER 8

Applying the Transtheoretical Model: Challenges With Older Adults From Diverse Ethnic and Socioeconomic Backgrounds

Sandra D. Saunders, Carol Ewing Garber, and Diane Martins

> "I cannot say whether things will get better if we change. What I can say is they must change if they are to get better."
>
> ~G. C. Lichtenberg

The focus of this chapter is the cultural, ethnic, educational, economic, and other sociocultural factors that impact on the design and provision of physical activity and health interventions in populations of diverse older adults. The issues of aging are viewed within the context of the more specific themes encountered in ethnically mixed groups, such as language barriers, distrust of the medical system, research and recruitment challenges, socioeconomic, educational, and literacy barriers. The application of the Transtheoretical Model (TTM) as a theoretical framework for behavior change in these populations is reviewed. Discussion of the topic is supplemented by case scenarios from the field that include low-income Black, Hispanic, Portuguese, and Cape Verdean elders, older adults with limited education, and those who have a primary language other than English.

Although health behavior change is a complex matter that requires several different kinds of efforts, individual responsibility tends to be the key factor emphasized by most health promotion programs. The nation's efforts have focused on individual change and individual health promotion and maintenance. It is believed that people should simply adopt healthier lifestyles. These beliefs result in blaming the victim (Ryan, 1971; Crawford, 1986) and do not address the social or environmental factors that may be relevant to the situation. Instead, the problem of poor health and the solution to improve health are solely the responsibility of the individual. Ideologies of individual responsibility have always been popular among health providers and academicians. Higher morbidity and mortality rates among the poor and minorities have traditionally been explained by lifestyle habits (Reissman, 1986; Crawford, 1986). This chapter proposes a dual approach that addresses not only changing behavior on the individual level, but also consideration of cultural and sociostructural factors that affect the health status and health decisions of the older adult.

ETHNICITY: A DEFINITION

Ethnicity involves a cultural identity linked to a common ancestry having shared national, religious, tribal, and linguistic origins often with common norms and values (Huff & Kline, 1999a; Nunnally & Moy, 1989; Paniagua, 1994). An ethnic group generally relates to its own culture differently than to the majority culture. The term ethnicity rather than race, a biological term, will be used here because it reflects a truer picture of the diverse multicultural older population as it exists and will evolve in the future.

DEMOGRAPHICS AND HEALTH OF THE OLDER ADULT POPULATION

Ethnicity

Approximately 16% of older adults aged 65 years and older belong to a recognized minority group (Federal Interagency Forum on Aging Related Statistics [FIFARS], 2000). However, the demography of the elderly population in the United States is undergoing dramatic change reflecting the shifting demographics in the population at large. These changes are expected to continue for decades to come, and by 2050, it is estimated that non-Whites will constitute approximately 35% of the elder population, an increase of 50% (FIFARS, 2000). The Hispanic population is expected to grow by 13 million by 2050, the largest growth in any ethnic group.

Roughly 1 out of 10 residents in the United States is foreign born (Spencer & Hollman, 1998), and more than 1 out of 8 older adults speaks a language other than English at home (U.S. Bureau of the Census, 1990a). Only some of these elders for whom English is not their primary language are members of officially recognized ethnic minority groups.

Life Expectancy

Life expectancy for older adults has increased, and a person who is 65 years old can expect to live an average of 18 more years (FIFARS, 2000). At age 85, the average life expectancy is 7 years for women and 6 years for men (FIFARS, 2000). There are differences in life expectancy among various minority groups, but these differences decline with age (FIFARS, 2000). At age 65, White elders can expect to live about 2 years longer than Black elders do, however by age 85, Blacks are more likely to live longer than Whites (FIFARS, 2000). Although the reasons for the striking differences observed in the health and mortality of ethnic minority groups are not fully understood, they suggest a combination of differential exposure to health-damaging and health-promoting factors, environmental and genetic factors, and characteristics of the health care system (Gould, 1999) including access and quality across age, gender, social class, and ethnic groups.

Health Status

Older Americans frequently rate their health as good, very good, or excellent, and there appear to be no differences in self-rated health by gender (FIFARS, 2000). The proportion of elders reporting good health declines with increasing age, and is lower in Black and His-panic male and female elders in every age group. Self-perceived health is important because good to excellent health has been related to lower mortality (FIFARS, 2000).

There are racial and ethnic differences in actual health as mea-sured by the percentage of older adults who have chronic conditions. Black elders are more likely to have arthritis, diabetes, stroke, coro-nary heart disease, and hypertension compared with Hispanic and White older adults, respectively (FIFARS, 2000). Cancer, however, is more common in White compared to Black and Hispanic elders (FIFARS, 2000).

Low Income and Poverty

Along with the growth of the over-65 minority population comes the potential for the development of additional inequity between rich and poor within that population. In every population group, lower income is directly related to poor health (FIFARS, 2000). Approximately 27% of older adults have low incomes and 11% of older adults live in poverty. The prevalence of poverty increases with increasing age; while 9% of those aged 65 to 74 years are impoverished, this proportion jumps to 15% in adults over age 85 years.

Poverty affects women and ethnic minorities disproportionately (FIFARS, 2000). Thirteen percent of older women and 7% of older men live below the poverty line (FIFARS, 2000). Approximately 20% of Hispanic and nearly a quarter of Black older Americans are impov-erished, compared with 8% of Whites (FIFARS, 2000). Divorced women are more likely to be poor than any other group, with nearly 50% of divorced Black older women living in poverty (FIFARS, 2000).

Living Arrangements

Living arrangements among elders differ by gender and ethnicity. Older adults living alone are more likely to live in poverty (FIFARS, 2000), and they are less likely to have the social support important for changing physical activity and health behaviors (Everard, Lach, Fisher, & Baum, 2000). Living arrangements are also related to economic status; nearly 50% of Black and Hispanic women and 19% of White women who live alone have incomes below the poverty line (FIFARS, 2000).

Older women are more apt to live alone, with 41% of women living alone compared to 17% of men. The proportion of older White and Black women living alone are similar, but only 27% of older Hispanic and 21% of Asian Pacific Islander females live alone (FIFARS, 2000). Black women who live alone are more often impoverished compared with White women (FIFARS, 2000).

Education

Educational attainment is related to both income and health status of older adults (FIFARS, 2000). Within the older adult population, the proportion of older adults who have not completed high school has decreased from 80% in 1950 to 18% in 1998 (FIFARS, 2000).

Approximately 67% of older adults have at least a high school diploma while an additional 15% have a bachelor's degree or higher. The proportion of older adults with at least a high school diploma, however, is considerably lower in Black and Hispanic elders, at 51% and 34%, respectively (FIFARS, 2000).

This review of demographics illuminates some of the dramatic differences between the lives of White privileged older adults and those of different ethnic and low income groups. Life expectancy and health status are generally reduced among those older adults who are non-White and/or poor. Living arrangements and education also reflect the social situations of this vulnerable group of older adults.

PHYSICAL ACTIVITY AND THE HEALTH STATUS OF OLDER ADULTS

It is clear that there are numerous benefits of physical activity for older adults, and that a physically active lifestyle promotes good health (American College of Sport Medicine [ACSM], 1998; United States Department of Health and Human Services [USDHHS], 1996; Larson, 1992). Participation in regular physical activity is associated with a variety of physiological and psychological benefits, and can improve strength, aerobic capacity, gait, balance, and functional status in older adults (ACSM, 1998; USDHHS, 1996; Larson, 1992). Exercise attenuates some effects of several chronic conditions common in older adults, thus improving disease management and decreasing morbidity (ACSM, 1998; Fletcher, 1997). In addition, physical activity is believed to play an important preventive role in reducing falls, which is a major source of mortality and morbidity in the elderly (ACSM, 1998; Myers, Young, & Langlois, 1996; Tinetti, Doucette, Claus, & Marottoli, 1995).

The benefits of regular physical activity has led the U.S. Surgeon General (USDHHS, 1996), the American College of Sports Medicine (ACSM, 1998), and the U.S. Preventive Services Task Force (1996) to recommend physical activity for older adults as a means to improve health and to attenuate the physical decline that occurs with aging. The recently released *Healthy People 2010* Health Objectives (USDHHS, 2000) has included physical activity as a health indicator for all adults, including the elderly, particularly among those where significant health disparities exist, such as those of minority or low socioeconomic status.

While it is clear that physical inactivity has many negative health consequences often limiting functional ability, the prevalence of physical inactivity increases with increasing age and affects about a third of men and 40% of women in older age groups (FIFARS, 2000; USDHHS, 1996). Even more worrisome is the fact that physical inactivity is more prevalent in older adults of minority status, particularly in Blacks and Hispanics, persons with lower income and educational levels, and those with arthritis and disabilities (USDHHS, 1996). Thus, the problem of physical inactivity is epidemic in older adults who fall into one or more of these population subcategories, and is a significant contributing factor to the health disparities seen among these population groups (USDHHS, 1996). While it is known that physical inactivity is more prevalent in older adults belonging to a minority group, until recently little attention has been paid to identifying factors that promote or impede physical activity participation in these subpopulations of elders.

Barriers to Physical Activity

Problems associated with longevity, chronic illness, and increasing disability as well as beliefs associated with being an older female, are frequently seen as barriers to participation in physical activity and health promotion interventions by older adults (Arean & Gallagher-Thompson, 1996; Clark, 1999). Even when the health benefits of physical activity are acknowledged, older women, more than men, perceive themselves as particularly vulnerable in exercise settings and find reasons not to take part (O'Brien Cousins, 2000). These concerns are attributed to an unfamiliarity with exercise, limited knowledge about health benefits, and lack of self-confidence in their ability to exercise (O'Brien Cousins, 2000).

Probably the greatest barrier to exercise participation in older adults is the fear that exercise will cause injury, pain, and discomfort or exacerbate existing conditions (Ferrucci et al., 1996; O'Brien Cousins, 2000). These can be very significant and often realistic fears that require careful consideration. Typically, older adults will spend several years of their later life with one or more disabling conditions that might limit their activity choices (Ferrucci et al., 1996).

Many older adults are very involved in individual, family, or community activities and see themselves as "too busy" to engage in health prevention behaviors such as regular physical activity. Surveys of the disincentives for exercise among older adults consistently report that time is considered a significant obstacle to regular physical activity (e.g., Richter, Marcera, Williams, & Koerber, 1993; Whaley & Ebbeck, 1997).

Costs associated with physical activity may present as a major barrier to physical activity, particularly to low-income elders. Often there is some cost associated with exercise such as memberships, shoes, and clothing. It is important that financial limitations be considered when developing and suggesting programs for the elderly.

Accessibility to appropriate physical activity facilities or programs can also make engaging in a regular physical activity program difficult for older adults. Inaccessibility is related to mobility limitations, transportation difficulties, safety issues, lack of appropriate programs, and financial restrictions. Even when physical activity facilities are located close by, the perception of older adults may still be that they are inconvenient or only offer classes or instruction at inconvenient times (Whaley & Ebbeck, 1997).

Lack of social support and increased social isolation can be a barrier to regular physical activity participation (Brenes, Strube, & Storandt, 1998; Courneya, Nigg, & Estabrooks, 1998). A strong social network that is supportive of physical activity behavior is an important predictor of physical activity levels (Brenes et al., 1998; Courneya et al., 1998). Exercise can prove a valuable source of affiliation and interaction for older adults, while simultaneously providing more resources to expand their social interactions (McAuley, Marquez, Jerome, & Blissmer, 2000).

Factors Associated with Exercise in Older African Americans

While a variety of factors have been associated with exercise participation in older adults, few investigations have examined the participation of older African Americans in exercise interventions. Studies that have included sufficient numbers of older African Americans generally have found that ethnicity plays no significant role in predicting participation in exercise and physical activity when other psychosocial, health status, exercise beliefs, and demographics characteristics are considered (Clark, 1999; Sharpe & Connell, 1992; Wolinsky, Stump, & Clark, 1995).

However, there is some evidence that older African Americans differ in their beliefs and perceptions about exercise. In examining beliefs about exercise and self-reported physical activity among older females, Fitzgerald, Singleton, Neale, Prasad, and Hess (1994) found that African American women were more likely to agree that older people should avoid vigorous exercise and more likely to find it difficult to adhere to a regular program of exercise. The study also found that older African American women were more likely to overestimate the number of days per week and the number of minutes per session needed to achieve aerobic fitness. In another study, Airhihenbuwa, Kumanyika, Agure, and Lowe (1995) explored perceptions and beliefs of African Americans toward exercise and found that most considered daily work to be a form of exercise. Specifically, older African American men reported that, after a lifetime of hard physical labor, retirement meant rest rather than leisure time physical activities. The retention of the work/rest dichotomy probably stems from a peasant/agricultural heritage where individuals who were physically able never retired, and now that older persons can retire, they feel that they "have earned it" (Purrell & Paulanka, 1998).

HEALTH BEHAVIOR CHANGE: RESEARCH DISPARITIES

In spite of the increasing proportion of older adults of minority status, there is very little scientifically based knowledge about how culture and socioeconomic factors influence health outcomes in old age (Ory, Lipman, Barr, Harden, & Stahl, 2000; Levkoff, Prohaska, Weitzman, & Ory, 2000). Recruiting and retaining older minority adults in studies has been historically difficult (Arean & Gallagher-Thompson, 1996; Prohaska, Walcott-McQuigg, & Peters, 2000). In recent years, several national initiatives have been created to address the health disparities and the underrepresentation of older ethnic, racial, and socioeconomic minorities in research (Ory et al., 2000). The Exploratory Centers for Minority Aging and Health Promotion (MAHP) was funded from 1993 to 1997 by the National Institute of Aging, National Institute of Health, and the Office of Research on Minority Health. The six interdisciplinary centers were established "to conduct research and related activities aimed at improving health status of older ethnic minority populations" (Ory et al., 2000, p. 11). In 1998 a new program, the Research Centers for Minority Aging Research, was developed to continue the work started by the MAHP. Additional programs, the Edward Roybal Centers for Research in

Applied Gerontology, the Claude D. Pepper Older Americans Independence Centers, and the Alzheimer's Disease Centers focus on
issues and research-related health promotion, disease and disability
prevention, life-style change, women's health, racial and ethnic disparities, and training of minority workers in the service and research
fields (Jackson & Curry, 1999). In April 2000 the American Public
Health Association (The Nation's Health, Oct. 2000) and the U.S.
Department of Health and Human Services formed a partnership
and the Initiative to Eliminate Racial and Ethnic Health Disparities
(APHA News, Oct. 2000). On November 22, 2000, President Clinton
signed the Minority Health and Health Disparities Research and
Education Act, which authorizes $150 million to be spent on minority
health and discrepancy research (The Nation's Health, Dec. 2000/
Jan. 2001). It is hoped that these efforts will lead to increased research
and improved intervention outcomes with these vulnerable
populations.

PHYSICAL ACTIVITY AND HEALTH PROMOTION IN THE CONTEXT OF ETHNICITY AND CULTURE

The consideration of cultural and social influences is important
when planning an intervention to increase physical activity in an
older multicultural population. Many factors make physical activity
and health promotion complex and often difficult in a culturally
diverse population. Attitudes and ethnocultural beliefs about health
causality and Western health care are often overarching determinants of participation in health-promoting activities (Huff, 1999;
Salembene, 2000; Leventhal, Leventhal, & Robitelli, 1998). Commonly held health beliefs and practices, or folk medicine, are important determinants of health behavior that are culturally specific
(Hufford, 1997; Pachter, 1994; Jack, Harrison, & Airhihenbuwa,
1994; Kramer, 1992; Huff & Kline, 1999a). Folk medicine beliefs can
facilitate or prevent participation in health promotion interventions,
and therefore must be considered in the development of a physical
activity or health promotion intervention.

"Traditional" interventions based on the norms, values, and beliefs
of the dominant White culture often do not address or meet the
needs of multicultural older persons (Arean & Gallagher-Thompson,

1996; Frankish, Lovato, & Shannon, 1999; Hudson, Leventhal, Contrada, Leventhal, & Brownlee, 2000). Additional time, money, and personnel may be needed during the design, planning, and implementation stages to ensure that all the elements of cultural and social influence are carefully taken into account and incorporated into the intervention. A successful intervention depends, in part, on a culturally sensitive evaluation of how the program is going to be perceived and accepted by the target population and the community. The challenge of a multicultural intervention is that what is acceptable and effective for one population subgroup may not be for another. The development of interventions that are generic enough to meet the needs of most of the population is the ideal, but often specific interventions targeted toward a particular group may be necessary to effect physical activity and health behavior changes. For a more detailed discussion of the many facets of promoting health in multicultural populations, the reader is referred to several comprehensive texts (Huff & Kline, 1999c; Levkoff, Prohaska, Weitzman, & Ory, 2000; Markides & Miranda, 1997; Martin & Soldo, 1997; Spector, 1996).

ATTITUDES OF HEALTH CARE PROFESSIONALS

The attitudes of health care professionals play an important role in their work with client populations. The majority of health professionals are White, financially secure, and well educated. The social dynamics of health provider and patient interactions places the health provider or researcher in the role with power (Brown, 1989). Furthermore, institutional settings impose their own organization on the social behavior of illness. There is control over the information that is shared and not shared with the client (Friedson, 1970). This is related to professional assumptions about clients and is based on the underlying, often unrecognized belief that clients are too limited in intelligence to comprehend the information they receive and will become too upset about their health problems to use the information rationally and in a responsible way (Glaser & Strauss, 1965). As medical dominance has increased, attention to social problems has decreased and the societal roots of personal troubles have become less apparent through stigma and labeling of patients. By responding in limited ways to social problems, health care providers tend to shift the focus of attention from societal issues to the individual (Conrad & Schneider, 1992; Zola, 1983). On the individual level, a paternalistic attitude on the part of the provider results in a lack of sensitivity to meanings attached to situations by clients; to the client's personal needs, values, and goals; and to the resources available to the client to carry out the health care provider's recommendations.

A critical theory perspective recognizes the broader socio-structural factors that are strongly integrated with the possibility of change. Once those factors are identified, the health care provider, in addition to acting on the individual level, would become involved in actions to change the socio-structural environment including the political, social, and economic environment. Efforts to empower the individual are also essential. The reality that health, health behaviors, and social problems are intricately linked cannot be ignored.

INTERVENTION CONSIDERATIONS

Several experts (Arean & Gallagher-Thompson, 1996; Huff & Kline, 1999c; Levkoff et al., 2000; Spector, 1996; Tripp-Reimer, Johnson, & Rios, 1994) have identified a number of population characteristics important in the development of interventions and evaluation in multicultural populations. These factors include age, gender, social class and status, educational attainment, literacy, language and dialect, spirituality and religion, income, acculturation and assimilation, and health beliefs and attitudes. These factors will be discussed in more detail in the following sections.

Age and Gender

Age and gender characteristics of the target population may be an important factor determining the success of participant enrollment in an intervention. In many ethnic groups, men are acknowledged as the decision makers in matters relating to the outside world, while women are expected to have a minor role in the family's interaction with the community at large (Ferrales, 1996; Purrell & Paulanka, 1998). Hazzuda et al. (2000) found that Mexican American husbands served as family gatekeepers influencing their wives participation in exercise and health promotion activities. Conversely, Fuller-Thompson, Minkler, and Driver (1997) note that many older African American women are in a matriarchal role, with men having minimal family, economic, and social contributions. Adult children may have the role of gatekeeper for their elderly parents influencing their willingness to participate (Hazuda et al., 2000). In other groups, the family's elders, who may still believe in traditional practices, are the decision makers for the family with regard to major health, legal, and financial matters (Huff & Kline, 1999c; Purrell & Paulanka, 1998; Ishida, Toomata-Mayer, & Mayer, 1996; Uba, 1992; Spector, 1996).

Public display of physical activity such as running or other vigorous activities may not be acceptable in some cultures, where modesty is the social norm for women (Mo, 1992). Vertinsky (1998) found that older women often refrain from exercise participation because of sexist and ageist attitudes related to a history of being labeled as the weaker sex. These pervasive attitudes often cause older women to overestimate the risks and devalue the benefits of exercise. In addition, some older women perceive exercise as having low social status which fosters nonparticipation (O'Brien Cousins, 2000). If not identified, cultural attitudes, gender, and decision-making roles, usually linked to degree of acculturation and assimilation in ethnic groups, may present barriers to consent and thereby influence decision making, recruitment, and participation in physical activity programs.

The physical activity experiences among older adults are marked by vastly different socialization and practical experiences in men and women. Older adult males, even those from other countries, were encouraged to engage in sports and physical activity throughout their youth, whereas older females in the United States rarely participated in strenuous physical activity when young. The non-strenuous activity patterns evidenced throughout adulthood are maintained into old age, with older women exercising less than older males (Jones et al., 1998; USDHHS, 1996). The discrepancy between the activity levels of older males and females may, in part, be explained by their own perceptions of which activities are appropriate for males and females. A survey of older adults found that older adults considered a variety of physical activities to be more appropriate for men than women across the age spectrum (Stead, Wimbush, Eadie, & Teer, 1997).

Social Class and Socioeconomic Status

Social class, occupation (current or former), and income often influence the willingness of potential participants to be involved in an intervention that involves changing health behavior, including physical activity (Huff, 1999; Ishida, Toomata-Mayer, & Mayer, 1996). For marginal low socioeconomic populations, a focus on health promotion behavior, an ideological purview of the present medical industrial complex, has no relevance (Minkler, 1992; Cockerham, 2000). Thus, programs that focus on healthy individual lifestyles and behavior change that are not tailored for the underserved and marginal populations may be ineffective (Minkler, 1992; Cockerham, 2000).

The more disadvantaged members of society are too concerned on a daily basis with the basic survival issues of finding food and shelter to even consider participation in a physical activity intervention that is seen as unimportant or "silly." Having a health club or gym membership or purchasing fitness equipment is unthinkable when there is not enough money for food. Even trips for medical care for acute and chronic health problems are difficult to plan when life is a day-to-day struggle for safety and physical health. Only when a person has a sense that they are safe and can physically survive, can they then focus on other's (e.g., health care providers') perspectives on their needs (Robert & House, 2000). Even when receptive to taking part in an intervention, participation may be difficult because it may require missing work (if they are still working), or there may be transportation difficulties or other obstacles that are difficult to overcome.

Literacy

Literacy rates play a critical role in planning a study within a multicultural population. A large proportion of older adults are functionally illiterate, that is, they do not have the ability to use reading, writing, and computational skills at a level adequate to meet the needs of everyday life situations (Kirsch, Jungeblut, Jenkins, & Kolstad, 1993). The National Adult Literacy Survey (Kirsch et al., 1993) reported that 71% of adults over the age of 60 years perform in the lowest two thirds of prose literacy, and 68% have difficulty in locating and processing numeric information. Illiteracy appears to be independent of visual impairments in older adults (Kirsch et al., 1993). Four out of five older adults have difficulty in filling out forms, reading and following directions, and using schedules. While functional illiteracy exists in all segments of society and in all geographic areas, particularly non-suburban areas (Kirsch et al., 1993), it is highly correlated with poverty, education, income, and occupation (Kirsch et al., 1993). In spite of these documented low literacy skills, most older adults with low literacy skills described themselves as reading and writing English well or very well (Kirsch et al., 1993), so it is important that health professionals develop strategies to assess literacy other than self-reported ability.

Many studies have demonstrated that the majority of current health education strategies and materials are not appropriate for a large number of older adults (Baker, Parker, Williams, Clark, & Nurss, 1997; Doak, Doak, & Root, 1995; Weiss, Reed, & Kligman, 1995; Weiss & Coyne, 1997). Even if written materials are at a grade level appropriate for elders with low literacy skills, factors such as the conceptual complexity, tone of the text, or visual layout of the passage may render the materials ineffective (Plimpton & Root, 1994). Taking into account the literacy level of many elders, intervention and evaluation materials and delivery channels need to be selected and designed with this subgroup of the population in mind. The reader is referred to recent publications for more detailed information in developing materials for low-literacy populations (e.g., Doak et al., 1995; Plimpton & Root, 1994; Weiss & Coyne, 1997).

Language

Language is a major part of culture. In immigrant populations, many older adults have never mastered English and older women, in particular, may have had few opportunities or need to communicate outside their home and their ethnic enclave. Older men may have learned enough English to "get by" on the job, but their wives may not have had the same need.

Being able to speak the language of the culture in which an individual lives helps to foster communication and increase understanding. Uba (1992) noted the importance of being able to speak and comprehend the language well enough to make medical appointments, convey symptoms, or understand instructions. Cultural barriers such as values, attitudes, and health beliefs and practices are difficult to convey with a restricted command and understanding of the language. Acquisition of language skills varies with the level of acculturation or adoption of the dominant culture.

In some immigrant populations, both recent and well established, there is a resistance to abandoning familiar cultural and social norms to adopt the values and language of the new culture (Locke, 1992). Many older people, especially women, live within such ethnic enclaves and exist with minimal English skills. Therefore, it becomes important in many multicultural settings to present linguistically and culturally appropriate advertising and educational materials to enhance participation, especially from the elderly. Materials with graphic or pictorial content may prove useful in a very diverse community. Similarly, verbally presented information is sometimes better understood that something in writing that is open to cultural interpretation (Huff & Kline, 1999b). In addition, one cannot assume that foreign speakers are literate in their own languages.

To allay misunderstanding and to create a positive working relationship, it may be critical to have culturally sensitive staff who are fluent in the language and dialect of the target populations. This becomes problematic when there are several spoken and written languages, often with different dialects, present in the community.

Communication barriers include not only issues with English as a second language or literacy, but the barriers to health care that may be related to the actual encounter between the health provider and the client. These encounters may involve class distinctions shown in utilization of language, ineffective and/or inappropriate vocabulary, mutual misunderstanding, and stigma and labeling messages given by the health provider or researcher (Habermas, 1984).

Spirituality

Spirituality is an important factor in the culture and lives of many people. Religious views may influence such varying areas as diet, dress, grooming, and the suitability of certain physical activities in daily life. Some individuals with strong cultural roots often see spirituality as an important part of health and the prevention and response to disease (Jack et al., 1994; Lassiter, 1995; Murray & Rubel, 1992; Waldfogel, 1997). Illness or disability may be seen by some groups as a problem of spiritual disharmony or being taken over by spirits (Fadiman, 1998; Kramer, 1992; Lyon, 1996; Waldfogel, 1997).

Understanding a group's religious or spiritual beliefs is very important because it may influence how information is explained and delivered. For example, it may be inappropriate to present a program on a certain day of the week, or a group may find some material offensive. It can be helpful to involve the local community's religious leaders at the planning stage to help avoid such problems.

Acculturation

Adoption of cultural traits or social patterns of a new society vary with the level of acculturation and assimilation of the individual (Huff & Kline, 1999c). Some immigrants focus on learning the language and customs of a new community as quickly as possible, while others cling to their old traditions tenaciously. In most immigrant communities, there is a spectrum ranging from those who eagerly adopt the new culture to those who reject everything that seems new and foreign to them. Often the first generation of immigrants remain more wedded to the old country's language and customs, while their children and grandchildren immediately engage in the mainstream culture and quickly become fluent in English. The health professional needs to understand this continuum of acculturation and how it may influence beliefs about health in the target community.

Residence Patterns

Residence patterns are closely related to issues of income, social class, and culture (Huff & Kline, 1999b). The environmental conditions of participants may be a significant influence on recruitment, retention, and participation. Researchers and project planners must consider the daily environmental realities of participants. There are many

questions to ask about the environment in which the target population lives: Are the residents living in high crime areas? Is personal
safety a concern? Are there accessible places to exercise nearby? Are
they in crowded housing, in rural areas, in suburbs, or in an inner
city? What public transportation is available? Does the residential
setting make the planned intervention impractical? What resources
are available where multicultural older adults feel safe and welcome?
To be successful, programs must be tailored to meet environmental challenges.

APPLYING THE TRANSTHEORETICAL MODEL TO
MULTICULTURAL OLDER POPULATIONS

Even with the knowledge of the potential benefits of increased physical activity and exercise in older adults, achieving long-term lifestyle
change remains as much of a challenge in older adults as it is in
individuals of all ages (Dishman, 1994; Sallis & Owen, 1999; Shepard,
1994). Attempts at physical activity and promotion delivered through
traditional methods have generally achieved disappointing results
and poor short- and long-term adherence (Sallis & Owen, 1999;
Shepard, 1994; Dishman, 1994).

Key constructs of the stage-based TTM (Prochaska & DiClemente,
1983) have been applied to exercise behavior in adult community
and work site-based adult populations by several researchers with
promising results (Prochaska & Marcus, 1994; Marcus et al., 1997;
Marcus et al., 1998; Marcus et al., 1992). The application of the
TTM in older adult populations has been limited, however, and
there still is much to be understood (Barke & Nicholas, 1990; Clark,
Kviz, Prohaska, Crittended, & Warnecke, 1995; Courneya, 1995;
Crane et al., 1998; Gorely & Gordon, 1995; Hellman, 1997; Nigg et
al., 1999; Rakowski et al., 1998).

Further complicating the application of the TTM is its lack of use
in underserved populations, such a minority groups and persons of
low income (Audrain et al., 1997; Kelaher et al., 1999; Lafferty,
Heaney, & Chen, 1999; Laforge, Velicer, Richmond, & Owen, 1999;
Lee, 1993; Ruggiero & deGroot, 1998). Even less attention has been
given to the adaptation and application of the TTM in multicultural
older adult populations (Lee, 1993). One pilot study used the TTM to

explore Mexican women's (over age 65 and of lower socioeconomic status) readiness to exercise and their multiple roles. Findings indicated that the majority of women fell in stages of precontemplation and contemplation with stages of change and role commitments not significantly related (Gonzalez & Jirovec, 2001).

As noted previously, most studies of physical activity behavior change have been in White, middle-class populations. Theoretical assumptions have been built and tested on well assimilated people of Western European background with minimal consideration of the additional variables of culture and socioeconomic status that is needed when attempting to influence change in a multicultural population. While the TTM is presented here as a sound, rational, and suitable framework to use in promoting healthy lifestyle behaviors among older adults who happen to be ethnically diverse, there is still a lack of experience in applying this theoretical model to diverse populations of both older and younger adults.

THE TRANSTHEORETICAL MODEL: APPLICATION AT SEVERAL SITES OF RESEARCH

Multiple challenges arise when applying models of behavior change to a diverse elder population. Most of these are addressed during the research design phase, while others require reassessment, attention, and adjustment during the intervention process. The following discussion will focus on the authors' experiences with some of the issues that surfaced in an effort to design and tailor culturally sensitive, behavior change/health promotion research for older adults with varied cultural heritage. Lessons learned from research are also relevant for practice as an exercise program was initiated as part of the research project.

Senior*cise*: A Pilot Study Promoting Health Behavior Change in Older Adults

An early pilot study using community-based exercise interventions presented by the interdisciplinary university research team met with some unexpected recruitment and data collection difficulties. The pilot study was based on the TTM model and was designed to address behavior change in several hundred older adults living in the community. Both urban and suburban housing complexes located around the small state of Rhode Island served as intervention sites.

The initial recruitment impact was positive in all enrolled sites with the exception of an urban site where resident composition revealed a more multicultural and economically disadvantaged population than the other sites involved in the study. Standard recruitment strategies did not work with the older residents living at this inner city high-rise. Regardless of the management's endorsement of the program, residents did not respond to our invitations to join the exercise program. It was difficult to get them to leave their apartments.

Issues of literacy, poverty, mental illness, safety, comorbidity, and conflict of values were some of the items that surfaced as barriers to participation in an exercise group for the inner city high-rise. The complex is one of many government subsidized, elderly housing sites that is required by law to reserve a certain percentage of the units for physically and mentally challenged residents of all ages. Soon after the study began, a murder occurred in one of the elevators, increasing anxiety and unwillingness to answer the door. Residents were concerned about whether it was going to be safe for them to leave their apartments, when the best time to leave would be, and who would be in the halls or lobby. Our group was unknown and new to the residents, although university nursing students were frequent visitors to the site and were currently providing services to the residents.

Many residents could not read, understand, or speak English, the language of the researchers. Most of those who had English as their first language had not finished the eighth grade. Having limited literacy skills was a handicap for those persons confronted with the highly structured, time-intensive TTM baseline assessment. Some were surviving substance abusers who had advanced into old age with the attitude, "I've made it this far, why should I change?" Some had worked hard physically throughout their lives and did not intend to exercise now when they could rest in old age. For many, living in poverty had limited their worldview and outlook for the future.

After further assessment of the project, it became apparent that economic, time, and sociocultural limitations had clouded the perception of the barriers faced at the site. The goal of gaining resident's acceptance and cooperation suffered under the veil of inadequate cultural assessment and planning. A mistaken assumption was that this site could be treated like any other site in the study. Even if successful at getting a small group together to exercise, behavior change with residents living there would have been negligible at best. From the perspective of the TTM, the residents may have all been in the precontemplation or contemplation stages because of overwhelming social and environmental barriers. Even completion of interviews and assessment of stages of change was difficult because of issues of language, meaning, mistrust, and fear. This situation did, however, create a significant educational opportunity for everyone involved in the pilot study. One conclusion was that the marginal populations that often live in urban, low-income housing need changes at the structural level to improve their health (Cockerham, 2000; Robert & House, 2000; Wallace, 2000). The ideological hegemony, or prevailing view, in the present medical industrial complex is that health promotion efforts should focus downstream, at the individual behavioral level. This is not what is needed first by vulnerable, high-risk populations who are not members of the dominant social classes. Programs that focus on healthy individual lifestyles and behavior change are not client-focused for the underserved and marginal populations that also happen to be older adults (Cockerham, 2000; Robert & House, 2000; Wallace, 2000). In such extreme situations, structural changes focused on broader issues of environmental safety, meeting survival needs, and access to health care must occur first.

The SENIOR Project: A Study of Exercise and Nutrition in Older Adults

Overview of Study

The SENIOR Project, or the Study of Exercise and Nutrition in Older Rhode Islanders, is a stage-based health promotion project with older adults that is currently underway. The study represents a partnership of the City of East Providence, the University of Rhode Island, and the National Institute on Aging (NIA). The goal is to apply the TTM to increase physical activity and promote the adoption of a diet high in fruits and vegetables in a manner appropriate for large numbers of older people. A large sample ($N = 1,300$) older adults is being recruited to participate in the study.

The intervention site, East Providence, Rhode Island, was chosen because of its significant proportion (20%) of older persons and large subgroups of multicultural and non-English speaking residents that exist in this elder population. The community has three major ethnic groups: Portuguese, Irish, and Italians, as well as smaller representations of other groups. People of Portuguese ethnicity and Cape Verdeans officially comprise slightly more than 40% of the total population. A working-class majority with basic educational achievement is suggested by the educational, occupation, and income data from the 1990 census, although there are pockets of affluent, well-educated elders in some areas of the city (U.S. Bureau of the Census, 1990b). Study participants are community dwelling older persons 65 years of age and older. All interviews are being conducted in person, mostly in the participant's residence, with the planned educational interventions being delivered by mail and telephone.

Meeting the Challenges of Community Acceptance and Cultural Sensitivity

As this project began, the immediate and ongoing challenge for the researchers was to allay mistrust, overcome the perceptions of being outsiders, and gain recognition with the ultimate goal of being accepted and embraced by the community. The significant endeavor to recruit and retain 1,300 older individuals will never be realized without the help of local advocates and community involvement.

One of the first steps in the long continuum of project planning and development was to add a cultural anthropologist to the research team. He served as an adviser to the team and staff on cultural issues and recruitment strategies and helped to expand cultural awareness and cultural competence. Campinha-Becote (1994) defines cultural competence as "a process of effectively working within a cultural context of an individual or community from a diverse cultural or ethnic background." This is necessary if successful research is to be conducted with multiethnic groups.

Another initial step was to meet with representatives of the East Providence community, including staff from the planning department, the senior center director and nurse, and other officials to discuss planning and development strategies. They also served as essential advisors to the research team. The establishment of a community advisory committee was seen as crucial both as a guide in cultural and community matters and as a community resource. Representatives from several organizations, agencies, associations, and community groups, including major cultural and ethnic groups are members. Both of these advisory groups will meet throughout the 4-year study.

A project site office was established and staffed in the central part of the city. Specific activities, lectures on health topics and blood pressure clinics, for example, are being offered to build visibility, credibility, and trust in the community.

Development and Adaptation of Intervention Materials

The development and adaptation of intervention materials began with focus groups and pilot surveys that were conducted in other comparable populations of older adults. Because the intervention targets the senior population, it was decided that the approach and materials must be generally directed at older adults and not overtly focus on any specific ethnic group, yet it was agreed they must be sensitive to ethnic interests. Originally, consideration was given to translating all materials into Portuguese to enable participation of non-English-speaking Portuguese and Cape Verdeans. It soon became apparent that within the ethnic groups, 78 various dialects of Portuguese were spoken, usually dependent on country of origin, and Creole, the spoken language of many Cape Verdeans, had no written language. Translation of the numerous TTM educational materials including manuals, newsletters, and expert system reports, in addition to having Portuguese-speaking interviewers and counselors available, would have been a significant expense with little guarantee of return.

Due to financial limitations, a compromise was reached regarding translation feasibility. Translating the assessment instrument to convey the intended meaning proved difficult because some of the words did not exist in Portuguese or carried several different meanings. The assessment questionnaire was translated and made available for use by the Portuguese speaking interviewers and as an aid to interpreting the TTM concept language for English-as-a-second-language speakers.

A decision was made to translate the recruitment brochure into Portuguese, with the intention of attracting Portuguese participants who could read some English, possibly with the help of a bilingual interviewer. When the Portuguese brochure was given to independent readers for feedback and reaction, the difficulties of cross-cultural translation again occurred as we tried to back-translate words such as "home" and "marketplace" and got a different interpretation from three independent translators. After much discussion, translation decisions were made and this brochure was used successfully.

SUMMARY

Providing physical activity and health promotion programs for populations of underserved older adults who belong to ethnic and cultural minority groups often presents a challenge to the health care professional. It is clear that program designs need to be culturally sensitive and delivered in a manner that will enhance the understandability and acceptance of the programs. However, theoretical models have not often been applied to these populations leaving the research and/or health care professional unable to draw on the experience of others in providing these programs. Thus, providers may feel as though they are marching through uncharted territory, hoping for the best results. To help meet this need, the Health Education Authority in Great Britain has produced a guide to promoting physical activity with Black and minority elders as part of its "Active for Life" program (Health Education Act, 1996). This is an example of an effort to address specific needs and barriers that may be experienced differently among a multiethnic population.

Providing population-based, community interventions is more difficult when the target population is multicultural. What may work with one group may be ineffective for another group, and it is often not possible to design several different programs to meet the needs of all. This leaves the professional with the challenge of trying to bridge the cultural gaps while developing one program that will have efficacy for the majority of the target population.

The prevalence of chronic issues and socioeconomic conditions such as poverty and social isolation is higher in many older adults who belong to minority groups; these factors further complicate the ability to provide programs that result in health behavior change. However, it is these very elders who most need health promotion interventions. The best the health professional can do is to draw on experience with various populations of younger adults and hope the information gleaned will apply to a target population of older adults who may be living in different circumstances and most certainly have different life experiences.

The challenge is clear, but there is reason for optimism. More research is being conducted in this underserved population of older adults and knowledge is being developed about the elements and factors that improve the effectiveness of health promotion programs. Behavioral approaches, including the TTM, appear to improve the adoption and maintenance of health behavior change in older adults. Sociopolitical interventions at the system level are needed to bring about necessary change.

It must be remembered, however, that the older adult population is changing dramatically, both in the proportion of older adults in the total population as well as the demographics of the elderly. These facts, interacting with rapidly changing culture and technology, means that future generations of older adults will come to old age with much different life experiences and expectations and be influenced by a significantly different cultural milieu.

REFERENCES

Airhihenbuwa, C., Kumanyika, S., Agure, T., & Lowe, A. (1995). Perceptions and beliefs about exercise, rest and health among African-Americans. *Journal of Health Promotion, 9*(6), 426–429.

American College of Sports Medicine: ACSM Position Stand on Exercise and Physical Activity for Older Adults (1998). *Medicine and Science in Sports and Exercise, 30*(6), 992–1008.

Arean, P., & Gallagher-Thompson, D. (1996). Issues and recommendations for the recruitment and retention of older minority adults into clinical research. *Journal of Consulting and Clinical Psychology, 64*(5), 875–880.

Audrain, J., Gomez-Caminero, A., Robertson, A., Boyd, R., Orleans, C., & Lerman, C. (1997). Gender and ethnic differences in readiness to change smoking behavior. *Womans Health, 3*(2), 139–150.

Baker, D. W., Parker, R. M., Williams, M. V., Clark, W. S., & Nurss, J. (1997). The relationship of patient reading ability to self-reported health and use of health services. *American Journal of Public Health, 87,* 1027–1030.

Barke, C. R., & Nicolas, P. R. (1990). Physical activity in older adults: The stages of change. *Journal of Applied Gerontology, 9,* 216–223.

Brenes, G. A., Strube, M. J., & Storandt, M. (1998). Application of the theory of planned behavior to exercise among older adults. *Journal of Applied Social Psychology, 28,* 2274–2290.

Brown, P. (1989). Psychiatric dirty work revisited: Conflicts in servicing nonpsychiatric agencies. *Journal of Contemporary Ethnography, 18*(2), 182–201.

Campinha-Bacote, J. (1994). Cultural competence in psychiatric mental health nursing: A conceptual model. *Nursing Clinics of North America, 29*(1), 1–8.

Clark, D. O. (1999). Physical activity and its correlates among urban primary care patients aged 55 years and older. *Journal of Gerontology Social Sciences, 54B,* S41–S48.

Clark, M., Kviz, F., Prohaska, T., Crittenden, K., & Warnecke, R., (1995). Readiness of older adults to stop smoking in a television intervention. *Journal of Aging and Health, 7*(1), 119–138.

Cockerham, W. C. (2000). The sociology of health behavior and health lifestyles. In C. E. Bird, P. Conrad, & A. M. Fremont (Eds.), *Handbook of medical sociology* (5th ed., pp. 159–172). Upper Saddle River, NJ: Prentice Hall.

Conrad, P., & Schneider, J. (1992). *Deviance and medicalization: From boldness to sickness.* Philadelphia: Temple University Press.

Courneya, K. S. (1995). Perceived severity of the consequences of physical inactivity across the stages of change in older adults. *Journal of Sport and Exercise Psychology, 17,* 447–457.

Courneya, K. S., Nigg, C. R., & Estabrooks, P. A. (1998). Relationships among the theory of planned behavior, stages of change, and exercise behavior in older persons over a three year period. *Psychology and Health, 13,* 355–367.

Crane, L. A., Leakey, T. A., Rimer, B. K., Wolfe, P., Woodworth, M. A., & Warnecke, R. B. (1998). Effectiveness of a telephone outcall intervention to promote screening mammography among low-income women. *Preventive Medicine, 27*(5 Part 2), S39–S49.

Crawford, R. (1986). Individual responsibility and health politics. In P. Conrad & R. Kern (Eds.), *The sociology of health and illness: Critical perspectives* (pp. 369–377). New York: St. Martin's Press.

Dishman, R. K. (1994). Introduction: Consensus, problems, and prospects. In R. K. Dishman (Ed.), *Advances in exercise adherence.* Champaign, IL: Human Kinetics.

Doak, C. C., Doak, L. G., & Root, J. (1995). *Teaching patients with low literacy skills* (2nd ed.). Philadelphia: J. B. Lippincott.

Everard, K. M., Lach, H. W., Fisher, E. B., & Baum, M. C. (2000). Relationship of activity and social support to the functional health of older adults. *Journal of Gerontology: Social Sciences, 55B,* S208–S212.

Fadiman, A. (1998). *The spirit catches you and you fall down.* New York: Farrar, Strauss, and Giroux.

Federal Interagency Forum on Aging Related Statistics. (2000). *Older Americans 2000: Key indicators of well being.* Hyattsville, MD: Author.

Ferrales, S. (1996). Vietnamise. In J. G. Lipson, S. L. Dibble, & P. A. Minark (Eds.), *Culture & nursing care: A pocket guide.* San Francisco, CA: UCSF Nursing Press.

Ferrucci, L., Guralnik, J. M., Simonsick, E., Salive, M. E., Corti, C., & Langlois, J. (1996). Progressive versus catastrophic disability: A longitudinal view of the disablement process. *Journal of Gerontology Series A-Biological Sciences & Medical Sciences, 51*(3), M123–M130.

Fitzgerald, J., Singleton, S., Neale, A., Prasad, A., & Hess, J. (1994). Activity levels, fitness status, exercise knowledge, and exercise beliefs among healthy, older African American and White women. *Journal of Aging and Health, 6,* 296–313.

Fletcher, G. F. (1997). How to implement physical activity in primary and secondary prevention: A statement for healthcare professionals from the task force on risk reduction, American Heart Association. *Circulation, 96,* 355–357.

Frankish, C. J., Lovato, C. Y., & Shannon, W. J. (1999). Models, theories and principles of health promotion with multicultural populations. In R. M. Huff & M. V. Kline (Eds.), *Promoting health in multicultural populations: A handbook for practitioners* (pp. 47–72). Thousand Oaks, CA: Sage.

Freidson, E. (1970). *Professional dominance.* New York: Atherton Press.

Fuller-Thompson, E., Minkler, M., & Driver, D. (1997). A profile of grandparents raising grandchildren in the United States. *The Gerontologist, 37,* 406–411.

Giger, J., & Davidhizar, R. (1999). *Transcultural nursing.* St. Louis: Mosby.

Glaser, B., & Strauss, A. (1965). *Awareness of dying.* Chicago: Aldene.

Gonzalez, B. C., & Jirovec, M. M. (2001). Elderly Mexican woman's perceptions of exercise and conflicting role responsibilities. *International Journal of Nursing Studies, 38*(1), 45–49.

Gorely, T., & Gordon, S. (1995). An examination of the transtheoretical model and exercise behavior in older adults. *Journal of Sport and Exercise Psychology, 17,* 312–324.

Gould, M. (1999). Care of black and ethnic minority elders. In S. J. Redfern & F. M. Ross (Eds.), *Nursing older people* (3rd ed., pp. 111–122). New York: Churchhill Livingstone.

Habermas, J. (1971). *Knowledge and human interests.* Boston: Bacon.

Habermas, J. (1984). *The theory of communicative action: Reason and the rationalization of society.* Boston: Beacon Press.

Hazuda, H. P., Gerety, M., Williams, J. W., Jr., Lawrence, V., Calembach, W., & Mulrow, C. (2000). Health promotion research with Mexican American elders: Matching approaches to settings at the mediator- and micro-levels of recruitment. *Journal of Mental Health and Aging, 6*(1), 79–90.

Health Education Authority. (1996). *Guidelines: Promoting physical activity with black and minority groups.* London: HEA.

Hellman, E. A. (1997). Use of the stages of change in exercise adherence model among older adults with cardiac diagnosis. *Journal of Cardiopulmonary Rehabilitation, 17*(3), 145–155.

Horkheimer, M. (1972). *Critical theory.* New York: Herder & Herder.

Hudson, S. V., Leventhal, H., Contrada, R., Leventhal, E. A., & Brownlee, S. (2000). Predicting retention for older African Americans in a community study and clinical study: Does anything work? *Journal of Mental Health and Aging, 6*(1), 2000.

Huff, R. M. (1999). Cross-cultural concepts of health and disease. In R. M. Huff & M. V. Kline (Eds.), *Promoting health in multicultural populations: A handbook for practitioners* (pp. 23–39). Thousand Oaks, CA: Sage.

Huff, R. M., & Kline, M. V. (1999a). Health promotion in the context of culture. In R. M. Huff & M. V. Kline (Eds.), *Promoting health in multicultural populations: A handbook for practitioners* (pp. 3–22). Thousand Oaks, CA: Sage.

Huff, R. M., & Kline, M. V. (1999b).The cultural assessment framework. In R. M. Huff & M. V. Kline (Eds.), *Promoting health in multicultural populations: A handbook for practitioners* (pp. 481–489). Thousand Oaks, CA: Sage.

Huff, R. M., & Kline, M. V. (1999c). *Promoting health in multicultural populations: A handbook for practitioners.* Thousand Oaks, CA: Sage.

Hufford, D. J. (1997). Complementary and alternative therapies in primary care: Folk medicine. *Primary Care; Clinics in Office Practice, 24*(4), 724–741.

Ishida, D. N., Toomata-Mayer, T. E., & Mayer, J. E. (1996). Samoans. In J. G. Lipson, S. L. Dibble, & P. A. Minarik (Eds.), *Culture and nursing care: A pocket guide.* San Francisco: USCF Nursing Press.

Jack, L., Harrison, I. E., & Airhihenbuwa, C. O. (1994). Ethnicity and the health belief systems. In A. C. Matiella (Ed.), *The multicultural challenge in health education.* Santa Cruz, CA: ETR Associates.

Jackson, J., & Curry, L. (Chairpersons). Involving older ethnic minorities in health related research. Preconference workshop presented at the Gerontology Society of America Meeting, November 19, 1999. Supported by a National Institute of Aging grant R13 AG17581-01.

Jones, D. A., Ainsworth, B. E., Croft, J. B., Macera, C. A., Lloyd, E. E., & Yusuf, H. R. (1998). Moderate leisure-time physical activity: Who is meeting the public health recommendations? A national cross-sectional study. *Archive of Family Medicine, 7,* 285–289.

Kelaher, M., Gillespie, A. G., Allotey, P., Manderson, L., Potts, H., Sheldrake, M., Young, M., & Joseph, L. (1999). The Transtheoretical Model and cervical screening: Its application among culturally diverse communities in Queensland, Australia. *Ethnic Health, 4*(4), 259–276.

Kirsch, I. S., Jungeblut, A., Jenkins, L., & Kolstad, A. (1993). *Adult literacy in America: A first look at the results of the national adult literacy survey.* Washington, DC: National Center for Education Statistics, U.S. Department of Education, U.S. Government Printing Office.

Kramer, B. (1992). Health and aging of urban American Indians. *Western Journal of Medicine, 157,* 281–285. (Special issue)

Lafferty, C. K., Heaney, C. A., & Chen, M. S., Jr. (1999). Assessing decisional balance for smoking cessation among Southeast Asian males in the U.S. *Health Education Research, 14*(1), 139–146.

Laforge, R., Velicer, W., Richmond, R., & Owen, N. (1999). Stage distributions for five health behaviors in the U.S. and Australia. *Preventive Medicine, 28*(1), 61–74.

Larson, E. B. (1992). Benefits of exercise for older adults, a review of existing evidence and current recommendations for the general populations. *Clinics in Geriatric Medicine, 8*(1), 35–50.

Lassiter, S. M. (1995). *Multicultural clients: A professional handbook for health care providers and social workers.* Westport, CT: Greenwood.

Lee, C. (1993). Attitudes, knowledge and stages of change: A survey of exercise patterns in older Australian women. *Health Psychology, 12,* 476–480.

Leventhal, E. A., Leventhal, H., & Robitelli, C. (1998). Enhancing self-care in research: Exploring the theoretical underpinnings of self-care. In M. G. Ory & G. DeFriese (Eds.), *Self-care in later life* (pp. 118–141). New York: Springer.

Levkoff, S. E., Prohaska, T. R., Weitzman, F. P., & Ory, M. G. (2000). Preface. In S. E. Levkoff, T. R. Prohaska, F. P. Weitzman, & M. G. Ory (Eds.), *Recruitment and retention in minority populations: Lessons learned in conducting research on health promotion and minority aging* (pp. 5–7). New York: Springer.

Locke, D. C. (1992). *Increasing multicultural understanding:* A comprehensive understanding. Newbury Park, CA: Sage.

Lyon, W. S. (1996). *Encyclopedia of Native American healing.* Santa Barbara, CA: ABC-CLIO.

Marcus, B. H., Banspach, S. W., Lefebvre, R. C., Rossi, J. S., Carleton, R. A., & Abrams, D. B. (1992). Using the stages of change model to increase the adoption of physical activity among community participants. *American Journal of Health Promotion, 6*(6), 424–429.

Marcus, B. H., Bock, B. C., Pinto, B. M., Forsyth, L. H., Roberts, M. B., & Traficante, R. M. (1998). Efficacy of an individualized, motivationally tailored physical activity intervention. *Annals of Behavioral Medicine, 20*(3), 75–86.

Marcus, B. H., Emmons, K. M., Simkin-Silverman, L., Linnan, L. A., Taylor, E. R., Bock, B. C., Roberts, M. B., Rossi, J. S., & Abrams, D. B. (1997). Evaluation of motivationally tailored vs. standard self-help physical activity interventions at the workplace. *American Journal of Health Promotion, 12*(4), 246–253.

Markides, K. S., & Miranda, M. R. (Eds.). (1997). *Minorities, aging, and health.* Thousand Oaks, CA: Sage.

Martin, L. G., & Soldo, B. J. (Eds.). (1997). *Racial and ethnic differences in the health of older Americans.* Washington, DC: National Academy.

McAuley, E., Marquez, D., Jerome, G., & Blissmer, B. (2000). Physical activity effects on social support: Generalized or specific? *The Gerontologist, 40,* A47.

Minkler, M. (1992). Community organizing among the elderly poor in the Unites States: A case study. *International Journal of Health Services, 22,* 303–316.

Mo, B. (1992). Cross-cultural medicine a decade later: Modesty, sexuality and breast health in Chinese Americans. *Western Journal of Medicine, 9,* 260–264.

Murray, R. H., & Rubel, A. J. (1992). Sounding board: Physicians and healers: Unwitting partners in health care. *New England Journal of Medicine, 326*(1), 61–64.

Myers, A. H., Young, Y., & Langlois, J. A. (1996). Prevention of falls in the elderly. *Bone, 18,* 87S–101S.

Nigg, C. R., Burbank, P. M., Padula, C., Dufresne, R., Rossi, J. S., Velicer, W. E., Laforge, R. G., & Prochaska, J. O. (1999). Stages of change across ten health risk behaviors for older adults. *The Gerontologist, 39,* 473–482.

Nunnally, E., & Moy, C. (1989). *Communication basics for health service professionals.* Newberry Park, CA: Sage.

O'Brien Cousins, S. (2000). "My heart couldn't take it": Older woman's beliefs about exercise benefits and risks. *Journal of Gerontology; Psychological Sciences, 55B*(5), P283–P294.

Ory, M. G., Lipman, P. D., Barr, R., Harden, J. T., & Stahl, S. M. (2000). A national program to enhance research on minority aging and health promotion. In S. E. Levkoff, T. R. Prohaska, F. P. Weitzman, & M. G. Ory (Eds.), *Recruitment and retention in minority populations: Lessons learned in conducting research on health promotion and minority aging*. New York: Springer.

Patcher, L. M. (1994). Culture and clinical care: Folk illness beliefs and behaviors and their implications for health care delivery. *Journal of the American Medical Association, 271,* 690–694.

Paniagua, F. A. (1994). *Assessing and treating culturally diverse clients: A practical guide*. Thousand Oaks, CA: Sage.

Plimpton, S., & Root, J. (1994). Materials and strategies that work in low literacy health communication. *Public Health Reports, 109,* 86–92.

Prochaska, J. O., & DiClemente, C. C. (1983). Stages and processes of self-change of smoking: Toward an integrative model of change. *Consultations in Clinical Psychology, 51,* 390–395.

Prochaska, J. O., & Marcus, B. (1994). The Transtheoreticl Model: Applications to exercise. In R. K. Dishman (Ed.), *Advances in exercise adherence*. Champaign, IL: Human Kinetics.

Prohaska, T. R., Walcott-McQuigg, J., & Peters, K. (2000). Recruitment of older African Americans into church-based programs. In S. E. Levkoff, T. R. Prohaska, F. P. Weitzman, & M. G. Ory (Eds.), *Recruitment and retention in minority populations: Lessons learned in conducting research on health promotion and minority aging*. New York: Springer.

Purrell, L. D., & Paulanka, B. J. (Eds.). (1998). *Transcultural health care: A culturally competent approach*. Philadelphia: Davis.

Rakowski, W., Ehrich, B., Goldstein, M. G., Rimer, B. K., Pearlman, D. N., Clark, M. A., Velicer, W. F., & Woolverton, H. (1998). Increasing mammography among women aged 40–74 by use of a stage-matched, tailored intervention. *Preventive Medicine, 27,* 748–756.

Reissman, C. (1986). Improving health experiences of low-income patients. In P. Conrad & R. Kern (Eds.), *The sociology of health and illness: Critical perspectives*. New York: St. Martin's Press.

Richter, D. L., Macera, C. A., Williams, H., & Koerber, M. (1993). Disincentives to participate in planned exercise activities among older adults. *Health Values, 17,* 51–55.

Robert, S. A., & House, J. S. (2000). Socioeconomic inequalities in health: An enduring sociological problem. In C. E. Bird, P. Conrad, & A. M. Fremont (Eds.), *Handbook of medical sociology* (5th ed.). Upper Saddle River, NJ: Prentice Hall.

Ruggiero, L., & deGroot, M. (1998). Smoking patterns of low-income ethno-culturally diverse pregnant women: Are we casting the net wide enough? *Addictive Behavior, 23*(4), 549–554.

Ryan, W. (1971). *Blaming the victim.* New York: Vintage Books.

Salimbene, S. (2000). *What language does your patient hurt in?: A practical guide to culturally competent patient care.* Amherst, MA: Diversity Resources.

Sallis, J., & Owen, N. (1999). *Physical activity and behavioral medicine.* London: Sage Publications.

Sharpe, P., & Connell, C. (1992). Exercise beliefs and behaviors among older employees: A health promotion trial. *The Gerontologist, 32*(4), 444–448.

Shepard, R. J. (1994). Determinants of exercise in people aged 65 years and older. In R. K. Dishman (Ed.), *Advances in exercise adherence.* Champaign, IL: Human Kinetics.

Skinner, C. S., Campbell, M. K., Rimer, B. K., Curry, S., & Prochaska, J. O. (1999). How effective is tailored print communication? *Annals of Behavioral Medicine, 21*(4), 290–298.

Spector, R. E. (1996). *Cultural diversity in health and illness* (4th ed.). Stamford, CT: Appleton & Lange.

Spencer, G., & Hollman, F. (1998). *National population projections, U.S. Census Bureau, the Official Statistics,* September 21, 1998. Washington, DC: U.S. Department of Commerce, Bureau of the Census.

Stead, M., Wimbush, E., Eadie, D., & Teer, P. (1997). A qualitative study of older people's perceptions of aging and exercise: The implications for health promotion. *The Health Education Journal, 56,* 3–16.

The Nation's Health: The Official Newspaper of the American Public Health Association. October, 2000.

The Nation's Health: The Official Newspaper of the American Public Health Association. December 2000/January 2001.

Tinetti, M. E., Doucette, J., Claus, E., & Marottoli, R. (1995). Risk factors for serious injury during falls by older persons in the community. *Journal of the American Geriatric Society, 43*(11), 1214–1221.

Tripp-Reimer, T., Johnson, R., & Rios, H. (1994). Cultural dimensions in gerontological nursing. In M. Stanley & P. G. Beare (Eds.), *Gerontological nursing.* Philadelphia: Lippincott.

Uba, L. (1992). Cultural barriers to health care for Southeast Asian refuges. *Public Health Reports, 107,* 545–548.

U.S. Department of Commerce, Bureau of the Census (1990a). *Social and Economical Characteristics of Selected Language Groups for U.S. and States.* Washington, DC: Author.

U.S. Department of Commerce, Bureau of the Census (1990b). *East Providence, Rhode Island Community Profile.* Washington, DC: Author.

U.S. Department of Health and Human Services. Public Health Service (2000). *Healthy People 2010, 2nd ed. With Understanding and Improving Health and Objectives for Improving Health.* Washington, DC: Author.

U.S. Department of Health and Human Services. Public Health Service (1996). *Physical Activity and Health: A Report of the Surgeon General.* Atlanta, GA: Author.

U.S. Preventive Services Task Force (1996). *Guide to clinical preventive services* (2nd ed.). Baltimore: Williams and Wilkins

Vertinsky, P. A. (1998). "Run, Jane, run:" Central tensions in the current debate about enhancing women's health through exercise. *Journal of Women & Health, 27*(4), 81–111.

Waldfogel, S. (1997). Complementary and alternative therapies in primary care: Spirituality in medicine. *Primary Care: Clinics in Office Practice, 24*(4), 963–976.

Wallace, S. P. (2000). American health promotion: Where individualism rules. *The Gerontologist, 40*(3), 373–376.

Weiss, B. D., & Coyne, C. (1997). Communicating with patients who cannot read. *New England Journal of Medicine, 337*(4), 272–274.

Weiss, B. D., Reed, R. L., & Kligman, E. W. (1995). Literacy skills and communication methods of low-income older persons. *Patient Education and Counseling, 25,* 109–119.

Whaley, D. E., & Ebbeck, V. (1997). Older adults constraints to participation in structured exercise classes. *Journal of Aging & Physical Activity, 5,* 190–212.

Wolinsky, F., Stump, T., & Clark, D. (1995). Antecedents and consequences of physical activity and exercise among older adults. *The Gerontologist, 35*(4), 452–462.

Zola, I. (1993). Problems with communication, diagnosis, and patient care. *Journal of Medical Education, 38,* 829.

CHAPTER 9

Applying the Transtheoretical Model: Behavior Change Among Family Caregivers and Nursing Staff

Cynthia A. Padula and Patricia M. Burbank

"If we don't change, we don't grow. If we don't grow, we aren't really living"

~Gail Sheehy

One of the critical questions in gerontology today is whether increasing life expectancy will result in improved or declined health and well-being among the aged. Older adults overwhelmingly desire to remain functionally independent within the community, and diminished functional health status is the primary cause of loss of independence. The illnesses of older people tend to be chronic in nature and chronic diseases represent the major underlying causes of physical disability (Fried & Guralnik, 1997).

Decreased functioning in either the physical, cognitive, or sensory domains can limit an older adult's ability to remain independent in the community (Fried & Guralnik, 1997). Physical disability has been identified as a major risk factor for loss of independence in functioning as well as for institutionalization (Feinleib, Cunningham, & Short, 1994; Fried & Guralnik, 1997). An important lifestyle contributor to the onset of physical disability is lack of exercise.

In the United States, more than 40% of people over the age of 65 do not participate in physical activity (United States Department of Health and Human Services [USDHHS], 1991). The American Colleges of Sports Medicine (ACSM) and the Centers for Disease Control (CDC) have recommended an accumulation of 30 minutes or more of moderate intensity physical activity on most (preferably all) days of the week (Pate et al., 1995). Older adults can benefit from regular physical activity, which does not have to be strenuous in order to provide health benefits (USDHHS, 1996a). Numerous benefits of exercise have been documented, including reduction of symptoms of many chronic diseases, improved health and functional status, enhanced quality of life and sense of well-being (Resnick, 2000: USDHHS, 1996b), decreased risk of falling (Province et al., 1995; USDHHS, 1996b), increased strength and aerobic capacity (Greene & Crouse, 1995), and improvements in functional abilities (McMurdo & Rennie, 1993; Skelton & McLaughlin, 1996). Additional benefits continue to be discovered (Marcus, King, Bock, Borrelli, & Clark, 1998). Despite popular belief, and contrary to common stereotypes, elderly persons encounter few complications associated with increased moderate intensity activity (Elward & Larson, 1992). Conversely, lack of exercise has been shown to be significantly associated with the onset of disability (Elward & Larson, 1992).

Despite the health benefits of physical activity, the majority of older adults remain sedentary (CDC, 1993). This finding is somewhat surprising, given that older people, particularly females, practice more health prevention strategies than younger people (Bausell, 1986; Leventhal & Prohaska, 1986). It has been suggested that physical activity can be viewed as a particularly challenging preventive health behavior because of the time and effort involved as well as the issue of regular maintenance (Marcus et al.,1998).

A major difference between younger and older adults is that about 50% of inactive older persons do not intend to start an activity program (Stephens & Craig, 1990). Difficulty with initiating and maintaining a physical activity regimen over time is further evidenced by high dropout rates from organized programs, which have been estimated at about 50% (Dishman, 1990). Positive effects have been demonstrated for short-term adherence to brief programs, but little success has been achieved in improving long-term maintenance (Dishman, 1988) across age groups, including older adults (Robinson & Rogers, 1994). However, individuals have been shown to be more likely to adopt and maintain moderate versus vigorous physical activity (Sallis et al., 1986). This is an important point because moderate activity is consistent with the recently revised joint ACSM and CDC guidelines. Clearly, innovative alternative strategies for behavior change are needed. The Transtheoretical Model of Behavior Change (TTM) offers an exciting alternative to traditional behavior change strategies.

THE TRANSTHEORETICAL MODEL OF BEHAVIOR CHANGE (TTM)

Traditional methods used to change health behaviors, including exercise, have focused primarily on education (Burbank, Padula, & Nigg, 2000). Strategies to increase physical activity need to incorporate an assessment of the needs as well as the barriers of potential participants (Marcus et al., 1998), and need to be individualized and tailored (Elward & Larson, 1992). Exercise behavior may be characterized by a multiple stage model requiring interventions targeted at an individual's stage of change (Dishman, 1990). The Transtheoretical Model of Behavior Change (TTM) (DiClemente et al., 1991; Prochaska & DiClemente, 1983) has been identified as a comprehensive and integrative model that offers a promising alternative to traditional methods. The TTM has been applied with success to numerous health behaviors, and more recently to exercise (Indledeiv, Markland, & Medley, 1998; Marcus et al., 1992; Nigg & Courneya, 1998). Though more limited, research to date has supported the application of the TTM to exercise in older adults (Courneya, 1995; Gorely & Gordon, 1995). A recent review of nine studies using the stages of change model validated that the same five stages of change exist for exercise in older adults (Nigg & Lees, in review).

Interventions based on the TTM tailor treatment to the individual's stage of change (Marcus et al., 1998). However, it must be recognized that individual health experiences are profoundly influenced by family relationships and dynamics. The social environment of older adults, which includes such components as family networks and supports, significant others, caregivers, and living arrangements, has a significant impact on the adoption (Padula, 1996) and maintenance (Murdaugh, 1998) of health behaviors. Some limited attempts have been made to integrate the role of social support into the TTM (Amick & Ockene, 1994), but clearly the impact of social context on individual behavior change is an important area of research that critically needs to be addressed.

When intervening with older adults, it is essential that a family-level perspective be incorporated throughout the process of planning, initiating, and evaluating a physical activity program. A serious limitation of most programs has been failure to recognize the tremendous impact that family and significant others have on a wide variety of lifestyle choices, including physical activity and other health-related issues. Interestingly, research has shown that important reasons for physical activity in older adults include receiving positive feedback from significant others (Duda & Tappe, 1988) as well as social interaction and improved mental health (Gill & Overdorf, 1994). Social support from family and friends has been consistently and positively related to regular physical activity (USDHHS, 1996a). That the immediate family and/or caregiving network would play a central role in health maintenance of the older person makes intuitive sense. Caregivers are integral to the well-being of most older people as they age.

CAREGIVING: INFORMAL AND FORMAL

Eighty-four percent of individuals over the age of 65 who are dependent in activities of daily living (ADLs) or instrumental activities of daily living (IADLs) reside in communities (Hing & Bloom, 1990); 95% of those have family members involved in their care (Administration on Aging, 1999). It is projected that by the year 2001, 2.1 million people over the age of 65 will require assistance with two or more daily activities, with fewer family caregivers available to provide care

(Robinson, 1997). The astounding fact that the overwhelming majority of functionally dependent older adults are able to remain in the community despite significant limitations is directly attributable to the family and the caregiving role. Clearly, most of the day-to-day management of care takes place in the home over an extended period of time, and occurs in the context of an evolving trajectory of care (Corbin & Strauss, 1991).

Informal Caregiving

Family caregiving can be categorized as an informal type of support, in contrast to formal support, supplied by health providers. Over 7 million people are informal caregivers; families have a long history and tradition of caring for impaired relatives at home (Administration on Aging, 1999; Shanas, 1979). It has been suggested that family caregiving has probably been in existence since the beginning of history (Robinson, 1997). Approximately 73% of the time caregivers are women (Stone, Cafferata, & Sangl, 1987), and spouses provide the most intense kind of care over longer periods of time, and with less resources (Montgomery & Datwyler, 1990). Spouses are also less likely to institutionalize (Seltzer & Li, 2000). A hierarchy of caregiving seems to exist (Cantor & Little, 1985) with daughters taking on primary responsibility when the spouse is deceased or unable to provide care (Dwyer, Henretta, Coward, & Barton, 1992).

Family caregiving has been conceptualized in numerous ways, including "the long haul" (Gaynor, 1990), as a career (Pearlin, 1992), and as a solitary journey (Boland & Sims, 1996), yet caregiving is often unplanned, unexpected, and not entered into totally by choice (Pearlin & Aneshensel, 1994). Aneshensel, Pearlin, Mullan, Zarit, and Whitlatch (1995) further identified caregiving as occurring in stages: preparation for caregiving, acquisition, caregiving role enactment, and role disengagement. This conceptualization is helpful in portraying the reality that caregiving generally occurs across a continuum of time and in the context of increasing caregiving demands. One thing is certain: The demands of caregiving increase over time in both a qualitative and quantitative sense. Yet, family caregivers often delay using formal as well as other informal services to provide assistance and support (Chenier, 1997). Families do not relinquish the caregiving role unnecessarily (Ory, Hoffman, Yee, Tennstedt, & Schulz, 1999), but sometimes caregiving demands simply exceed the resources available, and institutionalization in a long-term care facility becomes necessary. In reality, institutionalization is often a reasonable and necessary step in the caregiving trajectory, with the potential to provide the caregiver with much needed respite, and ideally to offer comprehensive, individualized, and family-oriented care.

Despite the many burdens and demands of family caregiving, nursing home placement is generally a very difficult decision (Chenier, 1997). As described by Aneshensel et al. (1995), contemplating the possibility of future nursing home admission requires that caregivers struggle through the process of disengagement from the caregiving role. This is particularly difficult because despite the many challenges and stressors of providing care on a day-to-day basis, caregiving in the home is often highly valued and viewed as a normalizing experience (Boland & Sims, 1996). Indeed, when family caregivers make the difficult and often painful decision to place a family member in a long-term care facility, they generally continue to visit regularly, provide support, and remain active participants in the delivery of care. Family members and care staff tend to have different expectations and beliefs about caregiving (Gladstone & Wexler, 2000), and difficulties in sharing caregiving roles (Kelley, Pringle-Specht, & Mass, 2000a) and implementing truly family-oriented and individualized care are evident.

Formal Caregiving in Long-Term Care Facilities

The importance of individualized care using tailored approaches that respond to the specific resident needs has become increasingly recognized (Werner, Koroknay, Braun, & Cohen-Mansfield, 1994), yet nursing homes have been and continue to be plagued by low nurse staffing levels. In 1995 the average registered nurse (RN), licensed vocational nurse (LVN), and licensed practical nurse (LPN) combined staffing levels were 72 minutes per day per resident, and the majority of care was provided by nursing assistants (NA) (Anonymous, 1998). Nursing assistants represent 70 to 90 percent of nursing staff in long-term care facilities. Extensive research has accumulated relating to the effect on quality of care of RNs providing training and guidance to NAs (Institute of Medicine, 1996), but training received by both NAs and the RNs who train them needs to be enriched (Anonymous, 1996). The nature and extent of employer support for education and training is an important factor influencing nurses' continuing education activities (Ryden & Krichbaum, 1996); unfortunately, overall there is a dearth of training in long-term care (Johncox, 2000). A recent analysis of several research studies indicated that insufficient time, lack of a team approach, unavailability of specific training or role modeling, limited participation of certified nursing assistants (CNA) in care planning, lack of respect for CNAs, and inflexible routines were frequently noted obstacles to implementation of individualized care (Curry, Porter, Michalski, & Gruman, 2000). Clearly, a philosophy of caring in long-term facilities is needed that embraces the essential contributions of all involved in the delivery of care: residents, family members, and all members of the health care team. Furthermore, the social environment of the individual nursing unit has been found to be an important contributor to residents' quality of life, as well as their interactions with other residents and the staff (Herzberg, 1997). The delivery of long-term care is a demanding and challenging responsibility; staff need to be empowered through education and training, reasonable workloads, institutional and peer support and recognition, and monetary compensation that is reasonably competitive with other health care systems. Espousing quality and verbalizing the need for individualized care are truly empty rhetoric without the institutional supports needed to truly effect change. Only then can individualized, family-centered care become a reality, in which family and providers unite to achieve mutually agreed upon goals.

Families bring their own expertise, often accumulated through years of experience, to the long-term care venue; family members highly value care and attention to themselves and their loved one, information, and opportunities to engage in joint problem solving (Gladstone & Wexler, 2000). Family members generally want to remain actively involved in the plan of care, yet truly actualizing that goal is extremely challenging given the multiple demands, time constraints, and shortage of professional nursing staff that tend to exist in long-term care. Many challenges face long-term care providers in their attempts to deliver quality, individualized care to residents, and while family can be viewed as tremendously helpful when staff and family goals are consistent, the opposite tends to be true if there is inconsistency of goals. Negotiation, clarification, and agreement on goals (Kelley, Pringle-Specht, & Maas, 2000b) is a necessary first step if family are to be effectively integrated into an individualized plan of care. Family members need to be viewed as having the potential to be powerful contributors to and supporters of the plan of care, if effectively integrated. The key lies in identifying family strengths and using them effectively in the delivery of care.

Summary and Conclusions

Physical activity offers many health benefits to older adults including increased ability to live independently and to perform activities of daily living, increased stamina and muscle strength, reduced symptoms of chronic diseases, and improved mood and feelings of well-being (USDHHS, 1996a). Traditional measures for encouraging the adoption and maintenance of healthy lifestyle practices, including physical activity, have been relatively ineffective. A new approach is needed—one that is capable of directing tailored intervention strategies to meet individual client needs, but comprehensive enough to support family/provider level intervention as well. The TTM represents an effective and readily applicable model for promoting health lifestyle changes in older adults (Burbank, Padula, & Nigg, 2000). Though the TTM has been most extensively applied to interventions at the individual level, it has also been applied to group-based interventions, most of which have taken place in on-site facilities (Marcus et al., 1998). More recently, the TTM was effectively used to assess organizational change in family service agencies (Prochaska, 2000).

In order to apply the TTM to family- and/or provider-level systems, it is essential that all members of the system be integrated into the intervention plan at some level. Two factors must be considered in this regard: (1) formal and informal providers need to be reasonably knowledgeable about the TTM, its major constructs, and how to use them to direct stage-based, individualized interventions; and (2) providers need to view behavior change related to fostering healthy lifestyles as a high priority item in their plan of care.

First, if formal providers are to be integrated into a TTM-based plan for behavior change, they need to be reasonably knowledgeable about major constructs, including stages of change, decisional balance, self-efficacy, and the processes of change. Most importantly, perhaps, they need to know how to tailor interventions to the particular stage-based needs of the individual. Numerous approaches have been used to train health providers, primarily physicians, to use the TTM to facilitate behavior change. Brief training programs for health professionals based on the TTM and including physicians (Bain & McKie, 1998; Health Education Authority, 1993), pharmacists (Sinclair, Bond, Lennox, Silcock, & Winfield, 1997), nurses and health visitors (Lennox et al., 1998), as well as diabetes educators (Edwards, Jones, & Bleton, 1999) have been positively evaluated by participants. It is important to note, however, that training health professionals in the TTM has not consistently produced the desired client outcomes. It has been suggested that training nurses, who have the needed expertise and may have more time to spend with clients, may be more effective than training physicians (Lennox et al., 1998). While there is evidence that health professionals can rather quickly grasp the major TTM constructs, the amount, intensity, and complexity of training required to develop skilled facilitator characteristics and specific intervention skills is less clear (Ashworth, 1997; Hall, James, & Roberts, 1997).

The challenges of incorporating informal/family providers, whose support is clearly needed to facilitate behavior change, would logically seem to be inherently more difficult. A necessary first step is to foster trust and understanding of the issues, as well as to emphasize the key role family members play in supporting behavior change. Family members' support for the TTM-based intervention plan should be actively enlisted whenever possible. Family members need to be provided with practical (versus theoretical) information about the TTM, focusing on what they need to know to optimally support intervention strategies. As identified by Kelley, Pringle-Specht, and Maas (2000b), family members and health professionals need to establish partnerships characterized by cooperation, negotiation, clarification, and agreement about goals. Caregiving needs to be supported by health professionals using a family-oriented perspective. Intervention programs need to focus on positive family outcomes and actively draw family into both formal and informal networks, including institutional care. Motivational interviewing, a directive client-centered counseling style, has been used effectively in conjunction with the TTM to facilitate behavior change in individuals (Noonan & Moyers, 1997; Rollnick, Heather, & Bell, 1992; Rollnick & Miller, 1995). Motivational interviewing is based on five general principles: express empathy, develop discrepancy, avoid argumentation, roll with resistance, and support self-efficacy (Miller & Rollnick, 1991). It can be used effectively by various health care providers after brief training (Stott, Rollnick, Rees, & Pill, 1995), and has been applied to family-level intervention (Zweben, 1991).

Second, simply offering educational strategies to providers does not assure that they will incorporate them actively into the delivery of care. Providers must identify health behavior change strategies as fundamental to the provision of comprehensive care, and as a means to potentially reduce care demands, which may be particularly problematic when intervening with older adults. Unfortunately, formal and informal providers often share the same biases as the lay public about the value of incorporating healthier lifestyles in those who have already reached old age. For example, research has demonstrated that physicians often do not routinely screen patients for preventive health activities (Dickinson, Wiggers, Leeder, & Sanson-Fisher, 1989; Owen, 1996). Clearly, research is needed to identify what motivates different health professionals to dispense advice about the importance of healthy lifestyles and the benefits of lifestyle change in general. A study of practicing nurses demonstrated that nurses who were themselves engaged in regular exercise were more likely to encourage physical activity than less active nurses (McDowell, McKenna, & Naylor, 1997). Further study is indicated.

APPLICATION OF THE TTM

Since exercise is such a critical component of preventive and treatment regimens for older adults, and the TTM is a useful tool for facilitating exercise behaviors, and expanding application of the TTM to family and staff caregivers is extremely important. Exercise counseling research among physicians found that although approximately 40% advised their patients to exercise more, only 15% regularly offered any exercise program to assist them. Physical activity was addressed in 21% of office visits (Russell & Roter, 1993). The Physician-based Assessment and Counseling for Exercise (PACE) program utilized the TTM to assist primary care providers in overcoming the barriers to exercise counseling. The program provided care providers with a tool to assess the stage of readiness for exercise and the risk of cardiac events, three structured counseling protocols related to the patient's stage, and an instruction manual. Evaluation was carried out with 27 providers to determine the program's feasibility for counseling use. In the 5 month follow-up, 78% of providers rated the program as good or very good, counseling was provided in less than 5 minutes by 70% of providers, and more than 50% reported that their patients became more active (Houde & Melillo, 2000). Since one of the goals in *Healthy People 2000* (USDHHS, 1991) was to increase, to at least 50%, the number of primary care providers who appropriately assess and counsel patients about physical activity, this type of program can make significant progress toward meeting that goal. Although more research is needed, lessons learned from the PACE program may also be relevant for application of the TTM with other health care providers and family caregivers as well.

No research was found that directly addressed the application of the TTM to informal family caregiving or formal care provider systems in long-term care settings. Therefore, two case studies were constructed to demonstrate practical rather than research-based application of the TTM to family and health care provider systems. For purposes of illustration, the first case study is focused on a family caregiving situation in the home, and illustrates application based on the pre-action stages of change (precontemplation, contemplation, preparation). In this case, TTM-based strategies are used by a health care provider who is knowledgeable about the TTM to actively involve a family caregiver in the plan of care. The second case takes place in a long-term care facility, and focus is on application of TTM principles by providers who are unfamiliar with the TTM. This scenario incorporates the stages of action and maintenance.

Case Study #1

Mrs. S. is a 76-year-old woman whose husband of 40 years died about 2 years ago. Mrs. S. and her husband were never physically active people.

Mrs. S. admitted to disliking most forms of physical activity, preferring to "work at home and do things around the house." Since her husband's death, Mrs. S.'s daughter Joan has noticed a decline in her mother's stamina and endurance, as well as increasing fatigue in performing her usual activities. Joan has become increasingly involved in her mother's daily care, and has taken on increasing responsibility in such areas as grocery shopping and meal preparation. Joan, in consultation with her mother, scheduled an appointment with the primary physician.

After completing an extensive assessment, the doctor concluded that Mrs. S. was "extremely healthy" for a woman of her age, and found no physiologic reason for her reported decrease in functioning. The doctor told Mrs. S. and her daughter that she needed to become more physically active, and instructed her to begin a walking program. Despite her daughter's coaxing and repeated attempts to convince her to start to walk regularly, Mrs. S. refused to change her daily activity patterns, stating "I'm simply too old to start exercising. What good will it do me at my age anyway?"

About a month later, Mrs. S. was hospitalized for a week because of a severe case of influenza, which was complicated by pneumonia. Prior to hospital discharge, Mrs. S. was referred to the visiting nurse service for continued cardiorespiratory assessment because of a perceived decrease in functional abilities while in the hospital.

At the time of initial nursing assessment performed in Mrs. S.'s home, which was also attended by her daughter Joan, Joan discussed her concerns about her mother's past and present reduction in stamina and endurance. She mentioned that her mother's doctor had told her to initiate a physical activity program. Mrs. S. responded angrily that she was tired of being told what to do, and that she simply did not like to exercise. She commented, however, that "If I thought that walking every day would help me to get stronger, then I might just consider it when I feel a little better."

Discussion and Application of the TTM

The first step in planning a behavior change program using the TTM is to assess the client's stage of change. Questions to assess stage of change related to physical activity are illustrated in Figure 5.1. It is important to note that these questions can be used to assess any behavior by simply substituting the targeted behavior for the words "physical activity" in each question. Though stage of change was not assessed during or after Mrs. S.'s appointment with her primary physician, her words indicate that she was in precontemplation, and did not intend to engage in regular physical activity in the next 6 months. It is important to note that the doctor did not discuss her needs, thoughts, and feelings, and did not address what barriers might exist. Rather, the physician simply told her what to do, without providing any rationale for that decision. In reality, providers frequently intervene with clients using action-oriented approaches, though most people who need to make lifestyle changes are in the pre-action (precontemplation, contemplation, preparation) stages (Prochaska, DiClemente, & Norcross, 1992). Furthermore, Joan's well-intentioned attempts to encourage her mother to start a walking program by coaxing her and repeatedly attempting to convince her were, in reality, counterproductive.

Using a stage-based approach, interventions can be targeted to the stage of change in order to facilitate behavior change. Goals, processes, and related strategies for each stage, using physical activity as the target for behavior change, are illustrated in Table 9.1.

The precontemplation stage is characterized by defensiveness about the issue, resistance to information, and reluctance to initiate behavior change; people in this stage are not ready to change (Bradley-Springer, 1996). Interventions during the precontemplation stage should be directed toward increasing awareness of the need to change; emphasis is placed on increasing awareness of the benefits (pros) of physical activity. Mrs. S. needed to be encouraged to begin to consider and think about the benefits of walking, so Joan's coaxing was simply not effective. Joan was a caring and interested caregiver, willing to support her mother in any reasonable way, so involving Joan in the plan of care would have been beneficial.

In evaluating the overall trajectory of Mrs. S.'s case, ideally the physician at the initial contact would have used the staging questions (see Figure 5.1) to determine Mrs. S.'s stage of change. If application of the TTM had occurred at that stage, the health care provider could have explained to Joan, in simple terms, what the stages of change are, as well as how using treatments based on the stage of change, and tailored to her mother's individual needs, would be useful. Ideally a goal would have been mutually developed, negotiated, and agreed upon, such as increasing Mrs. S's awareness of the benefits of increasing her daily activity. Briefly reviewing the choice

TABLE 9.1　Goals, Processes, and Related Strategies for Each Stage of Physical Activity (PA) Behavior Change*

Stage	Goal	Processes	Strategies
Precontemplation	Increase awareness of need to change	Consciousness raising	Focus on the pros (vs. cons) of PA
		Dramatic relief	Verbalize feelings about dislike of PA, reduced daily functioning
		Environmental re-evaluation	View documentary on benefits of PA
Contemplation	Increased motivation and confidence in ability to change	Consciousness raising	Discuss risks of PA and rewards of changing behavior
		Self-reevaluation	Challenge beliefs and expectations about PA: use imagery increase awareness
		Social liberation	Accept responsibility to integrate PA into life
		Self-liberation	Assist with decision-making around PA
Preparation	Negotiate plan for physical activity	Self-reevaluation	Create a new self-image: one involved with PA
		Helping relationships	Talk to friends about getting involved in PA
		Self-liberation	Find ways to integrate PA into everyday activities
Action	Reaffirm commitment and follow-up	Reinforcement management	Make a contract with yourself and with others
		Helping relationships	Start a walking routine with friends
		Counterconditioning	Find alternative ways to get PA
		Stimulus control	Confront excuses for not performing PA
Maintenance	Problem solving to maintain and prevent relapse	Counterconditioning	Use relaxation before PA to encourage a positive mindset
		Helping relationships	Join a PA group
		Reinforcement management	Reward self for PA accomplishments

*Modified from Burbank, Padula, and Nigg (2000).

of stage-appropriate strategies, and together identifying those that would likely be most effective would have been beneficial. Reminding Joan how important her support was, and specifically instructing her as to how she could facilitate each of the chosen interventions would be indicated. Joan's input in tailoring the specific strategies to her mother's interests and lifestyle would be invaluable, and Joan's continued support and follow-up essential.

Strategies based on the processes of consciousness raising, dramatic relief, and environmental reevaluation are appropriate in the precontemplation stage. Consciousness raising involves increasing information about the problem (DiClemente & Scott, 1997) so providing information to Mrs. S. in the form of direct feedback, through educational materials, or via the media, as well as an interpretation emphasizing the benefits (pros) would be indicated. Incorporating Joan in these discussions, answering any questions or concerns that she might have, and enlisting her support to actively reinforce this information would be essential. Dramatic relief involves expressing feelings about the problem and the solutions (DiClemente & Scott, 1997); examples would include encouraging Joan to provide her mother with opportunities to express her feelings about the loss of physical functioning that she had experienced, and what that loss meant to her. Environmental reevaluation involves assessing how one's problems affect the personal and physical environment (Prochaska, Redding, Harlow, Rossi, & Velicer, 1994). For this process, literature, media, or personal testimonies that illustrate the impact of loss of functional abilities on loved ones would be useful. Encouraging Joan to discuss with her mother how her decrease in functioning has impacted her life would be beneficial.

Mrs. S.'s comment after her illness that she might consider increasing physical activity in the near future if it would help her to regain strength was likely an indicator of movement toward the contemplation stage. Major life events that disrupt routines and habits can trigger a reassessment and offer opportunities to introduce the potential for change (Stead, Wimbush, Eadie, & Teer, 1997). In contemplation, the individual is considering the possibility of adopting a behavior change in the near future. They remain indecisive, however, and lack commitment but are aware that a problem exists and are open to new information (Grimley, DiClemente, Prochaska, & Prochaska, 1995).

Ideally, the nurse completing the home assessment would recognize Mrs. S's potential future interest in physical activity as a possible indicator of stage transition, and would seize the moment to assess the stage of change. Using the staging questions, the nurse would determine that Mrs. S. was indeed in the contemplation stage. She would briefly describe this stage to Mrs. S. and Joan, and together identify the goal of reinforcing Mrs. S's knowledge about the benefits of physical activity as well as providing information about the cons of not being physically active. In planning targeted interventions in this stage, the benefits (pros) of physical activity are still a major focus, but in this stage the risks or cons are also introduced. Again, it would be beneficial to explain each of the processes and related interventions in clear terms to Joan, determine together which would likely be most effective for Mrs. S., and encourage Joan's support and involvement.

Four processes are most useful in this stage: consciousness raising, self-reevaluation, social liberation, and self-liberation. Use of consciousness raising in this stage might include the nurse providing Mrs. S. with further education and information about the benefits of physical activity, but also expanding to include the potential risks of not being physically active. Joan would be included in discussions whenever possible, and encouraged to reinforce the information and provide needed feedback. Self-reevaluation involves the individual's assessment of how they feel and think about themselves with respect to the physical inactivity (Prochaska et al., 1994). Joan could be taught the technique of values clarification, which she could use with her mother. Given their strong relationship, Joan could be pivotal in helping her mother become aware of the apparent inconsistencies in her thinking: that she highly values health and independence, yet is unwilling to commit herself to a planned physical activity program that could help to her to maintain her health and independence. Social liberation involves increasing alternatives for non-problem behaviors available in society (DiClemente & Scott, 1997). An appropriate intervention for this process would be to encourage Joan to examine with her mother other people her age that are actively involved in physical activity, and empower her to explore ways to facilitate a walking program for herself and others. For example, she might be encouraged to consider going regularly to a mall with a companion, and purposely walking. Joan's support here could be essential; indeed Joan's willingness to share this activity with her mother could be a primary motivator. Self-liberation is the belief in the ability to change and making the commitment to act on that belief (Cassidy, 1997). An appropriate intervention would be for Joan to encourage her mother to make a realistic resolution to herself, a pact per se, and to stick with it. Joan's recognition and praise for any accomplishment achieved, no matter how small, would be invaluable.

Mrs. S. may or may not progress to the next stage of change, preparation. Movement through the stages of change has been described as cyclical (Prochaska et al., 1994), and progression often occurs very slowly. Indeed, not all clients will successfully progress through the stages of change, and many will slip back or relapse. Relapse needs to be seen in a more positive light so clients are encouraged to restart their progression.

In preparation, people have often begun to experiment with behavior change. They are preparing to make a behavior change within the next month, are establishing a firm commitment, and need to begin to develop a specific plan for action. Clients in this stage should be encouraged to set specific achievable goals and to experiment with new skills. In the event that Mrs. S. did progress to preparation, three processes would be relevant: self-reevaluation, self-liberation, and helping relationships. Both self-reevaluation and self-liberation processes were also used in the contemplation stage, and self-reevaluation in preparation might include identifying personal values about exercise and creating a new self-image as an exerciser. Joan's expressed recognition of her mother's increased activity and identification of her as a more active person would reinforce these principles. Self-liberation could be used by encouraging Mrs. S. to make a public announcement about what she intents to do in regard to physical activity. Joan could encourage Mrs. S. to express her intent to her closest friends, and then provide support, reinforcement, and positive feedback related to progress made. Finally, the process of helping relationships involves being open and trusting about problems with people who care (DiClemente & Scott, 1997). Helping relationships could be facilitated by Joan actively encouraging her mother's close friends to support Mrs. S's accomplishments, allowing her to express her feelings, and by challenging them to become more physically active themselves. Encouraging Mrs. S. to plan, in conjunction with her friends, an ongoing schedule of events that would involve physical activity would be useful.

Case Study #2

Mr. J. is an 80-year-old gentleman who was admitted to a long-term care facility after an acute hospitalization for repair of a fractured hip. Mr. J. had fallen from a ladder while trying to replace a bulb in a ceiling light.

Despite a past medical history of mild Parkinson's disease and a prior cerebrovascular accident (CVA) with residual slight left-sided weakness, Mr. J. had been able to remain living at home with his wife of 50 years. Mr. and Mrs. J. had no children and no living relatives nearby, but had numerous friends who were available for assistance. Mrs. J. rarely asked them for help, feeling that she didn't want to burden them. Mrs. J. described her husband as fiercely independent, always wanting to do things for himself. Having to accept her assistance over the last few years with grooming, and having to give up driving, had been very difficult for Mr. J., but he was able to maintain a positive attitude despite his limitations. Over the last 6 months, Mrs. J. had noticed increased forgetfulness in her husband, and found it necessary to frequently repeat herself. He had become totally dependent on her for instrumental activities of daily living (IADLs) and required increasing assistance with activities of daily living (ADLs). More recently, Mr. J. had developed urinary incontinence, especially during the night. Despite the fact that Mrs. J. was sleeping poorly and finding it increasingly difficult to care for her husband, she was unwilling to consider institutionalization unless it became "absolutely necessary."

Mr. J. had always been a very active man prior to the onset of chronic diseases; he golfed as much as possible and completed all the yard work and household maintenance. Mr. J. was forced to give up these tasks after suffering a CVA, but only more recently stopped golfing because of increased tremors secondary to Parkinson's disease. Mr. J. and his wife had continued to take their evening stroll every night until a few months prior to his recent hospitalization. Though Mr. J. loved these walks, they had become increasingly difficult for Mrs. J.: She had to repeatedly remind her husband where they were going and which route to take to get back home, and Mr. J. had begun to experience extreme fatigue with increasingly shorter distances.

While in the nursing home, Mr. J. was sometimes described by the nursing staff as "uncooperative," and concerns about safety were identified. Mr. J. became angry when the staff tried to assist him with hygienic care, but forgot what had been completed unless instructed in detail. He complained that "you don't help me like my wife does." Mr. J. frequently told the staff that he had to "get back on his feet"; he needed to be frequently reminded to ask for assistance when getting out of bed or ambulating, to stay within the activity guidelines provided, and to use his walker. Mr. J. got up to the bathroom one night, unassisted and without using his walker, and experienced a fall. No apparent injuries were noted. When asked why he didn't call for assistance, Mr. J. responded "I didn't know I had to . . . can't I even go to the bathroom by myself? How am I ever going to get better if you people don't let me do anything for myself?" When informed about the incident, Mrs. J. became angry with the staff for "not being there to prevent the fall." She was also very angry with her husband and reminded him that his "thick-headedness" had contributed to the fall that caused the broken hip, and that he needed to "do what he was told." Frustrated, Mrs. J. requested a family conference with the staff.

Discussion: TTM-based Staff Education

Mrs. J. was wise in requesting a team conference because clearly communication was needed. Interestingly, it would appear that the client, family, and staff had similar goals: safety as well as rehabilitation of Mr. J. to the highest level of functional ability possible. The complexity apparent in this case is not unusual in the long-term care setting; it is, in fact, the norm. Intervening effectively with individuals, most of whom are older adults with numerous comorbidities and functional limitations, is a considerable challenge. Another is the reality that long-term care facilities tend to be understaffed, have minimal numbers of multidisciplinary professionals employed, and for the most part use nursing assistants, often not enough of them, to deliver the majority of direct client care.

Use of TTM-based strategies can be viewed as an exciting alternative to traditional intervention plans. Although knowledge about the model is a necessary component, simply educating the staff about the TTM is not the answer. When a TTM-based educational program is initiated, administrators and staff members at all levels and across disciplines need to discuss their views about the value of health behavior change and healthy lifestyles for long-term care residents, as well as the importance of client and family involvement in care overall. The institution must support, through its mission and philosophy, the promotion, restoration, and maintenance of healthy client lifestyles, as well as the principle of active client and family involvement in care delivery. Without clear institutional mandates and tangible institutional support (for example, support for continuing education), attempts to educate staff about mechanisms to facilitate healthy behavior and behavior change will not be successful. All levels of staff also need to be motivated to think differently, and to be willing to try a new approach. This is not easily accomplished because change is always stressful. Staff need to be encouraged to discuss their feelings and concerns, and concretely shown how application of TTM-based principles can not only potentially improve care delivery and save time in the long run, but also assist them in their role as providers in the process.

Ideally, staff members at all levels need to be trained related to the TTM; practically, recruiting staff members who are especially interested in behavior change, and training them first, would be reasonable and cost effective. All attempts should be made to include nursing assistants in the initial training efforts as they clearly spend the most time at the bedside. Given positive outcomes, trained staff members could subsequently be used as informal peer trainers, facilitating the acceptance and application of the model throughout the system.

When planning a training session, it is important to assure that the level of content is appropriate for a wide array of staff, ranging from the nursing assistants to social workers and physicians. Content should focus on what staff members need to know and "how to's," and should include: a brief description of the TTM including its major constructs, examples of how it has been successfully applied in a related population, a discussion of how using the TTM could be beneficial to clients and staff, a description of the staging question and how to use it, discussion of the processes and how to select and apply them, and how to evaluate stage-based interventions. Case study scenarios and use of actual clinical situations is invaluable. Content should be delivered in an interactive format, encouraging dialogue and participation of staff, with use of illustrative audiovisual materials and detailed handouts whenever possible. Use of motivational interviewing during staff training is beneficial, emphasizing the potential benefits of mutually developed strategies for all involved, but focusing on the concrete rewards for staff, such as potential reduction in negative client behaviors. For purposes of illustration, Mr. J.'s case will be used to illustrate how staff educated in TTM-based interventions could apply the model.

Application of the TTM

Frustrated, Mrs. J. requested a team conference to discuss her husband's care. Using the TTM staging question, the nurse assessed Mr. J.'s stage of change, and found that despite his functional limitations he was in the action stage of physical activity. Prior to his acute injury and despite his physical limitations, Mr. J. had likely been in the maintenance stage, having maintained a regular schedule of physical activity for more than 6 months. The acute hip fracture and subsequent recovery process had forced a change in his regular pattern of activity, but clearly Mr. J. was very anxious to get back to a more active lifestyle.

The primary objective of the action stage is to support the change efforts, so it was imperative that the health care team develop innovative but realistic strategies to support Mr. J.'s intent to be physically active as he was able. A team conference was held, and the nurse identified that by gaining Mr. and Mrs. J.'s support and trust, their involvement in the plan of care could be facilitated as much as possible. This would not only improve care delivery, but could also be used as a means to appropriately reduce the demands on already limited staff time. Mrs. J. verbalized that she had hoped to take Mr. J. back home, but that she had come to accept that that would not be possible. The staff encouraged her to verbalize her feelings and supported her independent decision making. Discussion was then focused on the issue of safety and how it could best be facilitated. Through joint problem solving, the decision was made to move Mr. J. to a room directly across from the nurses' station to allow for more continuous observation. It was also agreed that Mr. J. would wear an audible alarm at all times while in bed, which would sound if it became disconnected. This would assist the nursing staff to recognize when Mr. J. might be attempting to get up without assistance. Mr. J. was also included in discussions about the need for hygienic care; Mr. and Mrs. J. and the staff negotiated for Mrs. J. to assist her husband with hygienic care whenever possible. Everyone agreed that allowing Mr. J. to do as much as possible for himself was an important goal in the attempt to increase his physical activity.

Processes of change appropriate to the action stage include reinforcement management, helping relationships, counterconditioning, and stimulus control. Reinforcement management is defined as the process of rewarding oneself or being rewarded by others for making changes (DiClemente & Scott, 1997). The health care delivery team realized that they could apply this process through development of a contingency contract. Dealing with the necessity of activity restrictions due to the hip fracture presented a challenging problem, because Mr. J. often simply did not remember the restrictions and was extremely anxious to "get back to normal." His objective was to be up and walking as much as possible. The staff had previously planned Mr. J.'s ambulation on a once- to twice-a-day schedule, as time and staffing levels allowed. The nursing assistants acknowledged that when they were able to get Mr. J. up more often, he was much less restless and tended not to try to climb out of bed himself. Mrs. J. was admittedly overcautious with respect to her husband's activity because she was afraid that he would fall and hurt himself again. Negotiation and compromise were needed in order to reach a mutually established goal. The staff developed an agreement with Mr. J. to get him up and out of bed at least three times per day. The staff recognized that the increased activity was beneficial for Mr. J., and that he had been less likely to try to get up himself when walked more often. In order to facilitate the increased activity, the staff asked Mrs. J. to enlist the help of friends, who had been frequently asking her what they could do to assist her and Mr. J. This also illustrates the process of helping relationships.

Counterconditioning is the process of substituting alternatives. The staff, after consulting with the physical therapist, presented Mr. J. with some alternative exercises that he could perform by himself while in bed or in the chair, and queried him as to which he would like to try. The nursing assistants suggested that written reminders be posted in the room to cue Mr. J. to do the exercises, since he was an avid reader and wanted to be involved; likewise Mrs. J. could actively reinforce them when she visited. Reminders from significant others are valuable additions to environmental cues (Murdaugh, 1998). The final action process, stimulus control, involves avoiding or countering stimuli that elicit problem behaviors (DiClemente & Scott, 1997). The staff noted that Mr. J. had been frequently trying to get up to the bathroom without his walker. In collaboration with Mr. J., the team agreed to leave the walker, along with Mr. J.'s slippers, at the immediate bedside at all times so they would be in sight. This would serve as a reminder for Mr. J. to use the walker.

Maintenance is reached after the target behavior has been sustained for 6 months. After several months, Mr. J. was able to increase his physical activity to ambulating several times a day with his walker without excessive fatigue. He became more involved in his daily care with his wife's assistance, and was able to complete at least some of his ADLs independently. The primary goal of the maintenance stage is to continue the behavior change and avoid relapse (Burbank, Padula, & Nigg, 2000). Three processes of change are of most importance in this stage: counterconditioning, helping relationships, and reinforcement management. The strategy of having Mr. J. perform alternative exercises during bed or chair rest had proven effective, but Mr. J. had tired of "doing the same things." Given his improved ambulation and overall functioning, the staff, after collaborating with the activities coordinator, decided to see if they could interest Mr. J. in some group activities to further enhance his physical activity. Mr. J. agreed and became involved in woodworking as well as indoor bowling, and continued to look for other activities. With the help of the staff and his wife, Mr. J. was also able to identify a small group of men who were interested in starting an informal exercise group. This is an excellent example of helping relationships. Finally, in terms of reinforcement management, the staff formally recognized Mr. J.'s progress made toward reestablishment of a physically active lifestyle, as well as the invaluable support provided by his wife.

SUMMARY

New approaches to encourage the adoption and maintenance of physical activity in older adults are needed. The TTM offers an exciting alternative to traditional behavior change strategies. The

TTM has been effectively applied to a wide variety of health behaviors, including exercise and physical activity in older adults. Application of the TTM to family and health care provider systems represents a necessary and innovative extension that holds promise to improve the quality and delivery of individualized, family-based care. Studies are needed to determine the most efficient educational process to teach caregivers to use the TTM, to assess what barriers are present among the caregivers or in the environment that make application of the TTM more difficult, and to examine the effectiveness of the TTM when used by care providers to change behavior.

REFERENCES

Administration on Aging. (1999). *Family caregiver fact sheet.* Washington, DC: United States Administration on Aging.

Amick, T., & Ockene, J. (1994). The role of social support in the modification of risk factors for cardiovascular disease. In S. Shumaker & S. Czajkowski (Eds.), *Social support and cardiovascular disease* (pp. 259–278). New York: Plenum.

Aneshensel, C., Pearlin, L., Mullan, J., Zarit, S., & Whitlatch, C. (1995). *Profiles in caregiving: The expected career.* San Diego, CA: Academic Press.

Anonymous. Nursing staff levels at U.S. nursing homes continue to be lower than recommended. *Research Activities, 222,* 12.

Ashworth, P. (1997). Breakthrough or bandwagon? Are interventions tailored to stage of change more effective than non-staged interventions? *Health Education Journal, 56,* 166–174.

Bain, N., & McKie, L. (1998). Stages of change training for opportunistic smoking intervention by the primary health care team. Part II: qualitative evaluation of long-term impact on professionals' reported behaviour. *Health Education Journal, 57,* 150–159.

Bausell, R. (1986). Health-seeking behavior among the elderly. *The Gerontologist, 26*(5), 556–558.

Boland, D., & Sims, S. (1996). Family care giving at home as a solitary journey. *Image: Journal of Nursing Scholarship, 28*(1), 55–58.

Bradley-Springer, L. (1996). Patient education for behavior change: Help from the Transtheoretical and Harm Reduction Models. *JANAC,* 7(Suppl. 1), 23–33.

Burbank, P., Padula, C., & Nigg, C. (2000). Changing health behaviors of older adults. *Journal of Gerontological Nursing, 26*(3), 26–33.

Cantor, M., & Little, V. (1985). Aging and social care. In R. Binstock & E. Shanas (Eds.), *Handbook of aging and the social sciences* (pp. 745–781). New York: Van Nostrand Reinhold.

Cassidy, C. (1997). Facilitating behavior change. Use of the Transtheoretical Model in the occupational health setting. *AAOHN Journal, 45*(5), 239–246.

Centers for Disease Control. (1993). Prevalence of sedentary lifestyle-behavioral risk factor surveillance system, United States, 1991. *Morbidity and Mortality Weekly Report, 42*, 576–579.

Chenier, M. (1997). Review and analysis of caregiver burden and nursing home placement. *Geriatric Nursing, 18*(3), 121–126.

Corbin, J., & Strauss, A. (1991). A nursing model for chronic illness management based upon the trajectory framework. *Scholarly Inquiry for Nursing Practice, 5*(3), 155–174.

Courneya, K. (1995). Perceived severity of the consequences of physical inactivity across the stages of change in older adults. *Journal of Sport and Exercise Psychology, 17*, 447–457.

Curry, L., Porter, M., Michalski, M., & Gruman, C. (2000). Individualized care: Perception of certified nurse's aides. *Journal of Gerontological Nursing, 26*(7), 45–51.

Dickinson, J., Wiggers, J., Leeder, S., & Sanson-Fisher, R. (1989). General practitioners' detection of patients' smoking status. *Medical Journal of Australia, 150*, 420–426.

DiClemente, C., Prochaska, J., Fairhurst, S., Velicer, W., Velasquez, M., & Rossi, J. (1991). The process of smoking cessation: An analysis of precontemplation, contemplation, and preparation stages of change. *Journal of Consulting and Clinical Psychology, 59*, 295–304.

DiClemente, C., & Scott, C. (1997). Stages of change: Interactions with treatment compliance and involvement. In L. Onken, J. Baline, & J. Boren (Eds.), *Beyond the therapeutic alliance: Keeping the drug-dependent individual in treatment* (pp. 131–156). NIDA Research Monograph 165. Rockville, MD: U.S. Department of Health and Human Services, National Institutes of Health.

Dishman, R. (1988). Exercise adherence research: Future directions. *American Journal of Health Promotion, 3*, 52–56.

Dishman, R. (1990). Determinants of participation in physical activity. In C. Bouchard, R. Shephard, T. Stephens, J. Sutton, & B. McPherson (Eds.), *Exercise, fitness, and health* (pp. 75–102). Champaign, IL: Human Kinetics.

Duda, J., & Tappe, M. (1988). Predictors of personal investment in physical activity among middle-aged and older adults. *Perceptual and Motor Skills, 66*, 543–549.

Dwyer, J., Henretta, J., Coward, R., & Barton, A. (1992). Changes in the helping behaviors of adults children as caregivers. *Research on Aging, 14,* 351–375.

Edwards, L., Jones, H., & Bleton, A. (1999). The Canadian experience in the development of a continuing education program for diabetes educators based on the Transtheoretical Model of Behavior Change. *Diabetes Spectrum, 12*(3), 157–160, 162–164.

Elward, K., & Larson, E. (1992). Benefits of exercise for older adults. *Clinics in Geriatric Medicine, 8*(1), 35–50.

Feinleib, S., Cunningham, P., & Short, P. (1994). *Use of nursing and personal care homes by the civilian population, 1987.* (AHCPR) 94006. Nation Medical Expenditure Survey Research Findings 23. Agency for Health Care Policy and Research. Rockville, MD: Public Health Service.

Fried, L., & Guralnik, J. (1997). Disability in older adults: Evidence regarding significance, etiology, and risk. *Journal of the American Geriatrics Society, 45,* 92–100.

Gaynor, S. (1990). The long haul: The effects of home care on caregivers. *IMAGE: The Journal of Nursing Scholarship, 22*(4), 208–212.

Gill, K., & Overdorf, V. (1994). Incentives for exercise in younger and older women. *Journal of Sport Behavior, 17,* 87–97.

Gladstone, J., & Wexler, E. (2000). A family perspective of family/staff interaction in long-term care facilities. *Geriatric Nursing, 21*(1), 16–18.

Gorely, T., & Gordon, S. (1995). An examination of the transtheoretical model and exercise behavior in older adults. *Journal of Sports and Exercise Psychology, 17,* 312–324.

Greene, J., & Crouse, S. (1995). The effects of endurance training on functional capacity in the elderly: A meta-analysis. *Medicine and Science in Sports and Exercise, 32,* 920–926.

Grimley, D., DiClemente, R., Prochaska, J., & Prochaska, G. (1995). Preventing adolescent pregnancy, STD and HIV: A promising new approach. *Florida Educator,* Spring, 7–15.

Hall, D., James, P., & Roberts, S. (1997). Evaluation of training in behaviour change counselling skills: The application of clinical-audit methodology. *Health Education Journal, 56*(4), 393–403.

Health Education Authority (1993). *Helping people change: Training course for primary health care professionals.* Oxford: HEA National Unit for Health Promotion in Primary Care.

Herzberg, S. (1997). The impact of social environment on nursing home residents. *Journal of Aging & Social Policy, 9*(2), 67–80.

Hing, E., & Bloom, B. (1990). Long-term care for the functionally dependent elderly. National Center for Health Statistics. *Vital Health Statistics 1990, 13,* 104.

Houde, S. C., & Melillo, K. D. (2000). Physical activity and exercise counseling in primary care. *The Nurse Practitioner, 25*(8), 8–39.

Ingledeiv, D., Markland, D., & Medley, A. (1998). Exercise motives and stages of change. *Journal of Health Psychology, 3,* 477–489.

Institute of Medicine 1996 report. Nursing staff in hospitals and nursing homes: Is it adequate? Excerpt from IOM summary. *Maryland Nurse, 15*(4), 6–8.

Johncox, V. (2000). Evaluability assessment of staff training in special care units for persons with dementia: Strategic issues. *The Canadian Journal of Program Evaluation,* Special Issue, 53–66.

Kelley, L., Pringle-Specht, J., & Maas, M. (2000a). Family involvement in care for individuals with dementia protocol. *Journal of Gerontological Nursing, 26*(2), 13–21.

Kelley, L., Pringle-Specht, J., & Maas, M. (2000b). Family involvement in care for persons with dementia: An intervention to promote quality outcomes for people with dementia and their care providers. *Old News, 3*(1), 8–10.

Lennox, A., Bain, N., Taylor, R., McKie, L., Donnan, P., & Groves, J. (1998). *Health Education Journal, 57,* 140–149.

Leventhal, E., & Prohaska, T. (1986). Age, symptom interpretation, and health behavior. *Journal of the American Geriatrics Society, 34*(3), 185–191.

Marcus, B., Banspach, S., Lefebvre, R., Rossi, J., Carleton, R., & Abrams, D. (1992). Using the stages of change model to increase the adoption of physical activity among community participants. *American Journal of Health Promotion, 6,* 424–429.

Marcus, B., King, T., Bock, B., Borrelli, B., & Clark, M. (1998). Adherence to physical activity recommendations and interventions. In S. Shumaker, E. Schron, J. Ockene, & W. McBee (Eds.), *The handbook of health behavior change* (2nd ed., pp. 189–212). New York: Springer Publishing Co.

McDowell, N., McKenna, J., & Naylor, P. (1997). Factors that influence practice nurses to promote physical activity. *British Journal of Sports Medicine, 31*(4), 308–313.

Miller, W., & Rollnick, S. (1991). *Motivational interviewing.* New York: Guilford Press.

McMurdo, M., & Rennie, L. (1993). A controlled trial of exercise by residents of old people's homes. *Age & Ageing, 22,* 11–15.

Montgomery, R., & Datwyler, M. (1990). Women and men in the caregiving role. *Generations, 14,* 34–38.

Murdaugh, C. (1998). Problems with adherence in the elderly. In S. Shumaker, E. Schron, J. Ockene, & W. McBee (Eds.), *The handbook of health behavior change* (2nd ed., pp. 357–376). New York: Springer.

Nigg, C., & Lees, F. (in review). The Transtheoretical Model applied to exercise: A review of the literature.

Nigg, C., & Courneya, K. (1998). Transtheoretical model: Examining adolescent exercise behavior. *Journal of Adolescent Health, 22,* 214–224.

Noonan, W., & Moyers, T. (1997). Motivational interviewing. *Journal of Substance Misuse, 2,* 8–16.

Ory, M., Hoffman, R., Yee, J., Tennstedt, S., & Shulz, R. (1999). Prevalence and impact of caregiving: A detailed comparison between dementia and nondementia caregivers. *The Gerontologist, 39*(2), 177–185.

Owen, N. (1996). Strategic initiatives to promote participation in physical activity. *Health Promotion International, 11*(3), 213–218.

Padula, C. (1996). Older couples' decision making on health issues. *Western Journal of Nursing Research, 18*(6), 675–687.

Pate, R., Pratt, M., Blair, S., Haske, W., Macera, C., Bouchard, C., Buchner, D., Ettinger, W., Heath, G., King, A., Driska, A., Leon, A., Marcus, B., Morris, J., Paffenbarger, R., Patrick, K., Pollock, M., Rippe, J., Sallis, J., & Wilmore, J. (1995). Physical activity and public health: A recommendation from the Centers for Disease Control and the American College of Sports Medicine. *Journal of the American Medical Association, 273,* 402–407.

Pearlin, L. (1992). The careers of caregivers. *The Gerontologist, 32,* 647.

Pearlin, L., & Aneshensel, C. (1994). Caregiving: The unexpected career. *Social Justice Research, 7,* 373–390.

Prochaska, J. (2000). A transtheoretical model for assessing organizational change: A study of family service agencies' movement to time-limited therapy. *Families in Society: The Journal of Contemporary Human Service, 81*(1), 76–84.

Prochaska, J., & DiClemente, C. (1983). Stages and processes of self-change in smoking: Towards an integrative model of change. *Journal of Consulting and Clinical Psychology, 51,* 390–395.

Prochaska, J., DiClemente, C., & Norcross, J. (1992). In search of how people change. *American Psychologist, 47*(9), 1102–1114.

Prochaska, J., Redding, C., Harlow, L., Rossi, J., & Velicer, W. (1994). The trans-Theoretical model of change and HIV prevention: A review. *Health Education Quarterly, 21*(4), 471–486.

Province, M., Hadley, E., Hornbrook, M., Lipsitz, L., Miller, J., Mulrow, C., Ory, M., Sattin, R., Tinetti, M., & Wolf, S. (1995). The effects of exercise on falls in elderly patients. *Journal of the American Medical Association, 273,* 1341–1347.

Resnick, B. (2000). Exercise and older adults. *Journal of Gerontological Nursing, 26*(3), 3.

Robinson, J., & Rogers, M. (1994). Adherence to exercise programs: Recommendations. *Sports Medicine, 17,* 39–52.

Robinson, K. (1997). Family caregiving: Who provides that care, and at what cost? *Nursing Economics, 15*(5), 243–247.

Rollnick, S., Heather, N., & Bell, A. (1992). Negotiating behaviour change in medical settings: The development of brief motivational interviewing. *Journal of Mental Health, 1,* 25–37.

Rollnick, S., & Miller, W. (1995). What is motivational interviewing? *Behavioural and Cognitive Psychotherapy, 23,* 325–334.

Russell, N. K., & Roter, D. L. (1993). Health promotion counseling of chronic disease patients during primary care visits. *American Journal of Public Health, 83*(7), 979–982.

Ryden, M., & Krichbaum, K. (1996). Employer support for the educational development of nurses in long-term care facilities. *Gerontology & Geriatrics Education, 17*(2), 3–19.

Sallis, J., Haskell, W., Fortmann, S., Vranizan, K., Taylor, C., & Solomon, D. (1986). Predictors of adoption and maintenance of physical activity in a community sample. *Preventive Medicine, 15,* 331–341.

Seltzer, M., & Li, L.W. (2000). The dynamics of caregiving: Transitions during a three-year prospective study. *The Gerontologist, 40*(2), 165–178.

Shanas, E. (1979). The family as a social support in old age. *The Gerontologist, 19*(2), 169–174.

Sinclair, H., Bond, C., Lennox, A., Silcock, J., & Winfield, A. (1997). An evaluation of a training workshop for pharmacists based on the Stages of Change model of smoking cessation. *Health Education Journal, 56,* 296–312.

Skelton, D., & McLaughlin, W. (1996). Maintaining functional ability in old age. *Physiotherapy, 82,* 11–20.

Stead, M., Wimbush, E., Eadie, D., & Teer, P. (1997). A qualitative study of older people's perceptions of ageing and exercise: The implications for health promotion. *Health Education Journal, 56,* 17–34.

Stephens, T., & Craig, C. (1990). *The well-being of Canadians: Highlights of the 1985 Campbell's survey.* Ottawa: Canadian Fitness and Lifestyle Research Center.

Stone, R., Cafferata, G., & Sangl, J. (1987). Caregivers of the frail elderly: A national profile. *Gerontologist, 27,* 616–626.

Stott, N., Rollnick, S., Rees, M., & Pill, R. (1995). Innovation in clinical method: Diabetes care and negotiating skills. *Family Practice, 12*(4), 413–418.

U.S. Department of Health and Human Services, Public Health Service (1991). *Health people 2000: National health promotion and disease prevention.*

(DHHS Publication No. PHS 91-50212). Washington, DC: U.S. Government Printing Office.

U.S. Department of Health and Human Services (1996a). *Physical activity and health. Older adults. A report of the Surgeon General.* Atlanta, GA: Centers for Disease Control and Prevention.

U.S. Department of Health and Human Services (1996b). *Physical activity and health. At-A-Glance. A report of the Surgeon General.* Atlanta, GA: Centers for Disease Control and Prevention.

Werner, P., Koroknay, V., Braun, J., & Cohen-Mansfield, J. (1994). Individualized care alternatives used in the process of removing physical restraints in the nursing home. *Journal of the American Geriatrics Society, 42*(3), 321–325.

Zweben, A. (1991). Motivational counseling with alcoholic couples. In W. Miller & S. Rollnick (Eds.), *Motivational interviewing* (pp. 225–235). New York: Guilford Press.

CHAPTER 10

Future Directions and Resources

Patricia M. Burbank and Deborah Riebe

> "It is not necessary to change. Survival is not mandatory."
>
> ~W. Edward Deming

Exercise is an important preventive and therapeutic strategy for everyone, especially older adults. It is important for older persons who are healthy as well as for those with physical and cognitive impairments. The effectiveness of exercise in slowing the deterioration associated with human aging is so marked that it is surprising it has not been embraced by more people. The challenge is to integrate regular physical activity into daily routines and to continue to exercise throughout life.

Changing behavior is a challenge for everyone. Habits of a lifetime are extremely difficult to change whether the person is 25, 50, or 75 years old. Many people believe the adage "you can't teach an old dog new tricks," putting further limitations on expectations of success in behavior change in later life. Once behavior patterns are established, it requires major lifestyle reorientation to alter them.

Over the years, many theories have been proposed to explain, predict, and control behavior. One of the most promising newer models, the Transtheoretical Model of behavior change (TTM) (Prochaska & DiClemente, 1983) incorporates several different theoretical perspectives. This book has reviewed the problem of lack of exercise among older adults, the benefits of exercise for this group, and presented the TTM as a method of behavior change most suitable for achieving success. Specific guidelines to assist the practitioner in applying the TTM to older individuals and their caregivers, both health care staff and family members, have been discussed. This chapter provides a short synopsis of each chapter and indicates future directions for research and practice. Because the purpose of this book is to discuss exercise behavior change rather than to present exercise programs suitable for older adults, no specific exercise guidelines have been included. This chapter does, however, include resources for health care professionals to utilize for more information about exercise and exercise programs for older adults.

In chapter 1, discussion of demographic changes and the prevalence of active versus sedentary lifestyles indicate a rapidly increasing population of primarily sedentary older adults. Because exercise is so beneficial to general health and maintenance of functional status, a sedentary lifestyle for older adults can result in a dramatic decline in quality of life in the later years. This puts additional strain on the already overburdened health care system. Specific age-related changes and the effects of exercise on musculoskeletal and cardiorespiratory systems among older adults are discussed, along with strength, flexibility, and balance as important skills necessary to maintain safe mobility. With aging, flexibility and balance also decline, putting the older person at higher risk for falls. Research is summarized on exercise programs that include strength and balance training, walking and weight transfer, and that have been found to reduce the risk of falling. Psychological effects of exercise include a well-documented relationship between depression and exercise and less well-established information about the effects of exercise on cognitive function, especially cognitive impairment. Chapter 1 concludes by stating that those older adults who exercise have improved quality of life, are able to complete the activities of daily living more effectively, and remain independent for a longer time. More intervention studies are needed to determine the effects of different types of exercise and the duration and intensity needed to produce optimal results. Special attention needs to be given to clarifying the effects of exercise on cognitive function and cognitive decline.

Many older adults do not exercise, or they stop exercising as they grow older for a variety of reasons. These factors include health, cognitive, behavioral, cultural, social, economic, and environmental issues that must be overcome if the person is to begin to exercise. Chapter 2 discusses these challenges of exercise in older adults and suggests solutions whenever possible. One of the barriers to exercise is the belief that it is unsafe for older adults or for those with cardiovascular disease. Current dilemmas and recommendations for screening and for exercise supervision are discussed to provide the health care professional with guidelines for safe exercise interventions. Other issues that may affect exercise in a negative way are reviewed including a lack of social support for exercise, cultural values promoting a sedentary old age, economic issues, low education and literacy levels, and gender issues are reviewed. External barriers to physical activity discussed include insufficient time to exercise, financial barriers, and lack of accessibility to physical activity facilities or to a safe place to exercise. Lack of social support, increased social isolation, lack of self-efficacy, and fear that exercise will cause injury or pain, or exacerbate an existing condition are described as common internal barriers. Because of the dynamic nature of behavior change, the motivational factors and barriers for each person must be assessed individually and frequently throughout the change process. The exercise program will be more successful if the interventions can then be tailored specifically to meet each individual's needs. To date, most studies in this area have been quantitative. Future directions for research include a need for more qualitative research to illuminate how older adults think about barriers and limitations they experience related to exercise. Assumptions have been made in designing studies that older adults think in the same ways younger adults do, however, the key to resolving some of these challenges may be to explore the thought processes used by older adults qualitatively. Future quantitative studies can then be built on this solid foundation to determine challenges and potential solutions that may be more effective for older adults.

Many models and theories have been developed over the years to try to explain and control behavior change. These have been accessible to academicians and researchers, however transfer of knowledge to practitioners for application has posed more of a challenge. In order to facilitate use of the TTM by health care professionals, chapter 3 includes historical background of the development of the TTM and a complete description of this model as it was first presented by Prochaska and DiClemente (1983) through its current state. Major components including the five stages of change, the ten processes of change that people use to move through the stages, decisional balance (weighing the pros and cons), and self-efficacy are described in detail. Clear information is given on the model to enable the health care professional to utilize it to change any behavior with any group, although the purpose of this book is to specifically apply it to exercise behavior in older adults. Limitations of the model, such as the need for more research to validate certain concepts and stages, for more studies that test the model in its entirety, and for resolution of apparently incompatible philosophical perspectives underlying the processes are discussed. In addition, comparatively few studies have evaluated use of the model across behaviors with older adults. Further research in this area is much needed.

Chapter 4 is an extensive review of literature applying the TTM to a wide range of behaviors other than exercise. This review gives the reader information about the many ways the model has been used and the results of the studies applying the model in a wide variety of population groups and behaviors. By carefully reviewing these findings, one can learn strengths and limitations of the model and determine in which situations the model seems to be most predictive and effective. It is not possible to generalize knowledge from these other behaviors to exercise because at this time, findings indicate that changing one health behavior does not necessarily mean that other behaviors can be changed in the same manner. Different processes may be used more frequently with some behaviors that with others. Many questions remain about how people think about change in a variety of areas of their lives. Further exploratory studies are needed to determine in more detail what actually happens and how people think and process information in the pre-action stages. Intervention studies are also needed to examine the effectiveness of stage-tailored interventions for a variety of behaviors. Some authors (Nigg et al., 1999) have indicated that there may be gateway behaviors, that is, key behaviors that if changed, facilitate behavior change to a healthier lifestyle in other areas as well. Further research is needed to determine if, in fact, gateway behaviors do exist and if so, more attention could be shifted to these behaviors by both researchers and health care providers.

Research on application of the TTM to exercise behavior among older adults is thoroughly reviewed from a historical perspective in chapter 5. Descriptive as well as intervention studies are reviewed and strengths and weaknesses of the studies described. Findings are summarized for each of the major constructs: stages of change, processes of change, decisional balance, and self-efficacy. Current research in the area at the University of Rhode Island is cited as a specific example of ongoing study in this area. A table summarizes the studies by author, sample, design, measurement, and results. Assessment tools for identifying a person's stage of change in both interview and questionnaire formats are included in this chapter. Unanswered questions in this area include knowledge about how older adults think about pros and cons of exercise in the precontemplation and contemplation stages. Qualitative studies that explore these thought processes used by older adults are needed. Interventions can then be designed and studied quantitatively based on this new knowledge about older adults.

Chapter 6 moves from research to practice by giving the reader specific guidelines about how to apply the model by tailoring interventions to stages of change for healthy older adults. Concepts of decisional balance (pros and cons), self-efficacy, and processes of change are clearly described and practically operationalized. Descriptions are given of each stage of change and processes that have been found to be successful in helping people in that stage. For each stage of change, specific examples of interventions that illustrate each process are given to assist the health care professional in utilizing the model successfully with older adults. Since the focus of this chapter is application, future research directions would entail evaluation research to determine the effectiveness of TTM-based program interventions on outcomes of stage progression and behavior change. Health care providers applying the model individually can keep anecdotal records about what seems to work and what is not as successful in helping older adults to change behavior. These notes can be very valuable in designing outcome-based research studies in the future.

Chapter 7 takes the reader further into application of the model with older adults, specifically applying the model with older adults who have chronic illnesses, who are physically or functionally impaired, or who are frail. A discussion of chronic illnesses and disability among this population reveals increasing prevalence of chronic illnesses and functional disabilities accompanying a growing aging population. Both physical and cognitive functioning are affected by this increase in chronic illness. Frailty, a term used to refer an increased state of physiological vulnerability, is also discussed. Research documenting the positive effects of exercise on physical, cognitive, and emotional functioning for these different groups of older adults is reviewed. Examples of exercise goals for these older people are presented with discussion of how the goals are different from those of younger people or healthy older adults. Finally, the TTM is applied in a stage-by-stage manner with examples of how processes may be used in each stage. Special attention is given to the pros and cons of this group of older adults, as they are different from those of healthier older persons. Because relatively little research has been devoted to behavior change in this population, much needs to be done. As with older adults in general, qualitative research on how this group of older adults thinks about barriers to exercise in relation to their illnesses would be especially useful. Studies with older adults who have maintained successful exercise programs in the face of debilitating chronic illnesses, and with caregivers who have been successful in assisting the older person to exercise regularly, would give insight into how the processes were used to accomplish these successes. Larger quantitative studies and intervention studies can then be designed based on this important foundational work.

One of the criticisms of the TTM has been its limited usefulness with people from diverse ethnic groups and of low socioeconomic backgrounds. Because the older minority population is increasing dramatically, it is imperative that the theories and models utilized be applicable to meet the special needs of this group as well. Chapter 8 addresses this issue by discussing not only individual factors but also socio-structural factors that affect the health status and health decisions of older adults. Research on beliefs about exercise among older African Americans, for instance, found that this group feels that older people should avoid vigorous exercise and that retirement meant rest rather than leisure time that included physical activity. Factors that must be considered when working with a multi-ethnic and/or lower socioeconomic group of older people are age and gender characteristics, social class differences, literacy, language issues, spirituality, degree of acculturation, and residence patterns. Examples of the authors' research applying the TTM to change exercise and nutrition behaviors among a group of older adults in multi-ethnic and low income communities is given with suggestions regarding steps that can be taken to improve application of the model with this most vulnerable group. Since the older adult population and minority populations are so heterogeneous, it is difficult to generalize research findings. Research is difficult with multi-ethnic groups for several reasons. One of the major barriers is that most researchers are White, well-educated, and English speaking. Cultural differences and language challenges often present difficult problems that affect the outcomes of the research. Research teams incorporating members of the communities being studied have been successful in helping to reduce some of these barriers. More collaboration of this sort is encouraged to facilitate research in this important area. In addition to interventions at the individual level, sociopolitical interventions are needed to increase cultural appropriateness of the health care system and address issues of poverty and limited access to services.

Because physically and cognitively impaired, and frail older adults often require care, chapter 9 discusses application of the TTM to family and professional caregivers. Informal and formal care giving is discussed along with an overview of the situation in long-term care institutions. Case studies are used to illustrate application of the TTM with family caregivers and with long-term care staff as well. A description is given of the Physical Activity Counseling for Exercise (PACE) model (Houde & Melillo, 2000) where professionals are trained in the TTM and then apply this training to the treatment of individual clients. Although research needs to be carried out to evaluate the use of TTM with long-term care staff, it is not too early to apply concepts of the TTM to change staff behavior and incorporate the much-needed exercise into daily care of residents. Health care providers and family caregivers who apply this model are again encouraged to keep anecdotal records of the process and outcomes to help evaluate the usefulness of the TTM at this level. Perhaps these anecdotal records could be summarized and shared in a publication that may serve as the basis for future research studies. Teaching the TTM to caregivers to use with the person who is changing the behavior is a diversion from usual applications of the model. Very few studies to date (the PACE model is one) have evaluated this application of the TTM, however, this area holds much promise for behavior change.

This book provides a strong case for applying the TTM of behavior change with diverse groups of older adults at all levels of health and illness, as well as their caregivers. A thorough description of the model itself and how to apply it is given so that readers can easily utilize it in their own practice settings. Once the model is understood and methods of application are determined, actual exercise programs individualized for older adult clients can be implemented. It is beyond the scope of this book to include suggestions for specific exercises, and the following section offers a selected bibliography of exercise books for older adults as well as a list of resources and organizations where additional information can be obtained.

RESOURCES

Books

Active Older Adults: Ideas for Action
Lynn Allen
Champaign, IL: Human Kinetics Publishers, 1999
ISBN 0-7360-0128-X

Exercise for Older Adults
Richard T. Cotton and Christine Ekeroth
Champaign, IL: Human Kinetics Publishers, 1998
ISBN 0-88011-942-X

SeniorCise: Exercise Your Way to Good Health
University of Rhode Island, 1999
Program in Gerontology

White Hall G-15
Kingston, RI 02881

Aging, Physical Activity and Health
Roy J. Shepard
Champaign IL: Human Kinetics Publishers, 1997
ISBN 0-87322-889-8

Exercise Activities for the Elderly
K. Flatten, B. Wilhite, and E. Reyes-Watson
New York: Springer, 1988

Safe Therapeutic Exercises for the Frail Elderly
O. Hurley
Center for Books on Aging, 1996

Senior Fitness Test Manual
Roberta Rikli and C. Jessie Jones
Champaign, IL: Human Kinetics Publishers, 2001
ISBN 0-7360-3363-7

Exercise Programming for Older Adults
Kay A. Van Norman
Champaign, IL: Human Kinetics Publishers, 1995
ISBN 0-87322-657-7

Strength Training Past 50
Wayne L. Wescott and Thomas R. Baechle
Champaign, IL: Human Kinetics Publisher, 1998
ISBN 0-88011-716-8

Yoga for the Young at Heart: Gentle Stretching Exercises for Seniors
S.W. Ward
Capra Press, 1996

Water Fitness After 40
Ruth Sova
Champaign, IL: Human Kinetics Publishers, 1995
ISBN 0-87322-604-6

Full Life Fitness: A Complete Exercise Program for Mature Adults
Janie Clark
Champaign, IL: Human Kinetics Publishers, 1992
ISBN 0-87322-391-8

Strength Training for Seniors
Wayne L Wescott and Thomas R. Baechle
Champaign, IL: Human Kinetics Publishers, 1999
ISBN 0-87322-952-5

Exercise, Aging & Health: Overcoming Barriers to an Active Old Age
S.O. Cousins
New York: Taylor and Francis, 1998

Exercise and Fitness for the Older Adult
W. H. Osness
Dubuque, IA: Kendall/Hunt Publishing Company, 1998

Still Kicking: Restorative Groups for Frail Older Adults
A. V. Brown-Watson
Baltimore, MD: Health Professions Press, 1999

Exercise: A Guide from the National Institute on Aging
Bethesda, MD: National Institute on Aging

Videos

Fitness Forever
Human Kinetics Publishers
ISBN 0-99-002393-1

SeniorCise: Exercise Your Way to Good Health
Video 1—*Overview of Exercise*
Video 2—*Basic Exercise*
Video 3—*Advanced Exercise*
University of Rhode Island
Program in Gerontology
White Hall G-15
Kingston, RI 02881

Organizations and Websites

American Heart Association
www.americanheart.org
American Heart National Center
7272 Greenville Avenue
Dallas, TX 75231
1-800-242-8721

National Institute on Aging
www.nih.gov/nia
1-800-222-2225

National Institute on Aging/NASA
http://weboflife.arc.nasa.goc/exerciseandaging

The Arthritis Foundation
www.arthritis.org

Shape Up America!
www.shapeup.org
6707 Democracy Blvd
Suite 306
Bethesda, MD 20817

AARP Fulfillment
601 E St., NW
Washington, DC 20049

The National Osteoporosis Foundation
www.nof.org
1232 22nd Street N.W.
Washington, DC 20037-1292
202-223-2226

The Foundation for Osteoporosis Research and Education
www.fore.org
300 27th Street
Oakland, CA 94612
888-266-3015

American College of Sports Medicine
www.acsm.org
P.O. Box 1440
Indianapolis, IN 46206
317-637-9200

REFERENCES

Houde, S. C., & Melillo, K. D. (2000). Physical activity and exercise counseling in primary care. *The Nurse Practitioner, 25*(8), 8–39.

Nigg, C. R., Burbank, P. M., Padula, C., Dufresne, R., Rossi, J. S., Velicer, W. F., Laforge, R. G., & Prochaska, J. O. (1999). *The Gerontologist, 39*(4), 473–482.

Prochaska, J. O., & DiClemente, C. C. (1983). Stages and processes of self-change in smoking: Towards an integrative model of change. *Journal of Consulting and Clinical Psychology, 51*, 390–395.

Index